THE PACEMAKER CLINIC OF THE 90'S

ESSENTIALS IN BRADY-PACING

Developments in Cardiovascular Medicine

VOLUME 175

The titles published in this series are listed at the end of this volume.

The Pacemaker Clinic of the 90's

Essentials in Brady-Pacing

Edited by

N. M. VAN HEMEL

Department of Cardiology,
St. Antonius Hospital,
Nieuwegein, The Netherlands

F. H. M. WITTKAMPF

Heart Lung Institute,
University Hospital Utrecht,
Utrecht, The Netherlands

and

H. ECTOR

Department of Cardiology,
University Clinic Gasthuisberg,
Leuven, Belgium

KLUWER ACADEMIC PUBLISHERS

DORDRECHT / BOSTON / LONDON

A C.I.P. Catalogue record for this book is available from the Library of Congress.

ISBN 0-7923-3688-7

Published by Kluwer Academic Publishers,
P.O. Box 17, 3300 AA Dordrecht, The Netherlands.

Kluwer Academic Publishers incorporates
the publishing programmes of
D. Reidel, Martinus Nijhoff, Dr W. Junk and MTP Press.

Sold and distributed in the U.S.A. and Canada
by Kluwer Academic Publishers,
101 Philip Drive, Norwell, MA 02061, U.S.A.

In all other countries, sold and distributed
by Kluwer Academic Publishers Group,
P.O. Box 322, 3300 AH Dordrecht, The Netherlands.

Cover design: Hein van Putten
Book used: *Die Unregelmässige Herztätigkeit*, by
K. F. Wenckebach and Hch. Winterberg, 1927,
Verlag von Wilhelm Engelmann, Leipzig.

Printed on acid-free paper

Printed in the Netherlands

To the memory of Bert Thalen
one of the European pioneers in cardiac pacing

• CONTENTS •

SECTION 1 : THE ANATOMICAL ELECTRICAL INTERFACE

Chapter 1 Cardiac Anatomy in Perspective of Cardiac Pacing 1
Anton E. Becker

Chapter 2 The Electrical Electrode-Myocard Interface 13
Fred H.M. Wittkampf

SECTION 2 : CONSIDERATIONS BEFORE IMPLANT OF A PACEMAKER

Chapter 3 Timing Cycles in Dual-Chamber Adaptive Rate Pacemakers and the Consequences for Programming 33
Jaap H. Ruiter and Jan P.M. Corstjens

Chapter 4 Pacing in Elderly Patients: Pre-operative Evaluation and Pacemaker Selection 55
Rob van Mechelen, Karel den Dulk and Hein J.J. Wellens

Chapter 5 Single Lead Atrial Synchronized Ventricular (VDD) Pacing 73
Jonathan C. Pitts Crick

SECTION 3 : PREVENTION OF PACEMAKER COMPLICATIONS

Chapter 6 Prevention and Treatment of Pacemaker Infection 81
Jo A.M.T. Defauw, Norbert M. van Hemel and Emile R. Jessurun

Chapter 7 Technical Follow-Up of Implanted Pacemakers 95
Peter van der Kemp and Lex Bakema

Chapter 8 A Stepwise Approach to Solve Pacemaker Problems 123
Berry M. van Gelder and Frank A.L.E. Bracke

Chapter 9 Cardiac Arrhythmias and the Interaction with Pacemakers 167
Luc Jordaens

SECTION 4 : MISCELLANEOUS ASPECTS

Chapter 10 Cardiac Stimulation as Nonpharmocological Treatment of Heart Failure 185
Patricia F.A. Bakker

Chapter 11 The Interplay Between Radiofrequency Catheter Ablation of Arrhythmias and Cardiac Pacing 199
Norbert M. van Hemel

Chapter 12 Cardiac Pacing in Children, Special Skills Needed? 215
Margreet Th.E. Bink-Boelkens and Gertie C.M. Beaufort-Krol

Chapter 13 Cardiac Pacing in Europe: Anno 1993 225
Hugo Ector and Giorgio A. Feruglio

Chapter 14 The Safety and Medico-Legal Responsibilities of the Pacemaker Implantation Team 239
Bas A.J.M. de Mol

Index 255

Hilbert J.Th. Thalen, MD

This book is a tribute to and in remembrance of Dr Hilbert J.Th. Thalen. Dr Thalen, born April 29, 1939, was one of the pioneers in the treatment of heart rhythm disturbances with the implantation of a pacemaker. Bert Thalen's dedication to this field of endeavour was total and his contribution in all aspects unlimited. He was active in the physiology of electric cardiac stimulation, the development and construction of a pacemaker and electrodes, various techniques for implantation, development of pacemaker control mechanisms, pacemaker clinics for follow-up of patients and, especially, sharing and promoting this knowledge and information through meetings, symposia and lectures all over the world.

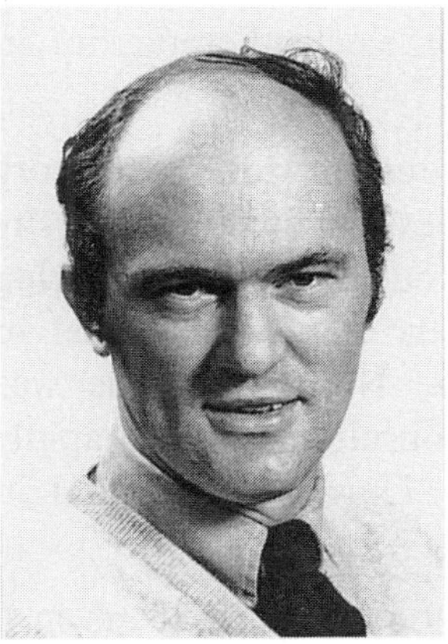

Bert Thalen was a man with a vision. He was highly motivated, inspiring, dynamic and a very well organized person. He radiated a feeling of urgency in his environment, as if he unconsciously knew, that his time to accomplish what he wanted, was limited.

As the surgeon who played a minor role in this research project, I must write this tribute partly from memory, because all the players of the first hour, such as Prof. Dr J.W. van den Berg, the physicist, and Prof. Dr J.J. Nieveen, the cardiologist, as well as Bert Thalen, are deceased.

When we started performing open-heart surgery with a heart-lung machine, developed in May 1957 by Dr Dorlas and myself, we realized the inevitable necessity to be able to stimulate the heart for longer or shorter periods of time. With this thought in mind, I started in 1960 -when I was still a trainee in general surgery- our investigation by creating heart blocks in dogs by an open direct vision method. We had learned this technique from closing atrial septal defects using hypothermia. Under direct vision, obtained by inflow occlusion, we could identify and ligate the bundle of His within 60 seconds of circulatory arrest. Professor van den Berg studied and researched information regarding the energy necessary for stimulation of the heart and how to do it. Then, in his own laboratory of medical physics, he constructed an implantable pacemaker, powered with mercury batteries and totally encapsulated in a soft, elastic, tissue friendly type of plastic.

In May 1962, after eleven successful implantations in dogs, we initiated the clinical application of our device. It was at this point that Bert Thalen, 24 years of age, came into the picture as student-assistant by our physicist, Prof. Dr J.W. van den Berg. The preparations for further research were complete. So to speak, the soil had been fertilized and Bert now started the real work of sowing, growing and harvesting the accumulated information. This work culminated in his academic thesis in 1969, 'The artificial cardiac pacemaker'. This thesis was published in a revised edition in 1975, and became at that time a standard reference work on the fast growing field of electrotherapeutics in cardiology.

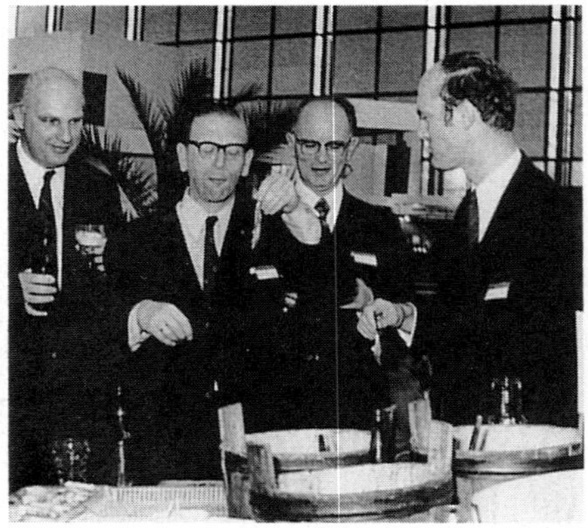

From left to right: Prof. Dr J.N. Homan van J.W. van den Berg and Dr J.H. Thalen, at the IVth International Symposium on The Netherlands

Dr Thalen finished his medical studies in 1969 and retired from the laboratory to the clinic. He studied cardiology under Prof. Dr J.J. Nieveen, at the University Hospital in Groningen. Additional experience was acquired in 1974-1975, during a clinical and research appointment at the Massachusetts General Hospital in Boston, Massachusetts, U.S.A. Upon his return to The Netherlands, he was appointed head of the Pacemaker Clinic and cardiac consultant of the rapidly expanding department of Cardiothoracic surgery at the University Hospital in Groningen.

Because it was impossible to produce a sufficient number of pacemakers in a laboratory, the Vitatron Pacemaker Company in Dieren was founded in order to produce the quantity of pacemakers needed. Due to his interest and work regarding pacemakers, of course Bert Thalen became their first advisor. It turned out to be a happy and fruitful marriage between research, industry and clinic. Many new ideas were developed and found to be clinically applicable, such as new pacemaker leads, new electrodes, P-wave triggered or R-wave inhibited pacemakers, to name a few. Although Thalen was active in all aspects of pacemaker therapy, his most visible and important contribution was the international sharing of his accumulated knowledge and clinical experience.

Following symposia in New York in 1963 and Monaco in 1970, Bert Thalen organized the IVth International Symposium on Cardiac Pacing in Groningen,

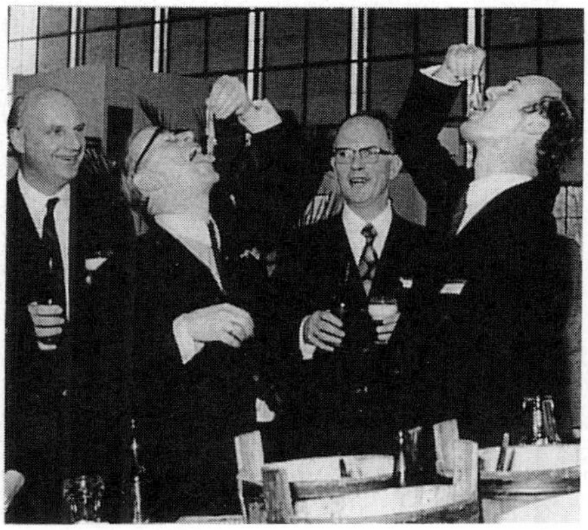

der Heide, Prof. Dr J.J. Nieveen, Prof. Dr tasting Hollands national delicacy, herring, Cardiac Pacing, April 1973, in Groningen,

April 1973. He played a prominent role as host and organizer, and shortly afterwards published the proceedings of this symposium: 'Cardiac Pacing'. In 1975 he organized an European pacemaker colloquium in Arnhem and after the Vth World Pacemaker Congress in Tokyo in 1976 he organized a second European colloquium in Brussels in 1977. The second colloquium resulted in a book in 1978: 'To pace or not to pace', edited by H.J.Th. Thalen and J.W. Harthorne. Both events were sponsored by the Vitatron Company. Following the VIth World Symposium on Cardiac Pacing in Montreal in 1979, he in co-operation with C.C. Meese edited another book based on the proceedings of his symposium: 'Fundamentals of Cardiac Pacing'. His last scientific contribution was a chapter on electrostimulation of the heart in a Dutch Textbook of Cardiology.

Bert Thalen became a fellow of the American College of Cardiology, a member of the European Work Group on Cardiac Pacing, a member of the International Society of Cardiac Pacing and he founded the Dutch 'Werkgroep Hartstimulatie'. As a recognized expert, he served on the editorial boards of the European Heart Journal, PACE, and Pacing and Clinical Electrophysiology. Bert Thalen was known world wide, not only for his fountain of publications but for his lectures and advice as he travelled around the world sharing his knowledge. We could call him the verbal 'globe-player' in pacemaker treatment.

Thalen's interest was not only cardiology, he also had a keen interest in sports. He accompanied student sport teams to world competitions, he was medical advisor to the soccer club F.C. Groningen in Groningen and he was cardiac consultant of the Dutch Society of Sports Medicine. Dr Thalen's family came from the province of Drenthe, and he was an active member of the annual family shoot. He was a good doctor for his patients and a trustworthy, loyal friend for those around him. He was an active member of the Remonstrant Congregation in Groningen. He was a man who said what he did, and did what he said! For those in his environment he seemed to possess a source of unlimited energy, as if he was automatically powered.

The combination of virtues, together with a keen interest in research and a rapid pen, made him the optimal candidate for the in 1982 vacant chair of Cardiology at the University of Groningen. As fate will have it, his destiny abruptly changed. In 1982, completely unexpected, Bert Thalen died at the age of 43, as a result of an uncontrolled diabetes. It was a tragic end to a brilliant career. At the Pacemaker Congress in Vienna, in May 1983, a 'Bert Thalen Memorial Lecture' was given by his friend J.W. Harthorne, and in honour of his memory a 'Thalen Young Investigators Award' was instituted.

Bert Thalen will be remembered as a dynamic pioneer of the second generation. A generation that made the pacemaker a safe, useful, reliable and long lasting tool in the armoury of cardiologists treating patients with rhythm disturbances. His candle burned on both ends and at the same time shed a clear light on its environment. Bert Thalen lived in style and according to the motto of my teacher Eerland: **'In serviendo consumor'.**

J.N. Homan van der Heide, MD
Emeritus Professor of Cardiothoracic Surgery
University of Groningen, The Netherlands

• ACKNOWLEDGEMENTS •

The basis of this monograph on pacing therapy and related topics was laid during the preparations of the one-day postgraduate seminar organized by the National Institute for Continuous Cardiovascular Education, director J. Herre Kingma, MD, on January 15th, 1995, in Utrecht.

The editors wish to thank Mrs Gerda van der Kuijl for camera ready preparation of the manuscript, illustrations and layout. Mrs Rosemery Lecluse-Ciarrocca, RNCCN, was of indispensable support for correction and editing of the English language of the manuscript.

Publication of this book became possible by educational grants of

INTERPACE
Nederland

and

STICHTING
ROGER CROWSON
FONDS

Roger Crowson Foundation
The Netherlands

• INTRODUCTION •

More than thirty years after the first implant, permanent pacing has become a worldwide established therapy for a symptomatic slow cardiac rhythm. After the initially simple ventricular pacemaker, the application of sensors, varying from the natural P wave to various biological signals to preserve mechanical atrioventricular synchrony as well as rate adaption, have widened impressively the therapeutical scope of bradycardia pacing in the eighties. Improved quality of leads, energy sources and other components of pacing devices and sophisticated tools for adapting pacemakers to individual needs, contribute today strongly to the well-being of pacemaker patients. In view of well-established guidelines for cardiac pacing and follow-up of paced patients, one can safely assume that current pacemaker therapy has achieved a high performance with a favourable cost/benefit ratio.

In the last twenty years, the magnitude of individuals receiving pacing therapy has shown large alterations. It is well recognized that today's elderly people, with ages above 70 years, enjoy much better mental condition and physical shape than comparable age groups thirty years ago. It has also been shown that their life expectancy has further increased by virtue of several causes. Dealing with an impressive growth of this population in western countries, it is to be expected that these elderly people will be forced to take care of themselves instead of being supported by governmentally organized day and night care. This obligatory independency requires optimal pacing therapy in pacemaker-dependent patients over many years. Therefore the question arises whether the initial pacing mode is sufficient in elderly people to answer all requirements and problems related to arrhythmias and cardiac changes arising in the following years of pacing. In other words, should we do more at the initial implantation procedure?

This concept of 'initial overtreatment' conflicts with the current tendency of decline in hospital budget. Moreover, recent audits have reported that in some western countries showing limited resources, physicians prefer restricting cardiac pacing to exclusively symptomatic patients, and omit implants for prophylactic reasons in asymptomatic cases despite well-estabished guidelines. One also has to accept that many patients of all ages do not receive appropriate pacing therapy in terms of restored mechanical atrioventricular synchrony or sufficiently paced ranges of heart rate due to deficient skill, effort and experience of hospital pacing teams. Finally, one also has to recognize that the natural course of the disease asking for cardiac pacing, is today still difficult to define in the individual patient. These reasons explain why the concept of an initial pacing mode with sufficient flexibility to cover all upcoming problems and changes encountered during pacing therapy, remains more a matter of belief than of practice although the eventual cost of therapy might be less.

The publication of this book was sparked by an one-day postgraduate course in January 1995, organized by the National Institute for Continuous Cardiovascular Education, and intends to refresh the knowledge of registered cardiologists, trainees in cardiology and associated professionals. This book also attempts to offer new insights in functional anatomy, pacing modes, paced ECG and miscellaneous topics, in order to achieve individualized pacing therapy. When the reader digests the presented experience and recommendations such that the concept of long-term flexible pacing therapy is gradually wining acceptance, all authors will have accomplished a great task. In that case the unlucky saying *one pacemaker suffices one patient* will get a complete different meaning.

Norbert M. van Hemel, MD
Fred H.M. Wittkampf, PhD
Hugo Ector, MD

• CONTRIBUTORS •

Lex Bakema
Head of the Pacemaker Department, Sint Antonius Hospital, Nieuwegein, The Netherlands

Patricia F.A. Bakker, MD, PhD
Department of Cardiopulmonary Surgery, Heart-Lung Institute, University Hospital, Utrecht, The Netherlands

Gertie C.M. Beaufort-Krol, MD
Division of Pediatric Cardiology Beatrix Children's Hospital, University of Groningen, The Netherlands

Anton E. Becker, MD, PhD
Professor and Head of the Cardiovascular Pathology Department, University of Amsterdam, Academic Medical Center, Amsterdam, The Netherlands

Margreet Th.E. Bink-Boelkens, MD, PhD
Division of Pediatric Cardiology Beatrix Children's Hospital, University of Groningen, The Netherlands

Frank A.L.E. Bracke, MD
Department of Cardiology, Catharina Hospital, Eindhoven, The Netherlands

Jan P.M. Corstjens
CPI Medical Devices and Diagnostics Divison of Elli Lilly Nederland B.V.

Jo J.A.M.T. Defauw, MD
Department of Cardiothoracic Surgery, Sint Antonius Hospital, Nieuwegein, The Netherlands

Karel den Dulk, MD, PhD
Department of Cardiology, Academic Hospital, Maastricht, The Netherlands

Hugo Ector, MD, PhD
Professor and Head of the Department of Cardiology, University Hospital Gasthuisberg, Leuven, Belgium. Chairman of the European Working Group on Cardiac Pacing (ESC)

Giorgo A. Feruglio, M.D.
Department of Cardiology, Regional Hospital, Udine, Italy. Director of the European Pacemaker Registration System, established by the European Working Group on Cardiac Pacing (ESC)

Berry M. van Gelder
Department of Cardiology,
Catharina Hospital, Eindhoven
The Netherlands

Norbert M. van Hemel, MD, PhD
Department of Cardiology,
Sint Antonius Hospital,
Nieuwegein, The Netherlands

Emile R. Jessurun, MD
Department of Cardiology
Sint Antonius Hospital,
Nieuwegein, The Netherlands

Luc Jordaens, MD, PhD
Professor and Head of the
Department of Cardiovascular
Diseases, University Hospital of
Ghent, Belgium

Peter van der Kemp
Interpace Nederland B.V.,
Ruurlo, The Netherlands

Rob van Mechelen, MD, PhD
Department of Cardiology,
Sint Franciscus Gasthuis,
Rotterdam, The Netherlands

Bas A.J.M. de Mol, MD, PhD, JD
Department of Cardiopulmonary
Surgery, Academic Medical
Center of the University of
Amsterdam & Safety Science
Group, Delft University of
Technology, The Netherlands

Jonathan C. Pitts Crick, MD, MRCP
Department of Cardiology,
Bristol Royal Infirmary,
University of Bristol, United
Kingdom

Jaap H. Ruiter, MD, PhD
Department of Cardiology,
Medical Center Alkmaar,
The Netherlands

Hein J.J. Wellens, MD, PhD
Professor and Head of the
Cardiology Department,
Academic Hospital, Maastricht,
The Netherlands

Fred H.M. Wittkampf, PhD
Heart Lung Institute,
University Hospital Utrecht,
The Netherlands

1 THE ANATOMICAL ELECTRICAL INTERFACE

Chapter 1

Cardiac Anatomy in Perspective of Cardiac Pacing

Anton E. Becker

Introduction

Pacing of the heart to overcome conduction and rhythm abnormalities has come a long way. Over the decade much progress has been made due in part to improvements in the understanding of mechanisms and, in part, to technical innovations. In the slip stream of these achievements the need is felt to review cardiac anatomy as it relates to cardiac pacing.

The Sinus Node and Atrial Anatomy

The sinus node, first discovered at the site of 'ultimum moriens' by Keith and Flack in 1907, is located lateral to the junction of the superior caval vein with the right atrium (figure 1). It is positioned on the epicardial side of the terminal groove, embedded within adipose tissue. Its position is often disclosed by a small but discrete fat pad, which overlies the body of the sinus node. The tapering extremities of the node are variable; the cranial extension may partially embrace the junction

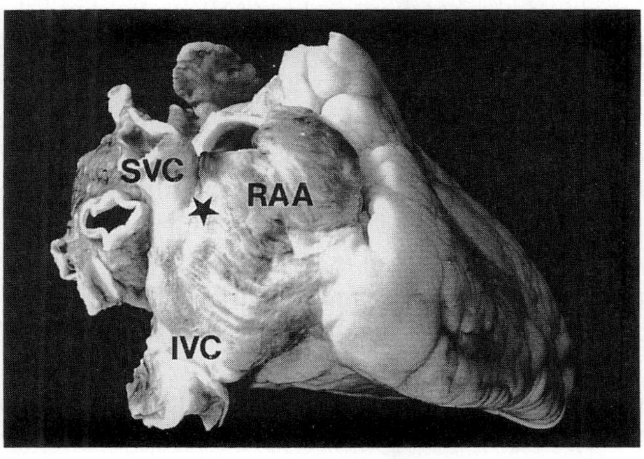

Figure 1. *Right-sided view of the heart. The sinus node(*) is located to the junction of the superior caval vein (SVC) with the right atrial appendage (RAA). It is positioned on the epicardial side of the terminal groove and may extend caudally towards the site of junction of the inferior caval vein (IVC) with the right atrium.*

with the superior caval vein anteriorly, while caudally the tail may extend along the terminal groove towards the site of junction of the inferior caval vein with the right atrium.

The arterial supply for the sinus node is provided by a large atrial branch, often known as the 'sinus node artery'. The usual site of origin is the most proximal segment of either the right coronary artery or the left circumflex artery. In the majority of hearts the 'sinus node artery' has extensive ramifications and collaterals with other atrial branches.

The sinus node itself is composed of nodal cells, grouped together in small interconnecting fasciculi, themselves embedded in a prominent fibrous tissue matrix. The latter increases with increasing age. The interweaving fasciculi of nodal cells make up the body and central portions of the node and, usually, surround the nodal artery. At the margins of the node, where nodal cells are contiguous with atrial myocardium, a small rim of transitional cells is present. The latter have characteristics intermediate between nodal cells and individual atrial myocardial cells.

Spread of Activation

Spread of activation from the sinus node onto atrial myocardium is determined largely by atrial architecture. The terminal groove, which harbors the sinus node, corresponds with the terminal crest at the inside. The terminal crest is an important landmark, which forms the boundary between the smooth-walled (sinus venosus) part of the right atrium and the trabeculated part (better known as the right atrial appendage). The crest is U-shaped with an anteromedial and a posterolateral descending limb (figure 2). The myocardial cells within the crest are parallel arranged and thus facilitate rapid spread of activation. The anterior limb descends towards the region of the atrioventricular (AV) node along the anteromedial wall of the right atrium, anterior to the oval fossa. The fibers, once approaching the atrioventricular septal junction (see below) fan out and in part insert into the base of the anterior leaflet of the tricuspid valve, anterior to the membranous septum, and, in part, contribute to the anterior input of the AV node. The anteromedial wall of the right atrium is in close apposition with the ascending aorta. This is an important topographic relationship with consequences for advancing age. In elderly people dilation of the ascending aorta may produce a distinct impression with atrophy of the corresponding atrial wall. This age-related phenomenon, therefore, could affect also the anterior inputs into the AV node.

The posterolateral descending limb of the terminal crest initially presents as a distinct ridge, but towards the site of junction of the inferior caval vein with the

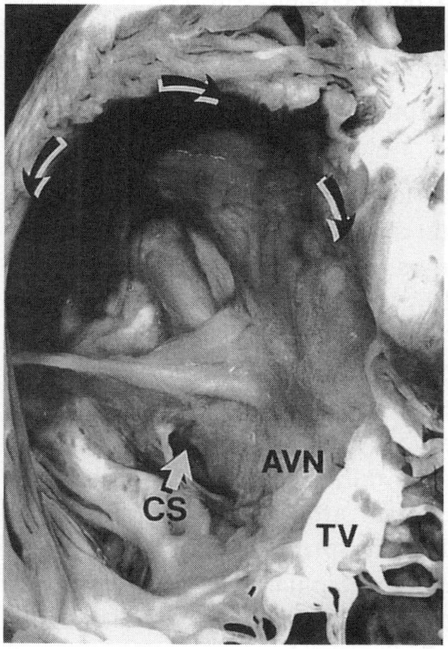

Figure 2. *Right-sided view of opened right atrium. The terminal groove corresponds with the terminal crest on the inside. The crest is U-shaped with an anteromedial and posterolateral descending limb (direction indicated by arrows). Fibers in both limbs approach the atrioventricular septal junction which contains the compact atrioventricular node (AVN). CS, os of coronary sinus; TV, tricuspid valve leaflet.*

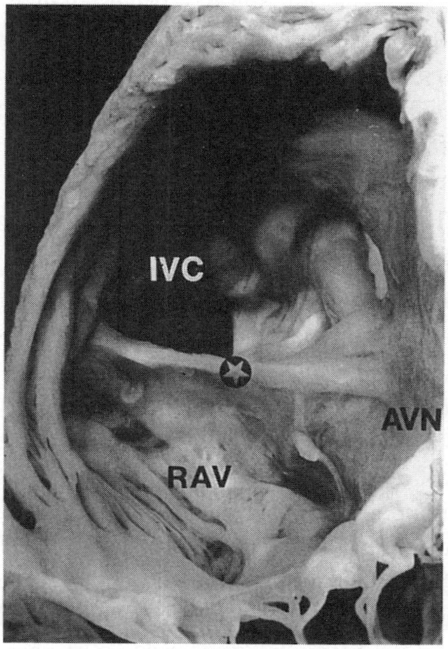

Figure 3. *Same heart specimen as shown in figure 2. The posterolateral descending limb of the terminal crest fans out into separate bundles towards the site of junction of the inferior caval vein (IVC) with the right atrium. One of these forms a distinct ridge between the IVC and the right atrial vestibule (RAV), known as the sinus septum (*). It runs anteriorly towards the site of the compact AV node (AVN) and contains the tendon of Todaro.*

right atrium the crest fans out into separate bundles. One of these continues lateral to the site of entrance of the inferior caval vein. It forms a distinct ridge between the inferior caval vein and the right atrial vestibule (figure 3). The bundle continues anteriorly and walls off the coronary sinus from the right atrial cavity. Viewed from the right side the structure seems to form the roof of the os of the coronary sinus. It is known as the sinus septum with parallel arranged myocardial fibers that run anteriorly towards the area of the AV node. The tendon of Todaro is embedded within this structure. Other bundles fan out from the terminal crest and contribute to the pectinate muscles that are present immediately posterior and lateral to the os of the coronary sinus. Viewed from the right side, some of these bundles continue anteriorly, underneath the os of the coronary sinus, and apparently contribute to the posterior input of the AV node. The pectinate muscles, which produce the characteristic anatomy of the right atrial appendage, are composed of distinct muscle bundles with a parallel orientation of the fibers, but the areas in-between are almost devoid of muscle. Only a small rim of muscle, sometimes only fibrous tissue, separates endocardium from epicardium.

Anterior to the junctional site of the superior caval vein, a muscular band crosses the interatrial groove and connects right atrial myocardium with left atrial myocardium. This band of muscle, known as Bachmann's bundle, contains parallel aligned muscle fibers. It is reinforced by myocardial fibers from the right atrial lateral free wall, which encircle the right atrial appendage from underneath and swing upwards along its medial wall. Posterior to the superior caval vein, however, there is no such connection. Once the epicardium is incised and the interatrial groove dissected, it becomes evident that right and left atrial myocardium are separated largely by fibro-fatty tissue and only a few bridging myocardial fibers. It appears also that the so-called intercaval area is mostly fibrous. The anatomy thus provides the substrate for the delay in spread of activation towards the left atrium, posterior to the superior caval vein. Similarly, inferior caval vein and coronary sinus are closely related and, in part, have fibrous continuity. When viewed from the right side, it appears as if a distinct bridge of muscle is present between both structures. In reality, however, this bridge of tissue is formed by ramifications of the terminal crest, such as the sinus septum. Once the superficial layer of muscle is removed, it shows that the 'isthmus', as it is known by electrophysiologists, is largely fibrous rather than muscular.

It thus appears that spread of activation from the sinus node takes preferential routes, dictated by the anatomy of the atria.

AV Node and 'Input' Anatomy

To understand the intricate anatomy of the AV node and its atrial inputs it is necessary to have good knowledge of the anatomy of the atrioventricular septal junction. The need for such understanding is exemplified by a current trend to subdivide this area into an anterior, middle and posterior part, apparently convenient to electrophysiologists exploring this area. However, what is fact and what is fiction?

The Atrioventricular Septal Junction

The area of the anticipated atrioventricular septal junction, viewed from the right side, presents important landmarks (figure 4). Anteriorly the atrioventricular

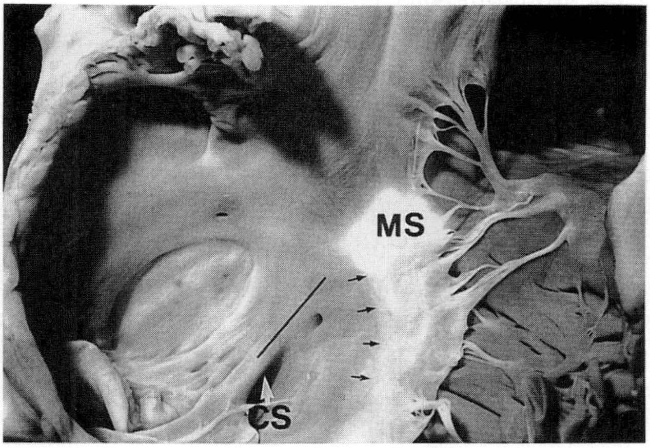

Figure 4. *Opened right side of the heart with transilluminated membranous septum (MS). The sinus septum contains the tendon of Torado (indicated by solid line), which together with the septal insertion of the tricuspid valve (indicated by arrows) forms the triangle of Koch with the compact AV node located close to its apex. CS, os of coronary sinus.*

membranous septum is such a structure. It is part of the central fibrous body and extends from the right fibrous trigone. Viewed from the right side, it is positioned at the site of the so-called septal commissure of the tricuspid valve. Viewed from the left side, it locates immediately adjacent to the zone of fibrous continuity between the anterior mitral valve leaflet and the non- and left coronary cusps of the aortic valve. From the left ventricular aspect, the atrioventricular membranous septum is a wholly ventricular structure, but on the right side the septal attachment of the tricuspid valve traverses the membranous septum, thus dividing it into an atrioventricular and an interventricular part.

In the light of a discussion of the atrioventricular septal junctional area, the membranous septum is important since it clearly delineates the anterior 'end' of the junction (figure 5). Anterior to the membranous septum, when

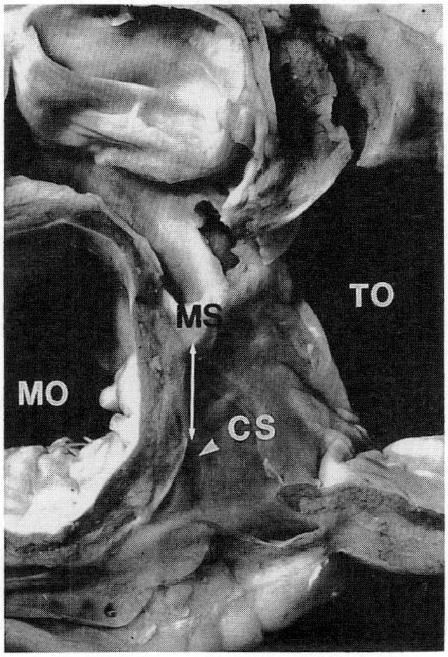

Figure 5. *Dissection of the atrioventricular septal junctional area. Note the narrowness of the true atrioventricular septum (white line), squeezed between the left ventricular outflow tract and the membranous septum (MS), anteriorly, and the os of the coronary sinus (CS), posteriorly. TO, tricuspid orifice; MO, mitral orifice.*

looked at from the right side, the atrioventricular junction is no longer septal but mural. This anatomic fact implies that the term 'anterior septum' is a misnomer for the atrioventricular junction anterior to the membranous septum.

Another landmark in considering the atrioventricular septal junction is the os of the coronary sinus. Some consider the area posterior to the coronary sinus as the 'posterior septum'. However, this again is a misunderstanding. The coronary sinus basically is an extracardiac structure, which runs in the atrioventricular groove separated from the left atrium by the mural left atrial wall (figure 5).

What is truly the atrioventricular septal junction is the area between the atrioventricular membranous septum anteriorly and the os of the coronary sinus posteriorly (figure 6). Basically this is a small zone, albeit quite variable in length from one individual to the other.

Not only is the atrioventricular septal junction much smaller than often thought of, it also has a complex topographic anatomy. Cross sections, perpendicular to the line of junction, show a considerable difference in the level of offsetting of the corresponding mitral and tricuspid valve leaflets. The septal attachment of the tricuspid valve is lower than that of the mitral valve. This creates a situation where the crest of the interventricular septum in part locates between the left ventricle and the right atrium. This structure is known as the muscular atrioventricular septum (figure 6). As a consequence, the anatomy is that of a composite of a thin layer of atrial myocardial fibers, whereas the bulk of muscle is formed by ventricular myocardial fibers as part of the crest of the interventricular septum. There is evidence that this particular anatomical configuration accounts for the recording of double potentials from this area. Understanding the topographic anatomy of the atrioventricular septal junctional area bears also on the understanding of the anatomy of the AV node and bundle.

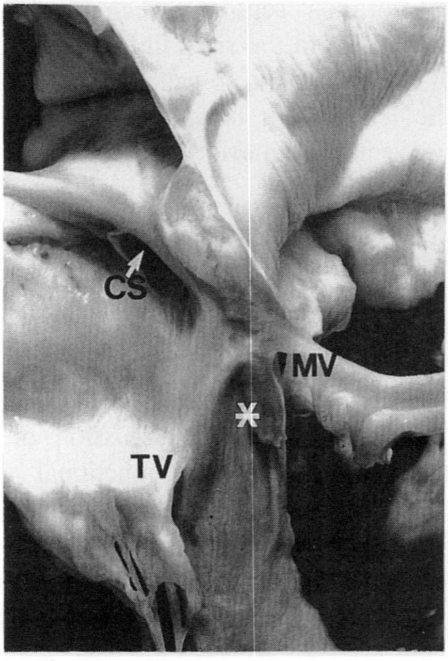

Figure 6. *Cross section through the atrioventricular septal junction, just anterior to the os of the coronary sinus (CS). The offsetting of the mitral (MV) and tricuspid (TV) valve leaflets are at different levels, thus creating a muscular septum between the left ventricle and the right atrium: the muscular atrioventricular septum (*).*

AV Node and Bundle

The compact AV node *(see below)* projects in the area of the muscular atrioventricular septum (figure 4). Its precise position is nicely delineated by the so-called triangle of Koch. This triangle is formed by the tendon of Todaro, which basically is a strand of fibrous tissue which continues from the Eustachian valve and is embedded in the sinus septum (see above), the atrioventricular membranous septum (in which the tendon inserts) and the line of attachment of the septal tricuspid valve leaflet (figure 4). The compact part of the AV node is located towards the apex of this triangle.

It is important to emphasize that the compact node is not confined to the very apex of the triangle of Koch, but rather occupies the area towards the apex. The total length of the compact part of the AV node may vary considerably and in some individuals the length of the compact AV node almost equals that of the atrioventricular septal junction as defined above. In other words, the compact AV node in some individuals may reach posteriorly almost as far as the os of the coronary sinus.

As a consequence of the characteristic shape of the muscular atrioventricular septum the compact AV node covers the right-sided slope of this septum (figure 6). The compact node itself is composed of interweaving slender nodal cells, producing a complex architectural structure. Posteriorly, the tail end of the compact node, tapers out often dividing into a left- and rightward extension. The length of these tail parts, once more, may vary considerably from one individual to the other. Anteriorly, the compact AV node continues as the nodal-bundle axis, which soon will be enveloped by the connective tissue of the central fibrous body and thus comes to run in the bottom part of the membranous septum. It is this fibrous tissue that isolates the nodal-bundle axis and compact node from the atrial myocardial fibers. The very site of the last atrial fiber contacting the nodal-bundle axis is considered the junction between AV node and penetrating (His) bundle.

The compact AV node is surrounded by cells that are transitional between the nodal cells and working myocardial cells. This adds to further heterogeneity with respect to the cellular component make-up of the zone that contains the compact AV node. Indeed, the more posterior, the more intermingling of transitional cells and working myocardial cells, which produce a layer of cells that cover the right-sided slope of the crest of the interventricular septum — the muscular atrioventricular septum as defined above.

The Atrial Inputs

As alluded to above the spread of activation from the sinus node takes preferential routes dictated by the geometry of the atria. Basically, there are three main inputs. First, through the anteromedial descending limb of the terminal crest. These fibers will reach the area of the AV node close to the site of the atrioventricular membranous septum. Some of these fibers will cross the sinus septum superficially and, for instance, have to be dissected away in order to expose the tendon of Todaro. The second major inputs into the area of the AV node are derived from the posterolateral descending branch of the terminal crest. The two major components are (1) the fibers that run within the sinus septum and (2) fibers that contribute to the pectinate muscles posterior to the os of the coronary sinus. From these sites myocardial cells are aligned parallel and directed towards the area of the AV node.

At present it remains uncertain still how atrial inputs, as alluded to above, precisely contact the AV node and, in particular, how these inputs relate to the zone of interposing transitional cells. Pain staking reconstructions of the site of the atrioventricular septal junction are mandatory to explore these aspects further.

Age-Related Changes

It is important that the area of the central fibrous body is changing with age. This can be understood easily if one considers that the right fibrous trigone and the atrioventricular membranous septum are located centrally, at the root of the aorta and the junction of the right and left atrioventricular annuli. Wear and tear, as part of the contractile force of the heart, causes molding of the connective tissues and this will affect the anatomy. The atrioventricular part of the membranous septum, for instance, is very small in the neonate but substantial in adults. These changes not only affect the detailed topographic anatomy of the AV node and bundle, but also atrial inputs such as the anteromedial extent of the terminal crest *(see above)*.

Intraventricular Conduction Tissues

The compact AV node is continuous with the His bundle, one of the historical contributions made by Tawara in 1906. The interlacing architecture of nodal cells, characteristic for the compact AV node, gradually changes to a more parallel alignment in the axis. The site of transition between the compact AV node and the penetrating (His) bundle has been defined as the site of the very last contact of atrial myocardial fibers with the nodal bundle axis. Serial sections of the area confirm Tawara's original illustrations in revealing that the compact node gradually 'sinks' into the connective tissue of the central fibrous body (figure 7). It becomes totally enveloped by connective tissue, thus being insulated from the overlying atrial myocardial fibers. At this stage it should be stressed that it is not uncommon in normal hearts, without any trace of conduction disturbance, to find connective tissue septa dividing the compact node and proximal part of the nodal-bundle axis into separate compartments. The importance of this connotation is based on the fact that occasional reports occur where such architectural aspects are linked to sudden and unexpected death. It is a pity to see that much of these reports lack adequate control studies.

The bundle 'penetrates' the connective tissue of the central fibrous body and thus courses towards the base of the membranous septum (figure 7). This particular segment of the axis is known also as the penetrating bundle. It soon 'rests' on the top of the crest of the interventricular septum and for some length may continue in that position without producing bundle branches. This segment, which varies considerably in length from one individual to the other, is known also as the non-penetrating/non-branching bundle. Both, the penetrating bundle and the non-penetrating/non-branching bundle may together be considered the bundle of His.

The bundle in this position is on the crest of the interventricular septum, but may be in a more left-sided position because of a right-sided septal muscle band, which reinforces the interventricular septum and at the same time 'pushes' the bundle towards the left. Obviously, this detailed anatomy depends highly on the presence and extent of the septomarginal trabeculation and, whether or not, this muscle band is hypertrophic. For example, in hearts with tetralogy of Fallot the posterior extent of the septomarginal trabeculation is always distinctly hypertrophic and well developed and, hence, the penetrating bundle is always left-sided when related to the midline of the interventricular septum.

Soon the non-penetrating/non-branching bundle will produce left bundle branches (figure 7) which cascade down the ventricular septum in subendocardial position. The length of the segment of take off of these left bundle branches may vary, but usually extends over a few millimeters. In the immediate subaortic area the endocardium overlying these proximal stems of the left bundle branches often is thickened, containing fibroelastic tissue. More apically this usually disappears leaving the endocardium much more thin and composed mainly of collagen fibers. Nevertheless, the left bundle branches that fan out over the left ventricular septal surface remain in subendocardial position embedded in connective tissue of the subendocardial space. This is one of the reasons why left bundle branches

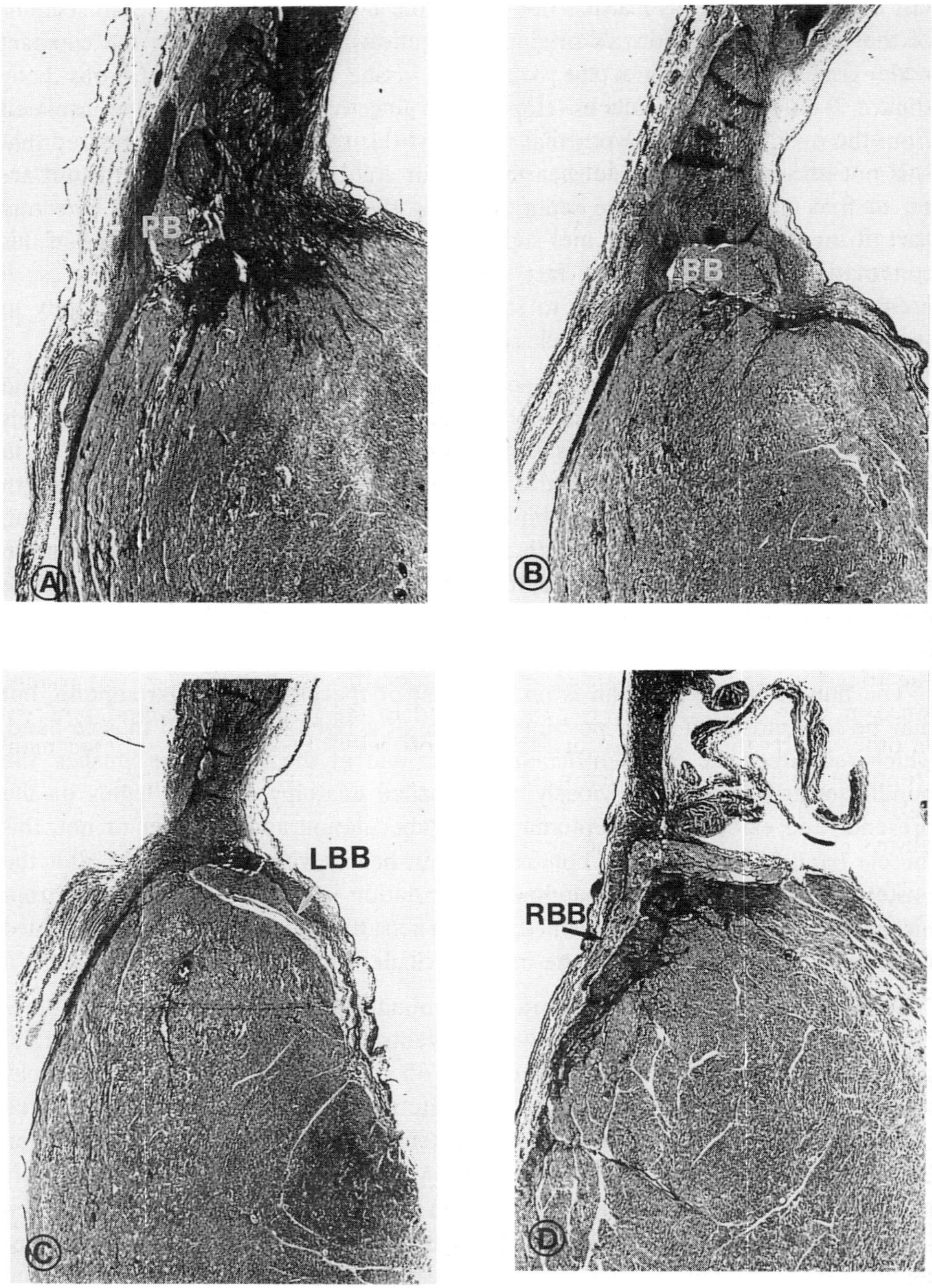
PB
A
LBB
B
LBB
C
RBB
D

can often be seen by the naked eye; strictly speaking it is not the bundle branch that is identified but the accompanying connective tissue. Along their course down the left ventricular septal surface the bundle branches rarely, if ever, produce ramifications that penetrate the underlying myocardium. It is only towards the apical part of the left ventricle that such ramifications appear. Regrettably, these ramifications can no longer be traced reliably in human hearts. There are no specific stains for these terminal branches of the conduction system and, therefore, the anatomical junctional characteristics of the peripheral Purkinje system with myocardial cells remain uncertain.

Once the left bundle branches have separated from the main conduction axis the latter continues as the right bundle branch. The proximal segment of the right bundle branch usually takes an intramural course, which is dictated largely by the presence of the septomarginal trabeculation. The right bundle continues in its intramyocardial position for a considerable length and eventually may surface to take a subendocardial position. This side usually relates to the position of the septal papillary muscle complex for the tricuspid valve. From there on the bundle usually continues in subendocardial position, and, like the left bundle branches, is embedded in connective tissue of the subendocardium. The right bundle branch continues its course superficially in the moderator band, which connects the septomarginal trabeculation with the base of the anterolateral papillary muscle of the tricuspid valve. The anatomy of the moderator band itself is quite variable, since in some hearts it may remain attached to the ventricular septum, whereas in other hearts there may be an early take off, with almost complete detachment from the septal surface, which results in a 'free floating' muscular trabeculation. Like with the left bundle branches, the peripheral ramifications appear late and always close to the apex of the right ventricle.

This particular anatomical configuration of the peripheral ramifications of the Purkinje system and the apparent insulation of the more proximal parts of the bundle branches may have consequences for the proper positioning of pacemaker electrodes.

← **Figure 7.** *Composite of micrographs showing the onset of the penetrating (His) bundle (PB) in A; the non-penetrating-non-bmaching bundle (BB), positioned on the crest of the interventricular septum at the base of the membranous septum, in B; the the origin of left bundle branches (LBB) in C; and the ultimate branching into the right bundle branch (RBB) in D. The orientation of the sections is the same from A-D, perpendicular to the atrioventricular septal junction with the tricuspid valve on the left-hand side.*

1 THE ANATOMICAL ELECTRICAL INTERFACE

Chapter 2

The Electrical Electrode-Myocard Interface

Fred H.M. Wittkampf

Introduction

Electrical effects at the interface between a pacemaker electrode and the heart affect current delivery to the myocardium and the detection of cardiac events necessary for an appropriate timing of those stimuli. In the following two sections, various important electrical aspects of the interface in relation to stimulation and sensing are described.

Stimulation

Ohm's Law. The most important law for all electrical phenomena and also for cardiac stimulation is Ohm's law. Voltage = Current x Resistance. With three parameters involved in this equation, the value of two must be known before the third can be calculated.

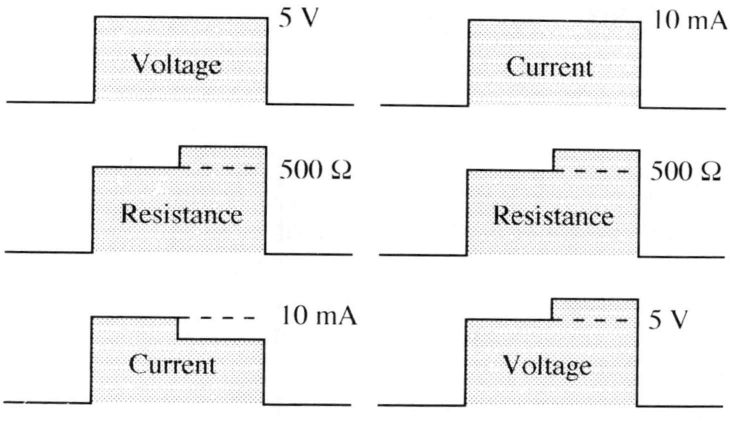

Figure 1. *Ohm's Law: Voltage = Current x Resistance or V = I x R*

Therefore, statements such as *'a smaller electrode has a higher current density'* are basically false. A smaller surface area usually causes a higher electrode-tissue interface resistance and thus less current drain with constant pacing voltage. A smaller surface area combined with a lower total current may therefore result in an equal and not necessarily in a higher current density. A smaller electrode causes a higher current density only if total current is kept constant which, however, is rarely the case.

To appreciate the effects of various parameters on cardiac stimulation we first have to understand the electrical behavior of an electrode in contact with the endocardium.

Capacitive Effects of the Electrode Double Layer

An important phenomenon with respect to pacing is the capacitive effect of the electrical interface between the pacing electrode and its surroundings. The electrode-tissue interface forms a double layer, with electron conduction on the electrode side and ion conduction on the blood-tissue side, and behaves like a capacitor. Such a capacitor can store charge, by binding positively and negatively charged 'particles' in a double layer. A capacitor can be charged by sending current through it.

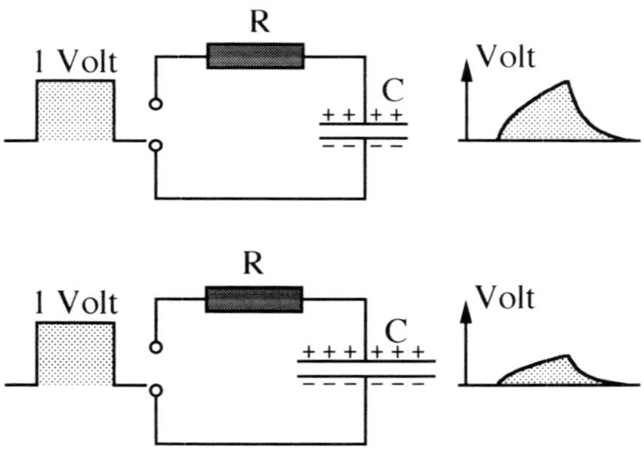

Figure 2. *Charging and discharging of a capacitor. With the same supply voltage, a larger capacitor results in a lower polarization voltage.*

In figure 2, a voltage source on the left is connected via a resistor to a capacitor. Electrons arriving at the capacitor on one side cause an equal number of electrons on the other side to leave. The double layer is charged (polarized) by an overdose of negatively charged electrons on one side and a depletion of electrons on the other side. Thus, while an electrical current flows through the capacitor with an equal amount of current entering and leaving the capacitor, the double layer is charged. With a lower voltage, a higher resistor, or a larger capacitor, a lower maximum voltage will be reached with the same stimulus duration.

At the beginning of the pulse, a capacitor behaves like a simple conductor with a very low resistance. Very soon, however, the capacitor becomes polarized and starts behaving like a battery itself, counteracting the stimulation voltage. Therefore, current flow will diminish during the stimulus by polarization of the capacitor. Thus, with the combination of resistors and capacitors as shown in figure 2, not only the amplitude (voltage) but also the duration of the impulse determines current flow. In that case, 'impedance' is a more correct term than resistance to describe the relation between voltage and current flow. An expression such as *'the impedance is 500 Ω'* is therefore improper. If it is indeed only 500 Ω, one should call the component a resistor. If there are capacitive properties involved one should specify their magnitude. Giving only the true resistive component of 500 Ω is incomplete information and often meaningless. Nevertheless the term *'impedance'* is often used for a pacemaker lead. It usually means that the lead, paced with a certain stimulus magnitude, draws an amount of current with an average value which is approximately equal to what is drawn by a simple resistor of 500 Ω.

The double layer at the electrode-tissue/blood interface is not a pure capacitor: once charged by a stimulus, it also discharges itself. In other words, the double layer capacitor leaks. As a first approximation this leak can be described by a resistor $R_{double\text{-}layer}$ across the capacitive (C) double layer (figure 3).

If we now follow the current path and leave the double layer we encounter the resistivity Rtissue of the surrounding tissue and body fluids.

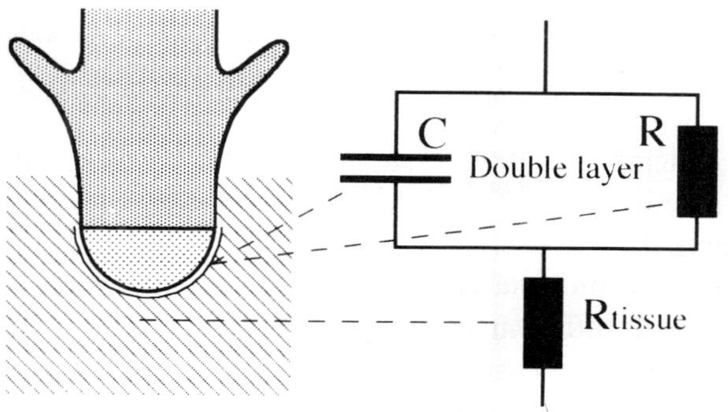

Figure 3. *Simplified diagram of the electrode-patient interface. Capacitive and resistive components of the double layer and the resistance of the tissue.*

Patient Resistance

For a pacing stimulus, the impedance of tissue and body fluids can be regarded as purely resistive as drawn in figure 3 as R_{tissue}. From figure 3 one should understand that all current flowing through the electrode-tissue double layer, via its capacitor or via its parallel resistor, also has to flow through the patient (R_{tissue}). The tissue will thus be affected (stimulated) by the total current flow through the electrode. The voltage present on the electrode, however, is not seen by the tissue since it is partly eliminated by the polarization voltage across the double layer. We will come back to that later.

Figure 4 illustrates that the apparent resistance of the electrode in-creases during the stimulus by the counteracting effect of polarization of the capacitive double layer. A lower stimulation voltage or a shorter pulse duration will cause less charging of the electrode-tissue interface double layer and thus lower the apparent average resistance. A higher voltage on the electrode will cause a faster charging of the double layer and thus increase the apparent average resistance. Therefore, the so called '500 Ω electrode impedance' is **only** true with a specific stimulation voltage or current **and** a specific duration of the stimulus.

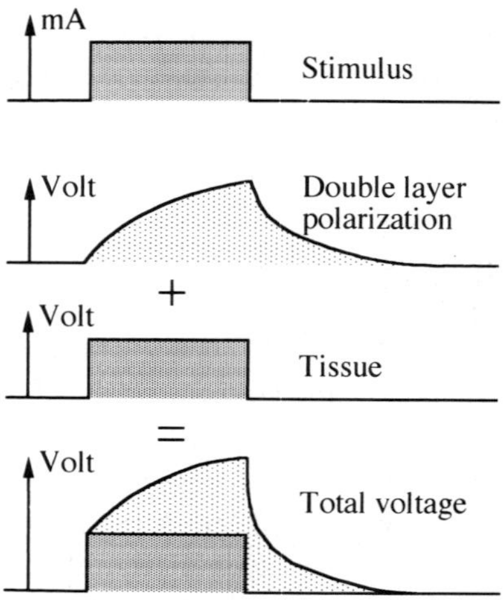

Figure 4. *The total effect of the components of an electrode in a patient can be demonstrated by the delivery of a current stimulus through the system. The resulting voltage between stimulating and indifferent electrode is mainly caused by the resistance of the tissue (R_{tissue}) and polarization of the double layer at the electrode surface.*

Measurement of Electrode Resistance

Some external stimulators or pacing system analyzers measure the average resistance during a stimulus. Others devices measure the resistance after a certain time duration. The apparent resistance will therefore often be different with different stimulators. If the average resistance during a stimulus is measured, value measured at a low stimulation voltage or short pulse duration (e.g. acute threshold) will be lower than with a higher stimulation voltage or longer pulse duration (e.g. chronic threshold).

Like the value of the two double layer components, the magnitude of the tissue resistance depends on the type and size of electrode and, because of a difference in resistance between tissue and blood, also on the intimacy of the electrode-tissue contact. The electrical current has to flow through tissue 'shells' with a small surface area close to the elec-

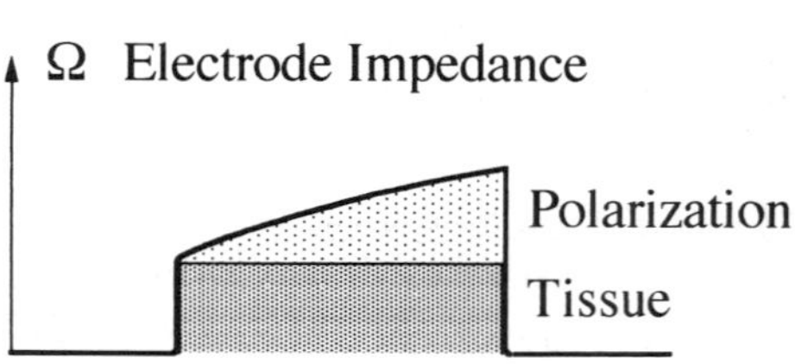

Figure 5. *The electrode impedance increases during the stimulus due to polarization of the double layer.*

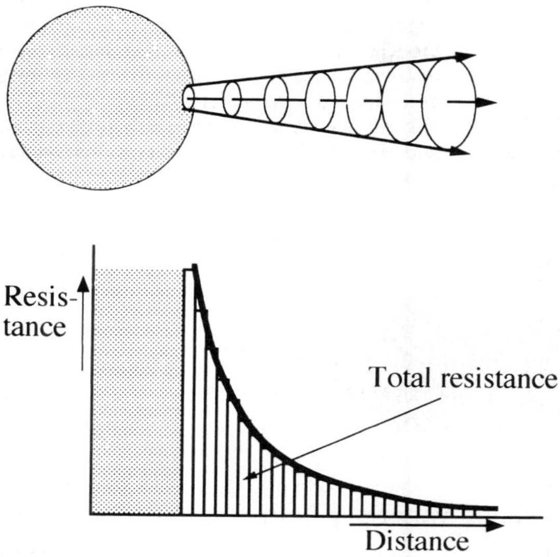

Figure 6. *With an electrode simplified as a sphere embedded in the issue, total electrode-tissue resistance is built up by an endless number of thin tissue 'shells' around the electrode, each with a resistance which decreases with the square of distance from the center of the sphere. The very first layers contribute most to total electrode-tissue resistance.*

trode. The surface area of each next shell becomes larger with the square of distance from the center of the electrode and the electrical resistance drops accordingly. Total tissue resistance equals the sum of all those tissue shells. Therefore, the resistive properties of the first shells are of greater importance for total resistance than the shells at greater distance with a much lower resistance, figure 6. Therefore, the material which is in very close proximity to the surface of the electrode is of major importance for total tissue resistance.

Influence of Electrode Size

The size of the electrode is the major determinant of total impedance. If electrode size in figure 6 is further decreased, one has to add smaller and smaller tissue shells with increasingly greater contribution to total resistance. Also the capacity of the double layer is proportional to electrode surface area, thus size. With a smaller surface area the capacity is lower thus causing an earlier charging and higher counteracting polarization voltage and therefore a higher average resistance for stimuli.

Electrode Surface Structure

Different types of surface structure also affect pacing impedance. An example is shown in figure 7. With an increased surface of the double layer as shown in figure 7, a larger capacity of the double layer is created. This lowers polarization of the double layer capacitor and thus lowers average resistance for a given

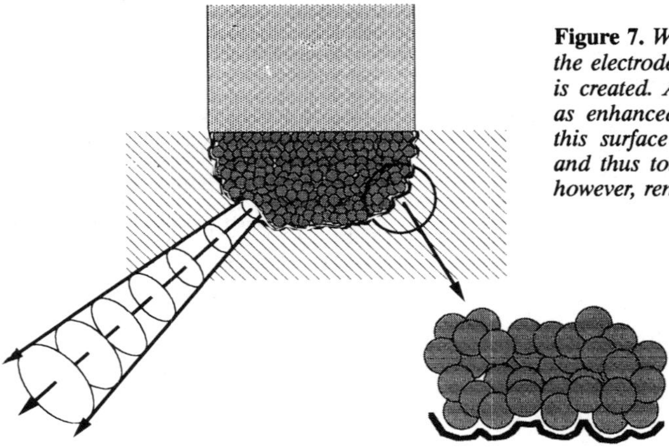

Figure 7. *With an increased micro-surface of the electrode, a larger capacitive double layer is created. Apart from medical aspects such as enhanced ingrowth and chronic fixation, this surface structure decreases polarization and thus total impedance. Tissue resistance, however, remains unchanged.*

stimulus magnitude. With a fixed stimulus voltage, a lower average resistance increases the amount of stimulation current. This will lower pacing threshold when expressed in voltage. To explain this we first have to understand some basic physics of cardiac stimulation.

Cardiac Stimulation

The double layer, with its capacitive and resistive properties, is located between the electrode with electrical conduction via electrons on one side and body fluids with conduction via ions on the other side. This double layer is thus **not** situated within the myocardium. The polarization voltage of the double layer is thus not noticed by the tissue. It does, however, affect stimulation efficacy! As described above, polarization voltage counteracts stimulation voltage so that less voltage is left over for cardiac stimulation. It thereby affects current drain during stimulation. As shown in figure 3, all the current flowing through the electrode eventually has to flow through the patient. Part of it will flow through blood or other non-excitable media and part of it will hopefully also flow through vital myocardium. During the short stimulus, the quality of the electrode contact with the myocardium is presumably stable. The shape of the current impulse through the myocardium will then be identical the shape of the total current flow through the stimulation electrode. The impulse seen by the myocardium is therefore directly proportional to total stimulation current and not to stimulus voltage. Therefore, stimulation voltage is not the parameter which stimulates cardiac tissue; it is the current flow through myocardium causing an electrical field stre-ngth which is the direct cause of stimulation. Also, the stimulation impulse that can be measured by a surface lead is a direct reflection of the current flow through the patient. This impulse, and its possible abnormalities in shape, reflect current flow through the patient and not stimulation voltage!!

Electrical Field Strength Within Tissue

At the beginning of this chapter we discussed Ohm's law: Voltage = Current x Resistance, V = I x R. A similar equation governs the electrical field strength: $E = i \times \rho$. This electrical field strength is expressed in voltage per distance or V/cm. In figure 8, the small cubic piece of myocardium is assumed to be homogeneous which, of course, is not correct. Extra- and intra-cellular fluids have

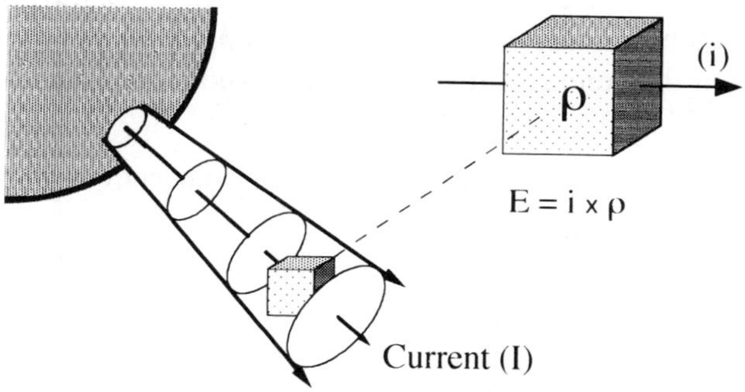

Figure 8. *With a certain amount of current flowing through the myocardium, cardiac cells are not directly affected by stimulus voltage but by current density. Field strength (E) within the myocardium equals current density (i) x specific resistance ρ.*

different ion contents, membranes have a higher resistance, blood and tissue are different and so on. The field strength across cell membranes is responsible for stimulation. This field strength, however, will be proportional to total field strength. Therefore, electrical field strength is a valuable parameter in the stimulation process. Also the direction of the field strength determines stimulation efficacy. Negative pulses are generally more effective (lower threshold) than positive pulses. This is probably due to the fast decrease in current density with increasing distance. At threshold level, stimulation will occur by a sufficiently large field strength across the closest cell membranes. A current flow towards the electrode (negative stimulus) will cause a net positive intra-cellular voltage across the cell membrane closest to the electrode. The negative voltage across the opposite membrane will be lower due to a lower current density at greater distance. Net intracellular voltage shift will then be positive. This is in concordance with the polarity of depolarization and may thus explain the difference in effectiveness between positive and negative stimuli.

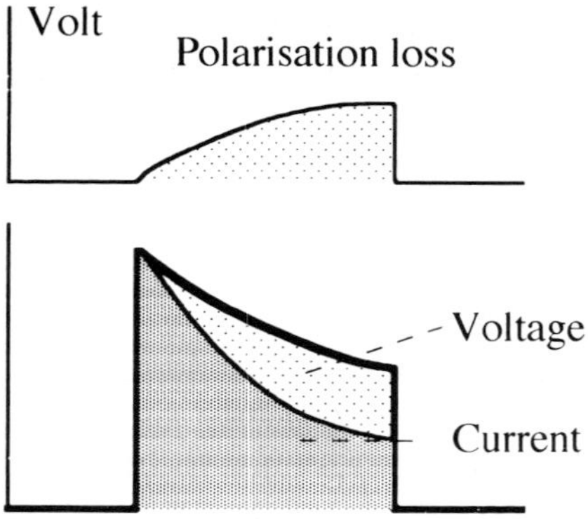

Figure 9. *Polarization of the electrode surface double layer causes a counter-voltage on the double layer capacitor. Consequently, the voltage across the tissue alone is different from the stimulation voltage applied to the electrode. According to Ohm's law, this causes a difference between the waveforms of stimulation voltage and current through the myocardium.*

As discussed above, the shape of the field strength impulse within the tissue, being proportional to current flow, is different from the shape of the stimulation voltage impulse as is shown in figure 9. Field strength, however, is not constant in the vicinity of the electrode. Current density and thus field strength decreases with the square of distance from the center of the electrode as shown in figure 10.

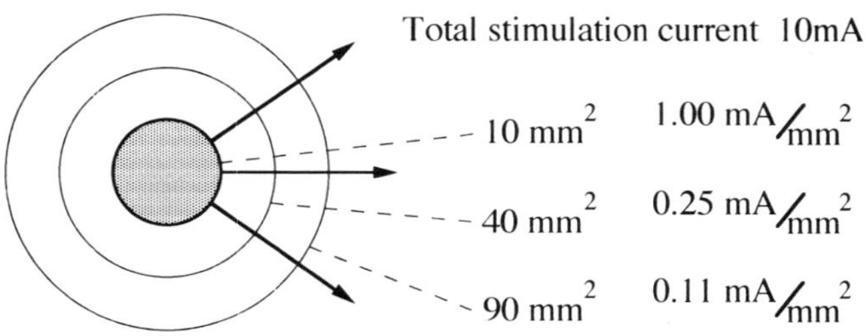

Figure 10. *With a spherical electrode embedded in homogeneous tissue, current density decreases with the square of distance from the center of the electrode and so does the resulting field strength.*

Moreover, current density at the surface of the electrode may be different at different sites on the surface of the electrode because a pacemaker electrode is not spherical. Sharp transitions at the electrode surface have a lower electrical resistance to tissue than relatively flat areas. As shown in figure 11, the surface area of successive tissue layers around the electrode increases more rapidly at the proximal edge of the electrode than at the distal end. Therefore, the electrical resistance will be lower and current density will be higher at those sharp transitions.

While the current density is very high at sharp edges initially, it also decreases more rapidly with distance than at other sites. Consequently, current density will be rather uniformly distributed at a few mm distance.

Figure 11. *Current flow in the vicinity of the electrode. At electrically sharp transitions, e.g. between tip and isolation, current density may by much higher than at relatively 'flat' parts of the surface.*

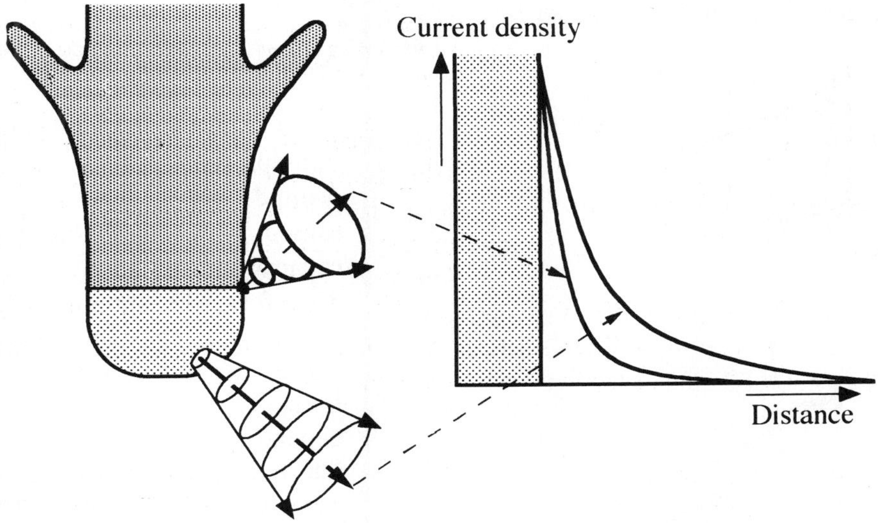

Chronaxy - Rheobase Curve

Stimulation threshold, whether expressed in voltage or current, depends on the duration of the stimulus. This relationship is expressed by the so-called chronaxy-rheobase curve, a plot of voltage threshold versus impulse duration as shown in figure 12. Generally, the total amount of energy consumed by the stimulus is lowest at the chronaxy point.

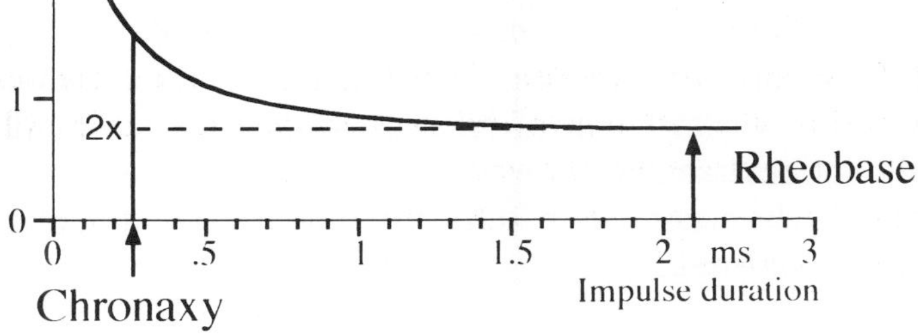

Figure 12. *The Chronaxy - Rheobase curve showing the relation between stimulus duration and stimulation voltage at threshold level.*

Clinical Implications

The basic principles described above have important implications for the clinical use of pacemaker technology.

Pacemaker Stimulus

As shown in figure 13, the stimulus delivered by an implanted pulse generator is caused by the discharge of a capacitor in its output circuit. Therefore, the stimulus does not have a constant voltage nor a constant current waveform. The voltage waveform depends on the magnitude of the pulse generator's output capacitor which varies per manufacturer but it also depends on the load. A large surface area electrode with a lower impedance will discharge the output capacitor more rapidly than a small surface area electrode, figure 13.

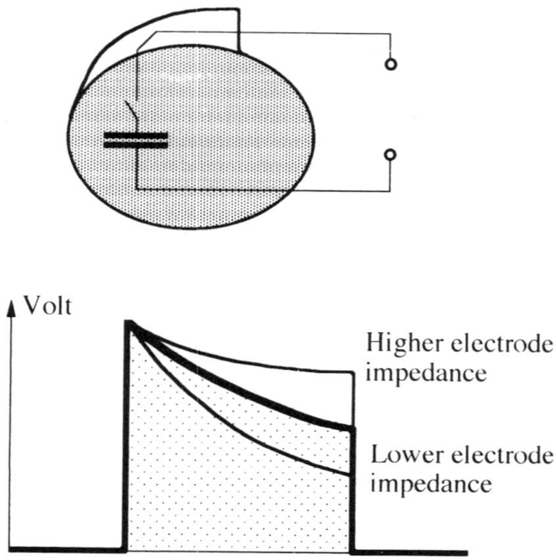

Figure 13. *The stimulus of the pulse generator is a capacitor discharge. The average amplitude depends on the impedance of the electrode.*

Moreover, the effective stimulus voltage further decreases by polarization losses as shown in figure 9.

Threshold Measurement

As described above, the magnitude of current flow during stimulation determines the effectivity of the stimulus. A different output circuit of, and waveform from, a stimulator will cause a different average magnitude of stimulation current and therefore a different threshold when expressed in stimulation voltage. Therefore, these different waveforms will result in a different reading for threshold values. The differences will not be dramatic but especially relevant when stimulation thresholds of different leads measured in different centers with different types of equipment are being compared.

Comparison of Stimulation Thresholds Between Different Leads

Whether stimulation threshold is measured in voltage or current is also important for the comparison of different electrode designs. If a polished platinum electrode is compared with a porous electrode with the same overall geometry, the difference in impedance between both is mainly caused by different properties of the double layer which, however, does not participate directly in stimulation. Tissue resistance will be approximately the same for both. In a comparison of for example acute stimulation threshold, we can not expect much difference if threshold is expressed in current (mA): an identical stimulation current and tissue resistance will cause the same field strength within the tissue. The porous electrode, however, will have a lower polarization voltage and thus a lower voltage threshold.

A second example is the comparison of stimulation threshold between two electrodes with a different surface area but the same surface structure, e.g. polished platinum.

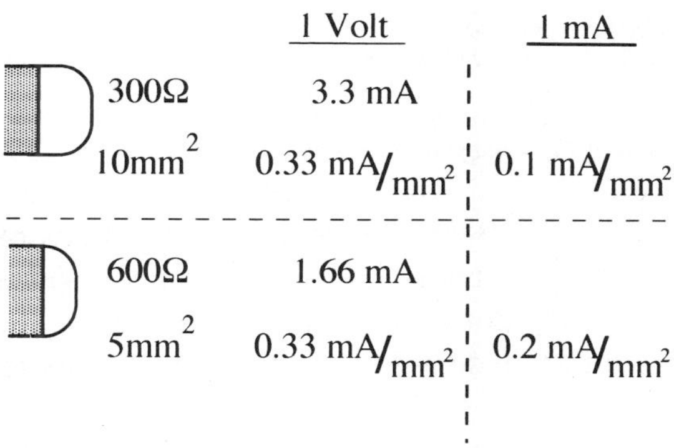

Figure 14. *Stimulation efficacy comparison between two different size electrodes. The smaller surface area electrode will have a higher average resistance. With the same voltage applied to both, approximately the same maximum current density is achieved at the surface of the electrodes. With the same total stimulation current through both leads, however, current density at the electrode surface is much higher for the smaller of the two electrodes.*

As shown in figure 14, the same voltage applied to both electrodes results in approximately the same current density at the surface of both electrodes. With the same total current, the current density at the surface of the larger electrode is much lower. Thus, in order to achieve the same current density within the tissue, the stimulus current must approximately be doubled for the larger of the two electrodes. Acute current threshold will therefore be much higher with the larger electrode whereas voltage thresholds will be similar. This is one of the reasons why acute stimulation threshold is most often measured in voltage: values are rather independent of electrode design and approximately the same threshold acceptance limits can be applied to different leads.

Stimulus Intensity

Once stimulation threshold is known, pulse generator output should be set at a higher level to ensure continuous stimulation.

As described above, stimulus intensity is directly related to stimulation current and duration. Effective stimulus magnitude is thus dependent of the surface area below the current impulse shown in figure 15. Because of a decay of stimulation voltage (pulse generator's capacitor discharge) and an even more dramatic decay of stimulation current (due to polarization) during the pulse, doubling of the duration of the stimulus does not result in a doubling of stimulus magnitude. Impulse duration should roughly be tripled to achieve a 50% safety factor as shown in figure 15. The same result is achieved by a twofold increase in stimulation voltage.

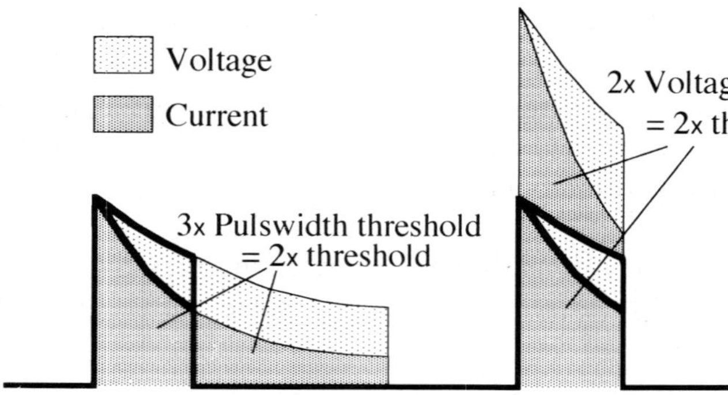

Figure 15. *Voltage and current waveforms at threshold (bold line) and a threefold increased impulse duration (left) and doubled amplitude (right). Because stimulation current is directly related to the electrical field strength within the tissue, one should double the content of the current stimulus waveform. This can be achieved by tripling the impulse duration or doubling the voltage of the stimulus.*

Stimulation Threshold Changes After Implant

Soon after implantation, the tissue starts reacting more or less aggressively to the foreign implant. The inflammatory reaction is known to cause an increase in stimulation threshold achieving its maximum approximately 2 to 3 weeks after implantation. After a few months, the situation has stabilized and the electrode is covered with fibrous tissue, figure 16.

Fibrous tissue lowers current density and field strength within the myocardium by increasing the distance from the electrode. This is the cause of an increase in

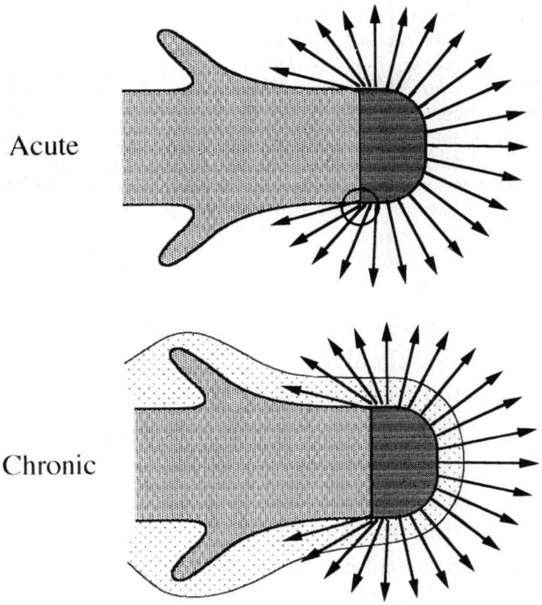

Figure 16. *Fibrous tissue increases the distance between the electrode and vital myocardium and thus lowers local current density. Local inhomogeneities in current density are reduced causing a more homogenous current density at the border with vital myocardium. This may shift the stimulation site.*

pacing threshold after implantation, figure 15. As shown in figure 11, the divergence of current is larger at the proximal edge of the electrode than at the distal site. Consequently, current density decreases more dramatically with increasing distance at those sharp edges. Therefore, the site of stimulation may also shift from the acute to the chronic situation. Attempts to reduce the foreign body reaction by means of steroid-eluting electrodes are very successful, but even then a thin layer of fibrous tissue will cover the electrode in the chronic situation. Besides this there are short term, daily variations in stimulation threshold and various studies have also indicated a very slow long term increase in stimulation threshold. These latter changes may also reflect changes within the myocardium with age rather than a reaction to the foreign implant. Nevertheless, pulse generator output has to be programmed to account for those changes and to ensure continuous cardiac stimulation. This should be done as shown in figure 15. However, by doing so, the effect of stimulus strength on pulse generator longevity should also be taken into consideration.

Pulse Generator Longevity

In figure 17, the effect of pacing voltage on battery current drain is illustrated. At 2.5 V and a 500 Ω lead, stimulation current is 5 mA. With a battery voltage of 2.5 V, which is the case in most pacemakers, the current of 5 mA is thus supplied directly by the battery. With one 0.5 ms stimulus per second, average battery current drain for stimulation is 0.5‰ of 5 mA thus 2.5 μA. If 2.5 V − 0.5 ms happens to be the chronic stimulation threshold and the policy is to set pacemaker output at twice threshold, one could either double stimulation voltage or triple

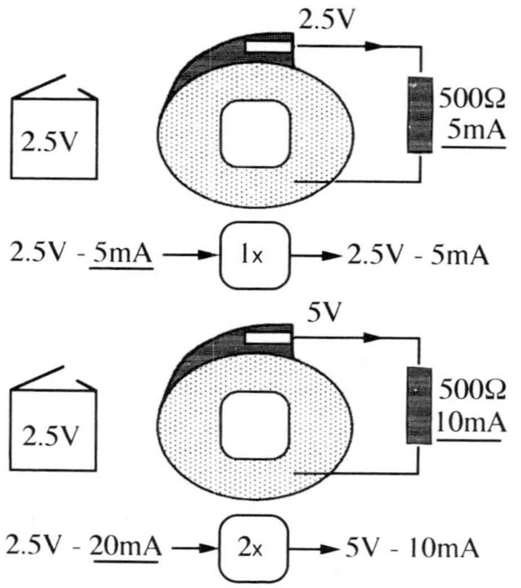

Figure 17. *Comparison of battery current drain with two different stimulation voltages. At 2.5 V output, 5 mA is delivered through a pacing lead with an average resistance of 500 Ω. Battery current drain during the stimulus is also 5 mA since battery voltage also equals 2.5 V. At 5 V output, stimulus magnitude is increased twofold to 10 mA. Due to the law of 'Conservation of Energy', battery current drain at 2.5 V, however, is increased fourfold from 5 to 20 mA during the stimulus.*

impulse duration. A twofold increase in stimulation voltage results in a fourfold increase in battery current drain as shown in the right hand panel of figure 17. Battery current drain would then increase to 10 μA. If this is applied to a dual chamber pacemaker with a basic circuit current drain of 10 μA, total battery current drain would thus increase from (10+2x2.5=) 15 μA to (10+2x10=) 30 μA. With a threefold increase in stimulus duration and thus one 1.5 ms stimulus per second, average battery current drain necessary for each of the two outputs will only double (figure 15) thus to 5 μA and total battery current drain to (10+2x5=) 20 μA. In this example, battery life with triple pulse duration would be 50% longer than with double stimulation voltage. When chronic stimulation threshold is rather low, e.g. 1 V/.5 ms, the difference between the two choices would affect battery life less because of the greater relative contribution of basic circuit current drain (10 μA) to total current consumption.

Summary:

- Stimulation causes polarization at the electrode-tissue interface.
- Polarization counteracts stimulation voltage.
- Therefore, the shape of the current impulse differs from voltage impulse.
- Current flows through myocardium where it creates a certain field strength across cell membranes.
- This field strength triggers myocyte depolarization.
- Negative stimuli are in general more effective than positive stimuli.
- The precise stimulation site may shift from acute to chronic.
- Comparison of stimulation threshold between different electrodes in voltage, current or both depends on electrode design. In general, voltage threshold is

implanted pacemaker may thus differ from the true amplitude, especially acutely. This also explains why, newer pulse generators designed for smaller electrodes, may sometimes detect cardiac signals less well than older units when connected to the same older chronic electrodes with relatively large surface areas.

The polarity of a bipolar electrogram can be either positive or negative. Amplifiers for bipolar pulse generators should therefore be equally sensitive for both polarities making them less specific. Far field signals, however, are eliminated more markedly by bipolar sensing which compensates for the lower detection specificity.

Judging Electrode Placement

A high frequency signal like the sharply negative deflection is a marker of good electrode-wall contact and may serve to position the electrode inside the heart. The filter in the pulse generator, however, is not optimally trimmed to that signal since its slew rate or frequency content is higher than in the chronic situation. The electrogram from an electrode with poor wall contact may also not show this negative deflection acutely and thus be equally effective for pacemaker sensing. In that case, however, stimulation threshold will often be unsatisfactory. This explains why good acute sensing does not guarantee a low pacing threshold. Alternatively, the example shown in figure 18 demonstrates that the true negative deflection may be reduced in amplitude by the acutely present lesion potential, especially in the case of electrodes with active fixation means. This may reduce electrogram amplitude temporarily whereas stimulation threshold may be quite low with such good wall contact. Therefore, measurement of both stimulation threshold and electrogram amplitude remains necessary to determine the quality of electrode tissue contact.

Summary:

- An endocardial electrode detects three kinds of signals: Far field electrogram, local depolarization and acutely a lesion potential.
- This lesion potential may affect electrogram amplitude temporarily.
- Morphology of bipolar electrograms varies more than that of unipolar electrograms from patient to patient, between different timing sequences, and between the acute and chronic situation. Changes in unipolar electrogram morphology are more predictable.
- Pacemaker filters affect electrogram detection.
- Pacemaker circuits are designed for a chronic lead which implies that the amplitude of the acute electrogram may be underestimated by the pacemaker.
- Good sensing does not ensure a low stimulation threshold.

2 CONSIDERATIONS BEFORE IMPLANT OF A PACEMAKER

Chapter 3

Timing Cycles in Dual-Chamber Adaptive Rate Pacemakers and the Consequences for Programming

Jaap H. Ruiter and Jan P.M. Corstjens

Introduction

With the development of new and more sophisticated pacing modes, understanding of pacemaker rhythms can be difficult and time consuming. A profound knowledge of the nomenclature and timing of dual chamber adaptive rate (DDDR) pacing is mandatory to program the parameters and special functions, in order to fine tune the pacing therapy for each individual patient. A DDDR pacemaker can control the cardiac cycle by processing the input of three sources, i.e. the atrium, the ventricle and a sensor circuit. Each of these three inputs impacts every subsequent cardiac cycle, as determined by the programmed timing intervals. Timing intervals are distinct periods that occur during the cardiac cycle and between subsequent cardiac cycles. Pacemaker timing intervals can be compared to the alarms of a clock. At the appropriate 'time', the pacemaker delivers a pacing pulse to either the atrium or ventricle, much the same way an alarm rings in a clock at a set time. Timing intervals can be triggered by atrial and ventricular events, both paced and sensed. In addition, timing intervals within and between subsequent cardiac cycles can be modified by sensor control.

Table 1 lists a series of abbreviations, used in the next sections to describe native and paced events and intervals of the timing cycle. It is important to note that the timing of pacemakers is based on intervals (ms) rather than on rate (bpm). Intervals are measured in milliseconds (= 0.001 second). For example, at a heart rate of 60 bpm the interval is 1000 ms. Most DDDR pacemakers timing intervals can be programmed over a wide range of settings with small increments. To interpret a DDDR pacing rhythm, information about the activity level of the patient, the sensor characteristics and programmed parameters is also needed.

Table 1.

P wave	:	a native atrial depolarization
R wave	:	a native ventricular depolarization
A	:	a paced atrial event
V	:	a paced ventricular event
PR interval	:	the interval between intrinsic atrial and ventricular depolarizations, as measured by the pacemaker
AVI	:	the interval from an atrial stimulus or P wave detection to the synchronized ventricular stimulus
AR interval	:	the interval from an atrial stimulus to the detection of a native R wave
VA interval	:	the interval from a ventricular stimulus to the detection of a retrogradely conducted P wave
AEI	:	Atrial Escape Interval. The interval from a paced or intrinsic ventricular event to the next intrinsic atrial event
VAI	:	Ventricular Atrial Interval. The interval from a ventricular paced or sensed event to the next atrial paced event at the lower rate limit
VEI	:	Ventricular Escape Interval. The interval from a paced or sensed ventricular event to the next intrinsic ventricular event
LRL	:	Lower Rate Limit. The minimum paced rate in atrium and ventricle, in the absence of intrinsic activity
MTI	:	Minimum Tracking Interval. Interval between two consecutive ventricular paced events at the Upper rate Limit
MTR	:	Maximum Tracking Rate. The maximum rate, at which 1:1 synchronization can occur (identical to URL)
MSR	:	Maximum Sensor Rate. Upper rate limit for sensor driven pacing
PVARP	:	Post Ventricular Atrial Refractory Period. Starts upon a paced or sensed ventricular event
TARP	:	Total Atrial Refractory Period. Equals the sum of AVI and PVARP
PAVI	:	Paced Atrio-Ventricular Interval. AVI following a paced atrial event (this actually is AVI)
SAVI	:	Sensed Atrio-Ventricular Interval. AVI following a sensed atrial event (= PAVI-pace/sense offset)
URL	:	Upper Rate Limit. The maximum attainable ventricular pacing rate in response to detection of faster atrial activity

The different modes of cardiac pacing are listed in table 2, using the NASPE (North American Society of Pacing and Electrophysiology) and BPEG (British Pacing and Electrophysiology Group) pacemaker code.

Table 2. NASPE Pacemaker Code

The NASPE pacemaker code uses the following characters to describe the pacing mode or pacemaker type. These characters are:

V - Ventricle
A - Atrium
D - Dual (atrium and ventricle)
T - Triggering (response)
I - Inhibition (response)
R - Adaptive Rate

The pacing mode is indicated by the following four letter code:

I Pacing	II Sensing	III Response to sensing	IV Adaptive Rate
V	V	I	
V	V	I	R
A	A	I	
A	A	I	R
D	D	D	
D	D	D	R

As most single chamber pacemakers can be used in both the atrium and ventricle, some manufacturers indicate the pacemaker type with the character S (single). Instead of VVI or AAI the code SSI is used. To indicate the pacing mode, S cannot be used.

Timing Cycles in Dual-Chamber Adaptive Rate Pacing

Dual-chamber adaptive rate pacemakers (DDDR) control the ventricular pacing rate during exercise by detection of intrinsic atrial activity and sensor control. In addition, new generation DDDR pacemakers incorporate features such as automatic mode switching, sensor controlled AVI and atrial refractory periods and algorithms for prevention of pacemaker mediated tachycardia.

The following timing cycles and features will be discussed in more detail:

- refractory and blanking periods
- atrio-ventricular interval (AVI)
- lower rate limit
- upper rate limit and upper rate limit behaviour
- sensor controlled intervals
- rate smoothing
- automatic mode switching
- pacemaker mediated tachycardia prevention

Refractory and Blanking Periods

After any cardiac depolarization no stimulus, regardless of it's strength, can provoke another depolarization during a brief period. This period is called the absolute refractory period. Similarly after a sensed or paced event, the pacemaker is refractory or unresponsive to any cardiac or noncardiac stimulus. Refractory periods prevent the sensing of pacemaker stimuli, the evoked cardiac depolarization and repolarization. During the noise sampling window, which falls inside the refractory period, the sensing circuit must be able to discriminate non-physiological signals such as magnetic, electrical and electromagnetic noise from spontaneous depolarization. Noise of sufficient strength and frequency content, similar to electrophysiologic signals, can otherwise interfere with proper pacemaker function. Blanking periods are used to prevent sensing of the pacing stimulus, delivered to the other heart chamber during dual-chamber pacing. The inappropriate detection of the atrial stimulus in the ventricle and detection of the ventricular stimulus in the atrium is referred to as 'cross talk'.

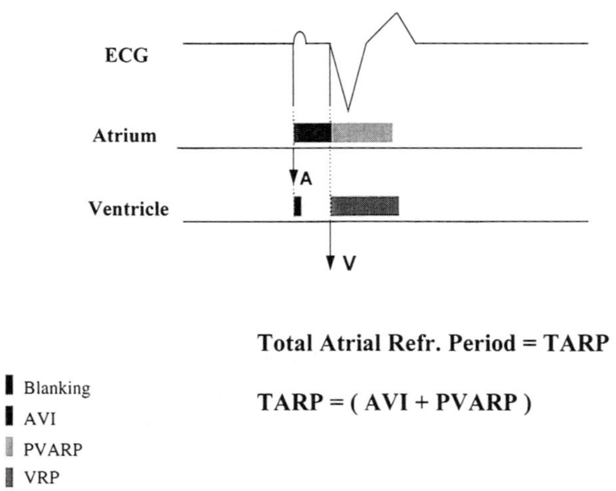

Figure 1 shows a schematic representation of the atrial and ventricular refractory and blanking periods. The atrial refractory period (PVARP) is defined as the period after a ventricular event, either paced or sensed, when activity in the

Figure 1. *The total atrial refractory period (TARP) equals the sum of the AV Interval (AVI) and post ventricular atrial refractory period (PVARP).*

atrium does not inhibit an atrial stimulus nor trigger a ventricular stimulus. The atrial refractory period starts at the ventricular event, to avoid far-field sensing of electrical signals coming from the ventricle. By selection of an appropriate PVARP, pacemaker mediated tachycardia, triggered by retrograde VA conduction, is usually prevented. The use of a long atrial refractory period lowers the maximal atrial rate that can be detected and thus limits the level of atrial tracking during exercise. In patients with atrial tachyarrhythmias, the atrial refractory period should be as short as possible to reliably detect the tachyarrhythmia and facilitate adequate mode switching (if available) into a non P wave synchronous mode, to avoid ventricular pacing at unwanted high rates. The initial part of the PVARP consists of a blanking period (programmable in some devices), followed by the relative refractory period. Atrial sensing can occur inside the relative atrial refractory period, however, this will not trigger a ventricular stimulus.

In DDD(R) pacemakers with the mode switching function, signals inside the relative part of the PVARP are monitored by the tachycardia detection algorithm to facilitate reliable atrial tachyarrhythmia detection. In DDDR pacing mode, sensor controlled atrial pacing can occur inside the PVARP, if the sensor rate is programmed sufficiently high. In some pacemakers, the duration of PVARP can be changed by sensor control. In such pacemakers, programmed to dual-chamber pacing modes, the adaptive PVARP can be as short as the programmable atrial blanking period. In DDD(R) pacing, the total atrial refractory period (TARP) equals the sum of atrioventricular interval (AVI) and post ventricular atrial refractory period (PVARP). The TARP limits the maximal atrial rate that can be detected by a DDD(R) pacemaker and limits the maximal rate at which the ventricle can be paced during P wave synchronous pacing in the absence of a separate MTR (figure 2).

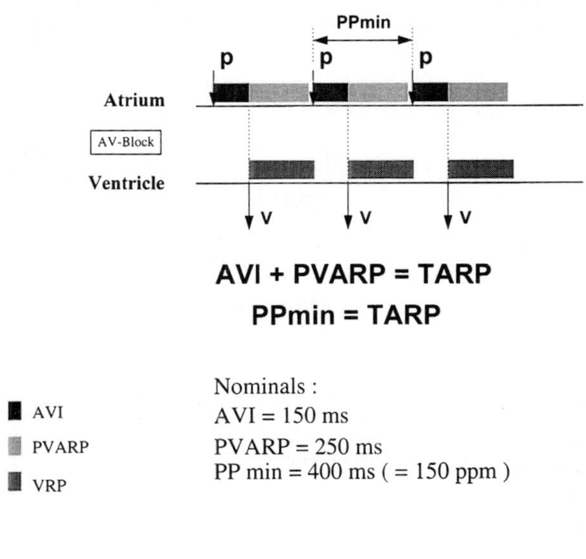

Figure 2. *The total atrial refractory period (TARP) limits the maximal atrial rate (or minimum PP interval) that can be detected by a DDD(R) pacemaker.*

The ventricular refractory period (VRP) follows any ventricular event. The VRP is programmable and consists of an absolute refractory period, a noise sampling period, and the remaining relative refractory period. The VRP prevents detection of the evoked ventricular depolarization and subsequent repolarization (T wave). In a ventricular based timing system, the VA interval starts after either a paced or a sensed ventricular event to control lower rate timing. The PVARP coincides with the initial part of the VA interval.

▸ *Blanking Periods.* During a blanking period, the sensing circuit of one channel ignores sensed electrical activity generated by a pacing stimulus, delivered in the other chamber. Ventricular pacing, if sensed in the atrium, would result in an inappropriately high ventricular pacing rate in an attempt to maintain AV synchrony. Atrial pacing, if sensed in the ventricle, would inhibit ventricular output, thereby potentially causing symptomatic ventricular pauses. An atrial stimulus synchronously triggers AVI and the ventricular blanking period. Electrical activity, sensed inside the blanking period, is ignored by the pacemaker so that ventricular inhibition due to detection of the atrial stimulus cannot occur. Some pacemakers have a feature called ventricular safety pacing. At the delivery of an atrial stimulus, the ventricular blanking period is followed by a cross talk sensing window. When electrical activity is detected inside the cross talk sensing window, the pacemaker is committed to deliver a ventricular stimulus at the end of the ventricular safety pacing window. The ventricular safety pacing window is usually fixed at a nominal value of 100 ms. If a ventricular premature beat or AV nodal escape beat coincide with an atrial stimulus and are sensed inside the ventricular safety pacing window, this will result in the delivery of a ventricular stimulus inside the absolute refractory period of the ventricular depolarization (figure 3).

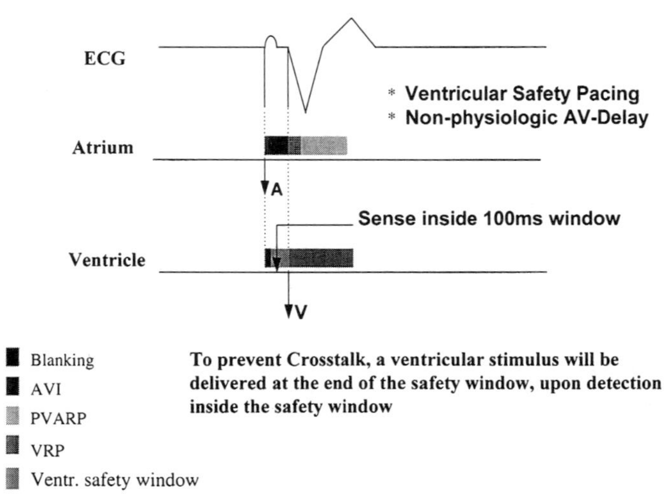

Figure 3. *The ventricular safety window starts in the ventricular channel upon delivery of an atrial stimulus. If, inside the safety window, electrical activity is detected, a stimulus will be delivered to the ventricle at the end of the safety window to prevent potential inhibition due to cross talk.*

The Atrio-Ventricular Interval

The atrio-ventricular interval (AVI) starts at the atrial stimulus or the onset of P wave detection and ends with the delivery of a synchronized ventricular stimulus. During the AVI, the atrial sensing circuit is refractory. The AVI provides the delay needed for ventricular filling after an atrial contraction. In DDD(R) pacing, AVI is programmable over a wide range and in small increments (i.e. 60-300 ms in 10 ms increments). In patients with intact AV conduction, AVI needs to be programmed long enough to facilitate spontaneous AV conduction. Atrial activation originating from the sinus node has a different intra-atrial conduction time (IACT) than paced atrial beats. Intrinsic atrial activity only can be detected after some atrial tissue has depolarised, since the tip of the atrial lead is positioned remote from the sinus node. A paced atrial beat originates at the atrial lead tip, and therefore no delay occurs between the delivery of an atrial stimulus and the start of AVI. In some pacemakers the AVI can independently be programmed for paced and sensed atrial events to obtain optimal hemodynamics. Programming the sensed AV interval (SAVI) shorter than the paced AV interval (PAVI) will compensate for the intra-atrial conduction delay between sinus node and electrode tip. AV nodal conduction is influenced by the autonomic nervous system and during exercise or emotions the PR interval shortens. Some DDD and DDDR pacemakers have a rate adaptive AVI (dynamic AV interval) for both sensor-driven and P wave synchronous pacing, including the differentiation between SAVI and PAVI. Dynamic AVI shortening may be gradual and coupled to heart rate (AVI as a percentage of cardiac cycle length) whereas in other pacemakers it may adapt in a stepwise fashion.

Lower Rate Timing

Current DDD(R) pacemakers use two basic types of timing systems:

1. Ventricular-based timing (V-V timing), with or without modification
2. Atrial-based timing (A-A timing), with or without modification

▸ *Ventricular-based timing systems and DDD mode.* A paced or sensed ventricular event starts the lower rate interval timer (LRI), (figure 4). After a ventricular event (paced or sensed), in absence of intrinsic atrial activity, an atrial stimulus is delivered at the end of the VA interval. The VA interval is fixed and will also be triggered by the detection of a premature ventricular beat (PVC). In DDDR mode, the VA interval interval can shorten due to sensor drive during exercise. The AVI follows the VAI and represents the last portion of the LRI. Thus the LRI is the sum of AVI and VA interval. The interval between a ventricular

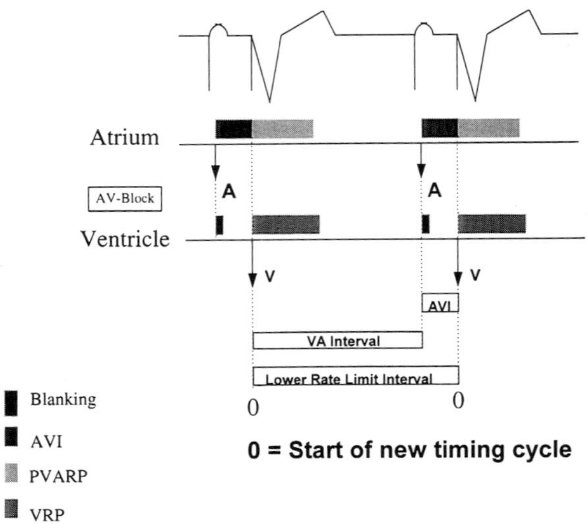

Figure 4. *The Lower Rate Limit interval (LRI) in ventricular-based timing systems.*

event (paced or sensed) and a spontaneous atrial event is called the atrial escape interval (AEI). In case of intrinsic AV conduction, the actual ventricular rate is faster than the programmed LRI. The interval after an atrial pace to a sensed R wave (AR interval) is shorter than the programmed AVI, which results in an actual LRI that is (AVI-ARI) shorter than the programmed LRI. If the sensed AV interval (SAVI) is programmed shorter than the paced AV Interval (PAVI), small LRI variations can occur when the spontaneous sinus rate approaches the lower rate limit. Shortening of the LRI can be caused by intrinsic AV conduction, ventricular safety pacing, dynamic AVI operation and programmed differences in paced and sensed AVI. In patients with 2:1 AV block and pacing at the lower rate limit, the ventricular cycle length will alternate between the LRI and a slightly faster rate, which is LRI-(AVI-ARI). Thus, in V-V timing the lower rate limit can change, depending on the condition of the AV conduction. However, the VA interval remains constant.

▸ *Atrial-based timing systems and DDD mode.* In atrial based timing, the interval between a sensed or paced atrial event until the following atrial paced event (LRI or A-A interval) is fixed. The LRI (A-A interval) equals the sum of AVI and VAI. In atrial based timing systems, the timer can be reset by both atrial and ventricular events. As a consequence, a ventricular premature beat starts a new A-A interval, resulting in a ventricular interval after the PVC that is longer than the LRI. The interval between a PVC and the following ventricular event equals the sum of LRI (= A-A interval) and AVI (figure 5). During AV conduction or AV block, the LRI does not change, as the PR interval or AVI fall inside the A-A interval. In atrial based timing systems, the LRI (or A-A interval) is fixed. Consequently the VA interval must change to keep atrial cycle lengths equal during intrinsic AV conduction or AV block. For instance, if an atrial event (paced or sensed) is followed by intrinsic AV conduction, the VAI will prolong

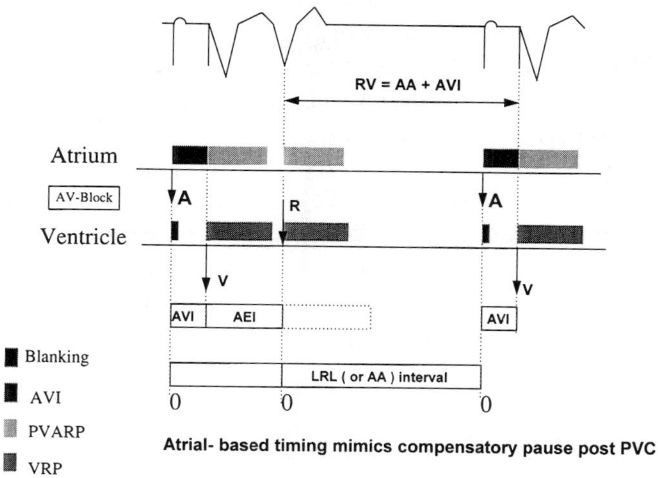

Figure 5. *Post PVC response in pacemakers with atrial-based timing systems.*

with the difference between the programmed AVI and intrinsic PR or AR interval. Theoretically, atrial based timing systems mimic natural sinus rhythm more closely than ventricular based systems. It is important to note, however, that in atrial based timing, the lower rate limit can be violated in the ventricle, if AV block follows a previous cardiac cycle with intrinsic AV conduction (figure 6).

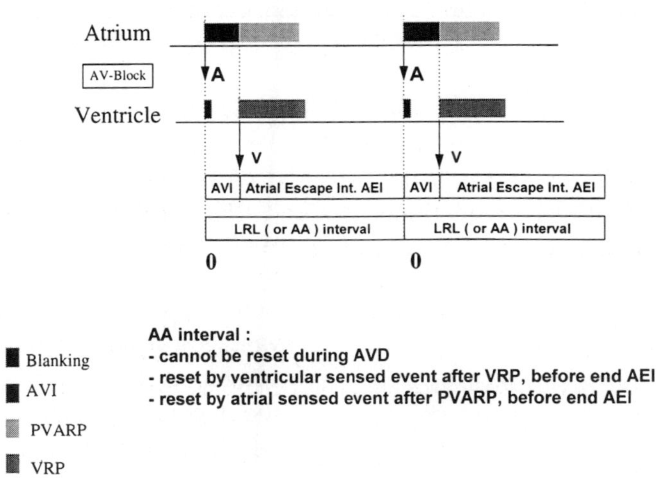

Figure 6. *The Lower Rate Limit or AA interval in atrial-based timing systems.*

Consequently, during 2:1 block pacing at the lower rate limit, alternating ventricular intervals above and below the lower rate limit will occur. Pure atrial based timing is not used in recent DDD(R) pacemakers due to the violation of LRL after a PVC. Most contemporary atrial based timing systems use V-V timing in response PVC detection.

▸ *Modified atrial-based timing systems.* To eliminate the post PVC pause as seen with conventional atrial based timing systems, a modification of this system was implemented. In response to detection of a PVC the subsequent A-A interval is reduced by the AVI, thereby eliminating the long ventricular interval after a PVC (figure 7). The post PVC response is equal to the response in ventricular based timing systems. However, the alternating ventricular intervals during 2:1 block and pacing at the LRI, and thus violation of the LRI, still can occur.

Table 3 shows the type of timing systems of several contemporary pacemaker manufacturers.

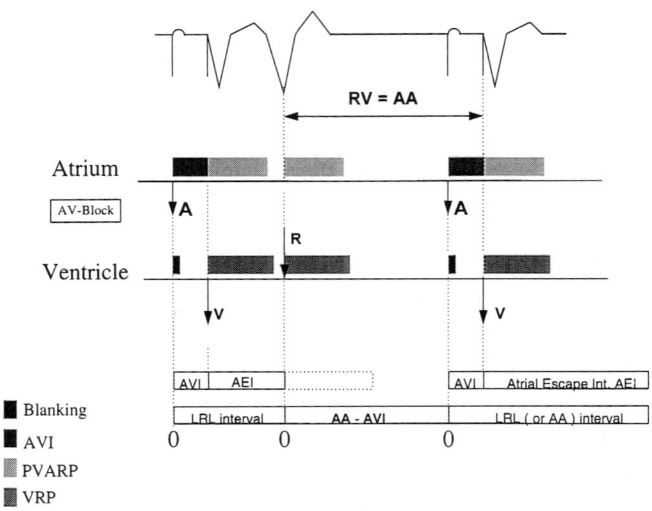

Figure 7.
Post PVC response in pacemakers with modified atrial-based timing systems.

Table 3.

Ventricular timing (± modification)	**Atrial timing** (± modification)
CPI	Medtronics
Vitatron	Intermedic
Pacesetter/Siemens	Biotronik
Telectronics	

New pacemaker designs combine ventricular based and atrial based timing systems, resulting in modified timing systems. As such, advantages of both timing systems are combined. It is mandatory to read the technical manuals carefully to be familiar with the functional characteristics of the pacing devices used.

Upper Rate Timing in DDD(R) Pacemakers

In the first generations of DDD pacemakers the maximum pacing rate was limited only by the duration of the total atrial refractory period (TARP = AVI + PVARP). If the intrinsic atrial interval becomes shorter than the TARP, every second P wave will fall inside the PVARP, resulting in a 2:1 block response (figure 8).

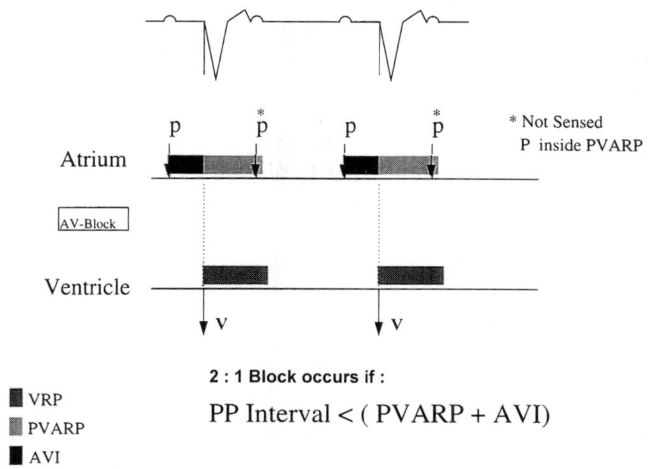

Figure 8. *Mechanism of 2:1 block pacing in DDD(R) pacemakers.*

If the atrial rate increases further, higher grade AV block such as 3:1 AV block can occur. It's obvious that an abrupt 2:1 block during exercise, particularly in otherwise healthy pacemaker patients, will result in significant symptoms and can severely limit their exercise capacity. To avoid this nonphysiological upper rate limit behaviour, the second generation of DDD pacemakers incorporated a separate upper rate limit (URL) also called maximum tracking rate (MTR). The MTR or URL determines the maximal rate, at which the ventricle can be paced in response to atrial sensed events. In almost every dual-chamber pacemaker the URL is programmable over a wide range of values, with small increments (e.g. 80-180 bpm and 5 bpm increments). During atrial tracking between the LRL and URL, every intrinsic P wave will stop the VA timer and initiate the AVI. Whenever intrinsic atrial activity occurs at a rate greater than the programmed MTR, a progressive prolongation of the AV interval occurs until a P wave falls inside the PVARP and a ventricular output is omitted (figure 9). If a P wave falls inside the PVARP, it is ignored by the pacemaker for timing purposes and the LRI interval

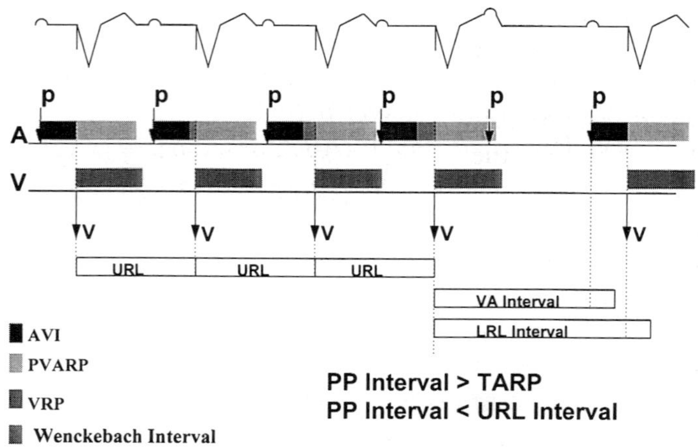

Figure 9. *Pseudo Wenckebach block in DDD(R) pacemakers.*

timer will complete its cycle. The difference between the TARP and minimum tracking interval (MTI) represents the Wenckebach interval. The 2:1 block rate (typically 150 bpm) is often higher than twice the lower rate limit (typically 60 bpm). Thus the next P wave will occur before time-out of the VAI timer and start the AVI timer, followed by a paced or sensed ventricular complex. Unlike a native Wenckebach pattern, where consecutive ventricular intervals become shorter, the intervals between consecutive ventricular paced complexes are constant (at the MTI). Therefore this is called a pseudo Wenckebach type upper rate limit behaviour. Programming of the URL below the 2:1 block rate will not prohibit the occurrence of 2:1 block once the atrial interval becomes shorter than the TARP (figure 10).

For rates between LRL and URL no difference in timing exists between ventricular-based, atrial-based or modified timing systems. In contrast with the DDD mode, in DDDR pacemakers atrial pacing can occur at rates above the LRL, depending on the sensor indicated rate. As was the case for rates near the lower rate limit, also at sensor driven high rates near the MSR, timing differences exist between atrial based and ventricular based timing systems. In a standard ventricular based timing system, the actual atrial pacing rate can be significantly higher than the programmed MSR if intrinsic AV conduction exists. The increase in actual atrial pacing rate above the MSR can even be more pronounced due to the effect of sympathetic drive on the intrinsic AV conduction. However, due to implementation of adaptive rate (or dynamic) AVI, the difference between AVI and AR interval is minimal, thus limiting the phenomenon of atrial pacing above MSR during AV conduction. With modified ventricular based timing systems, the difference between AVI and AR interval is added to the VA interval to eliminate unwanted fast atrial pacing rates during periods of AV conduction. In atrial based timing systems during sensor tracking and AV conduction, the atrial paced rate will not exceed the MSR, as the A-A interval is not influenced by AV block or AV conduction. In DDDR pacing mode, the pacing rate is determined by a comparison of the intrinsic atrial rate and the sensor-indicated rate. The rate arbitration algorithm is such, that the fastest of the two rates will control the pacing rate. The programmable maximum sensor rate (MSR) limits the maximal pacing rate during sensor-driven pacing. In most DDDR units, MTR and MSR can be programmed separately. For instance, the maximal tracking rate (MTR) can be programmed below the MSR. If the minimum sensor interval (MSI) is shorter than TARP, in other words, if the maximum sensor rate (MSR) is programmed above the 2:1 block rate, sensor-driven atrial pacing inside the PVARP may occur. With sensor-driven intervals shorter than TARP, P wave detection is impossible, as the atrial sensing window is closed. As both intrinsic atrial rate and sensor-indicated rate are used for rate arbitration, sensor-driven rate smoothing can occur near the URL. Pseudo Wenckebach block will not occur if the sensor indicated rate is close to the intrinsic atrial rate and both are slightly above the URL. Instead of waiting for the next P wave to arrive after a pseudo Wenckebach block, the DDDR pacemaker will deliver an atrial and ventricular stimulus at the sensor-indicated interval. In addition to Wenckebach block, 2:1 or higher block and thus periods of AV dissociation will also be prevented. Moreover, exercise induced atrial tachyarrhythmias may be prevented. Whether competitive atrial rhythms induce atrial tachyarrhythmias, due to pacing in the atrial vulnerable period, is still a matter of debate (figure 11). Optimal sensor-driven rate smoothing requires precise programming of MTR, MSR and the sensor parameters (figure 12). If sinus rate increases during physical exercise,

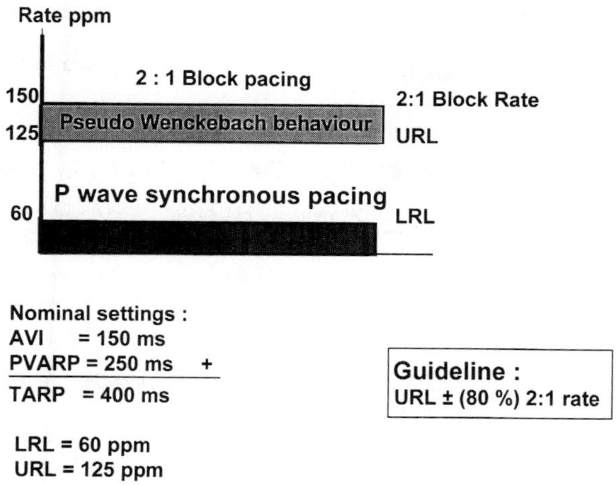

Figure 10. *Different rate limits in DDD(R) pacing.*

the rate arbitration algorithm will determine whether P wave tracking up to the MTR or sensor tracking up to the MSR occurs.

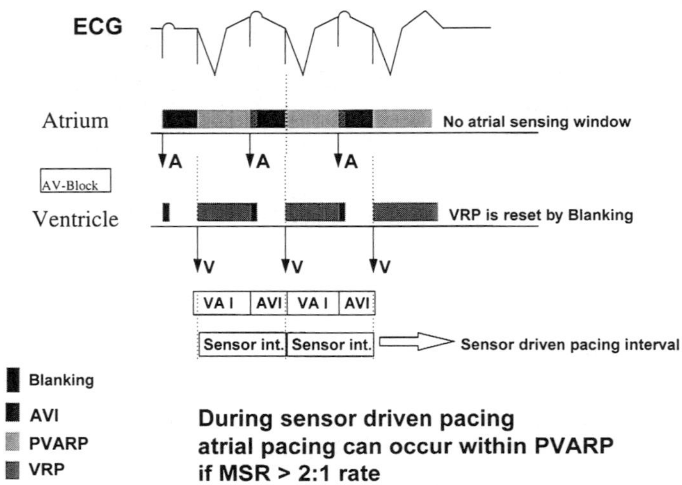

Figure 11. *Sensor driven atrial pacing inside PVARP.*

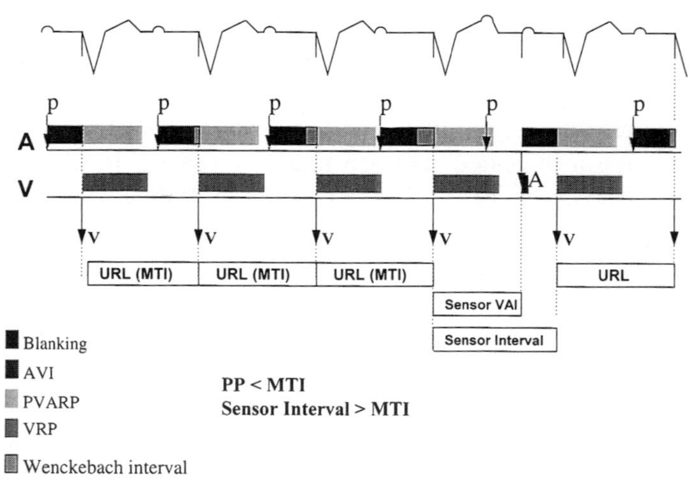

Figure 12. *Sensor driven rate smoothing at the URL (MTR).*

Rate Smoothing

Rate smoothing is designed to eliminate rapid cycle to cycle variations, as occurs with 2:1 block, at the onset of PAT or pacemaker mediated tachycardia, PAC, sinus arrhythmia and compensatory pauses post PVC. Guided by the programmed rate smoothing values, the most recent ventricular interval is used to calculate the atrial and ventricular windows for the next cardiac cycle. Rate smoothing is often programmable and can separately be selected for increasing and decreasing rates. If the intrinsic atrial rate increases faster than the programmed percentage of upward smoothing, the ventricular stimulus is delayed and AV dissociation will occur. If the intrinsic atrial rate tends to decrease faster than the programmed downward smoothing, AV sequential pacing will occur with a rate decreasing at the programmed smoothing percentage towards the LRI. This is the only situation in which a DDD pacemaker can pace the atrium at a rate above the LRL.

Mode Switching (Automatic Mode Change)

Mode switching is a feature that, during episodes of supraventricular arrhythmias, implements the automatic mode change from a P wave tracking to a nontracking mode, such as DDI(R), VDI(R) and VVI(R). This feature eliminates the phenomenon of pacing at the MTR due to tracking of atrial tachyarrhythmias. When an atrial arrhythmia is detected, the device will pace the ventricle at the LRL or at a sensor-indicated pacing rate. When the patient is at rest, the sensor-indicated rate is near the LRL. In that case, an automatic mode change decreases the ventricular pacing rate from the MTR towards the programmed LRL. The rate of decrease is controlled by the programmed fallback time. The pacemaker algorithm must be able to adequately detect a supraventricular tachyarrhythmia before a mode switch can happen. In some pacemakers, an atrial tachycardia is confirmed once 8 atrial cycles are counted above the URL, and in others after detection of an atrial rate faster than 180 bpm. Some pacemakers incorporate a programmable delay (duration), that upon detection of the atrial tachyarrhythmia determines when the actual decrease in ventricular pacing rate starts. The pacemaker reverts back into DDD or DDDR mode once a sequence of atrial cycles (<10) are counted below the MTR, or once a sequence of several sensor driven atrial stimuli have been delivered. In several DDD and DDDR systems, the automatic mode change has clinically proven to reliably detect atrial tachycardias, atrial flutter and fibrillation, and to appropriately switch to a non P wave tracking pacing mode if the tachycardia is sustained.

Pacemaker Mediated Tachycardia

Algorithms have been designed to terminate or break pacemaker mediated tachycardia (PMT), also called the endless loop tachycardia. The VA conduction pathway constitutes the retrograde limb and the DDD(R) pacemaker establishes the anterograde limb of the re-entry circuit (figure 13).

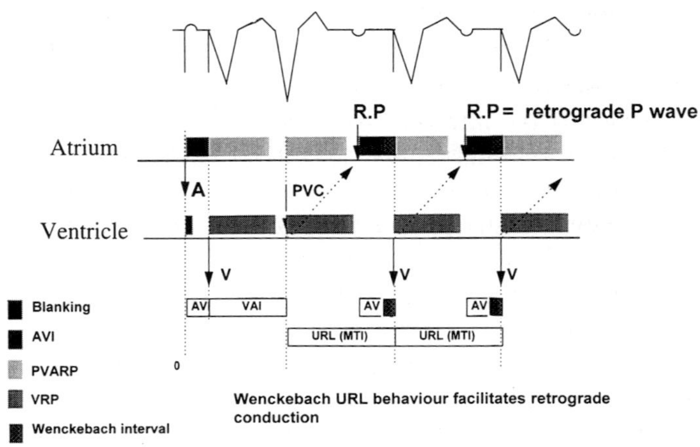

Figure 13. *Pacemaker mediated tachycardia.*

A retrograde P wave can occur once AV synchrony is lost. This most frequently occurs after a premature ventricular contraction, loss of atrial capture and detection of myopotentials in the atrial sense circuit. Several studies have shown, that programming the PVARP longer than the VA conduction time is a safe and effective strategy to prevent PMTs in most patients during long-term follow-up. However, in patients with slow VA conduction and thus selection of a long PVARP, limited maximal tracking rates result. In newer generations of dual-chamber pacemakers the PVARP extends during one cardiac cycle, once loss of AV synchrony or a PVC has been detected (PVARP extension). If PMT occurs despite the availability of PVARP extension, the PMT only will break spontaneously once the retrograde limb of the circuit dissipates. Several DDD(R) pacemakers can break an initiated PMT by using algorithms to identify a PMT and break the re-entry circuit for one cardiac cycle, after which an AV sequential pacemaker-escape will start a normal sinus or AV sequential rhythm. The PMT is no longer a clinical problem in today's DDD and DDDR pacemakers.

Programming of DDD(R) Timing Intervals

In the current DDD(R) pacemakers a wide range of timing intervals can temporarily or permanently be programmed, such as LRL, URL, MSR, AVI, PAVI, SAVI, PVARP, PVARP extension, VRP etc. Programming of the sensor and matching rate response to workload will not be discussed in this chapter. It is striking to observe that many DDDR pacemakers function their entire life-time in the nominal settings, determined by the manufacturer. This may indicate that all pacemaker patients are considered equal, which is probably not the case, or that physicians are not able to keep up with the increasing complexity of the DDDR pacing systems. As in other fields in cardiology, it requires more than a superficial interest to maintain proficiency with the newest advances of pacing. It is important to realise that pacemaker patients constitute only 4% of the cardiology patient population of a general hospital. However, pacemaker patients require more than 4% of the available time of a cardiologist.

In our department of cardiology in 1994, almost 3000 patients were admitted, of which 110 (3,7%) underwent implantation or replacement of a pacemaker and another 10 patients (0,3%) had pacemaker-related problems. In our outpatients' clinic 18000 patient visits were registered, of which 1200 pacemaker follow-up visits (6,6%). Fortunately, many Dutch pacemaker implanting hospitals have well trained technicians to give the cardiologist the necessary technical support. Nevertheless, according to law, pacemaker programming is a medical proceeding and thus should remain prescribed or authorized by a physician.

Lower Rate and Upper Rate Limit

In programming the lower and upper rate of a DDDR pacemaker the patient's age, activity and the presence of ischaemic heart disease should be taken into account. All these variables should be known before the implantation of a pacemaker. It is mandatory to study the patient's sinus node function for the presence of chronotropic incompetence, long pauses and the symptoms before implantation. In patients with normal sinus node function the LRL can be set low; we prefer a lower rate limit of 50 bpm in young and active patients and of 60 bpm in older and less active patients. However, age by itself is less important than physical fitness. It is always worthwhile to preserve intrinsic rhythm. Competition between sinus rhythm and lower rate pacing should be avoided. In some patients with frequent episodes of atrial arrhythmias, atrial overdrive pacing can suppress the occurrence of atrial tachyarrhythmias. Typical vagal induced atrial arrhythmias are rare and in our experience, the effectiveness of atrial overdrive suppression in these patients cannot be predicted by clinical variables.

The presence of ischaemic heart disease associated with symptomatic angina pectoris never may be a reason to deny patients DDD or DDDR pacing. Several studies have shown a better quality of life for DDD(R) patients compared to single chamber ventricular pacing, presumably due to superior hemodynamics associated with AV synchrony. A prospective study demonstrated a poorer survival of patients with coronary disease and a ventricular pacemaker, compared to a matched patient group with DDD(R) pacemakers.

The upper rate limit sets the maximum ventricular pacing rate in response to detection of intrinsic atrial detection. Before programming the upper rate limit, a clinical assessment of the patient is necessary. The most important clinical variables to evaluate are summarised in the table below:

Variables Determining the Selection of the Upper Rate Limit

- Age
- Daily activities
- Underlying rhythm
- Chronotropic incompetence
- Atrial arrhythmias
- Antiarrhythmic medication
- Coronary artery disease
- Heart failure

For children the desired upper rate limit is between 175-200 bpm, for active adults between 150-175 bpm and for the typical pacemaker patient 125-150 bpm. In our department, the typical pacemaker patient is a 70 year-old male with, as measured by holter, a heart rate above 100 bpm, only 5% of the time. In only 0,5% of the duration of the day, upper rate tracking was observed. To program the upper rate limit, it is important to first calculate the 2:1 (or fixed) block rate. In DDD(R) pacing, the maximum atrial rate that can be detected by the pacemaker, is limited by the duration of TARP, i.e. the sum of AVI and PVARP. Every P wave falling inside the PVARP will not result in a synchronized ventricular stimulus. For example, if we program AVI at 150 msec and PVARP at 250 msec, TARP = 400 msec and thus, 2:1 block will occur at a rate of 150 bpm. The rate adaptive or dynamic AV interval, a feature that shortens AV interval during sensor driven and/or atrial synchronous pacing at increasing rates and in some pacemakers the rate adaptive PVARP feature, shortening the PVARP at increasing pacing rates, allow the pacemaker to sense faster atrial rates.

The impact of a rate adaptive AV interval alone is substantial. For example, if the PAVI shortens from 150 msec at rest to 75 msec at maximal exercise, the

TARP shortens from 400 msec to 325 msec, obtaining a 2:1 block rate of 184 bpm. Literature indicates that in most patients, if present, the VA conduction time usually is between 170 and 230 msec. To prevent PMTs in patients with retrograde conduction, PVARP must be programmed longer than 230 msec. Prevention of PMTs is always preferred to PMT intervention. If the URL is programmed below the 2:1 block rate, a zone for pseudo Wenckebach behaviour is created. As a general rule the upper rate limit should be programmed at 80% of the 2:1 block rate. In our example, where the 2:1 block rate is 150 bpm, URL should be programmed at 120 bpm. In pacemakers with adaptive/dynamic AV interval, the URL can be programmed equal to the calculated 2:1 block rate at rest. In most DDDR units the URL and the MSR can be programmed independently. For instance, in very active patients the maximum sensor-driven rate can be programmed above the URL. In addition, sensor-driven pacing can smooth or eliminate pseudo Wenckebach block while pacing at the URL. In clinical practise, limitations for the programming of a high upper rate limit no longer exist.

AV Interval

The most optimal atrial pace to ventricular sense interval (AR interval) has been determined to be 125-150 msec at rest. The benefits of spontaneously conducted ventricular contractions compared to ventricular paced beats, at rest, are well documented. If AV conduction is normal, the pacemaker should preferably be programmed in the AAIR mode, or in the DDDR mode with a long AVI and with the dynamic AV interval feature turned off. If AV-nodal conduction only is normal at low heart rates, the dynamic AV interval feature can be programmed to on. During exercise, the increase in sympathetic tone shortenes the PR interval. Several studies in healthy volunteers and in pacemaker patients with normal AV conduction demonstrated an almost linear relationship between the increase in heart rate and the shortening in PR interval. This linear relationship is applied in several pacemaker algorithms to create the rate adaptive/dynamic AV interval. In some pacemakers, the rate at which the AVI shortening starts is programmable, in order to extend the benefits of spontaneous conduction as long as possible. Programming the sensed AVI (SAVI) shorter than the paced AVI (PAVI) can accommodate for the difference in intra-atrial conduction time between sensed and paced events. Most studies show a difference in intra-atrial conduction time of 30-50 msec, thus the sensed interval should be programmed at 30-50 msec shorter than the paced AV interval. The difference in paced and sensed AVI also exists during exercise, when rate adaptive AVI is active.

Hemodynamic studies in resting conditions and if possible during exercise may be necessary in pacemaker patients with angina pectoris, hypertrophic obstructive cardiomyopathy and severe heart failure, to determine optimal hemodynamic results with the pacing therapy. Most studies of patients with HOCM and severe congestive heart failure show positive results with AV sequential pacing using short AV intervals (80-110 msec).

Additional Timing Algorithms

Pacemaker Mediated Tachycardia Prevention/Termination

PMT termination algorithms, if available, preferably are programmed on in all patients with intact AV conduction. In current pacemaker types, VA conduction time can easily be measured by using the telemetered intracardiac electrogram (EGM) or an event marker channel. AV dissociation and consequential VA conduction can be facilitated by programming the pacemaker to VDD mode and a lower rate limit above the intrinsic sinus node rate. If VA conduction is short or absent, the nominal PVARP value can be accepted. With this technique also PMT termination algorithms can be tested. Otherwise, programming of a PVARP extension (post PVC) can prohibit initiation of PMTs in case VA conduction time is longer than the programmed PVARP.

Automatic Mode Switch

Automatic mode switch is indicated for use in patients with atrial tachyarrhythmias. In the early days of DDD pacing, the occurrence of paroxysmal atrial tachycardia was considered to be a contraindication for pacemakers with atrial tracking. We have learned that the alternative of ventricular pacing is certainly not a remedy against paroxysmal fibrillation; on the contrary, as a result of the dissynchrony between atrium and ventricle many patients may develop chronic atrial fibrillation. Maintaining AV synchrony as long as possible is considered to be an effective tool to reduce the incidence of atrial tachyarrhythmias. DDD(R) pacing with automatic mode change can reduce symptoms in these patients and may make the need for RF ablation of the His bundle redundant. The automatic switch from an atrial tracking mode to a nontracking mode during episodes of atrial tachyarrhythmia, has been proven to be of great clinical value for these patients.

Summary

In the table below you will find the values of the DDD(R) timing intervals, as most frequently programmed in our institution:

Timing Intervals in Patients with Abnormal AV Conduction
(pacing rate values in bpm)

Patient	LRL *	URL *	MTR *	PAVI +	PVARP +	MSR +
Active: young	50	150-175	175-200	75-125	225	175
older	60	125-150	160-180	100-150	225	160
Sedentary	70	120-130	150-170	100-150	250	150

* LRL, URL, MTR, MSR in beats per minute
\+ PAVI and PVARP in msec

References

1. Markowitz HT. Ventricular- and atrial-based timing in rate responsive dual chamber pulse generators. Technical concept paper. Minneapolis, Medtronic Inc., 1989.
2. Barold SS, Falkoff MD, Ong LS. A-A and V-V lower rate timing of DDD and DDDR pulse generators. In: Barold SS, Mugica J (eds), New Perspective in Cardiac Pacing. 2. Mount Kisco, NY, Futura Publishing Co., Inc., 1991, pp 203-47.
3. Hayes DL. Timing cycles of permanent pacemakers. Cardiol Clinics 1992;10:593-608.
4. Hayes DL, Levine PA. Pacemaker timing cycles. In: Ellenbogen KA (ed.), Cardiac Pacing. Boston, MA Blackwell Scientific Publications, 1992, pp 263-308.
5. Hayes DL, Ketelson A, Levine P. Understanding timing systems of current DDDR pacemakers. Eur JCPE 1993;3:70-86.
6. Furman S. Comprehension of pacemaker timing cycles. In: Furman S, Hayes DL, Holmes Jr DR (eds), A Practice of Cardiac Pacing, 3rd ed. Mount Kisco, NY, Futura Publishing Co., Inc., 1993, pp 135-94.
7. Merillat JC. Understanding and assessing DDDR pacing systems. In: Rate-Adaptive Pacing: Perspective in Cardiac Rhythm Management. St Paul, MN, Cardiac Pacemaker, Inc., 1993, pp 53-85.
8. Chu-Pak Lau. DDDR Pacing: Lower and upper rate behaviors. In: Rate Adaptive Cardiac Pacing: Single and Dual Chamber. Mount Kisco, NY, Futura Publishing Co., Inc., 1993, pp 271-91.
9. Barold SS. Ventricular- versus atrial-based lower rate timing in dual chamber pacemakers: does it really matter? PACE 1995;18:83-96.
10. Barold SS, Wenckebach upper rate response of dual chamber pacemakers: A reappraisal and proposed new terminology. PACE 1995;18:244-52.

2 CONSIDERATIONS BEFORE IMPLANT OF A PACEMAKER

Chapter 4

Pacing in Elderly Patients - Preoperative Evaluation and Pacemaker Selection

Rob van Mechelen, Karel den Dulk and Hein J.J. Wellens

Introduction

Much of today's planning for elderly people is based on the theory that although lethal conditions might be postponed as medical technology improves, the incidence of degenerative diseases will be unaltered. This theory predicts that people in their nineties suffer from more diseases and have a greater chronic disability than do people in their seventies or eighties. If this theory were true, then the continued increase in the size of the oldest old population would portend a significant burden of poor health among the oldest members of our society.[1-4]

The discovery that many people over age of 90 have no previous history of heart disease, cancer or stroke and have a good physical condition may mean that planning for the health care of the oldest old need to be revised (figure 1).[2,3] Although cause-of-death statistics for centenarians are sparse, available information suggests that the usual causes are acute illnesses such as pneumonia, as opposed to longstanding lethal conditions frequently observed in people dying in their seventies or eighties.[3]

In recent times we have learned much about health and how to maintain it. We have devised thousands of specific treatments for specific diseases and disabilities. Yet, nature has not allowed us to increase the maximum length of our life span (figure 2) shows that the average human lifetime was about 22 years in ancient Rome, was about 50 in the developed countries in 1900 and now stands at 75 in Europe and the U.S. Despite this increase each curve seems to stop sharply nearly 115 years. Centuries of improvement in health care does not affect that maximum.[3]

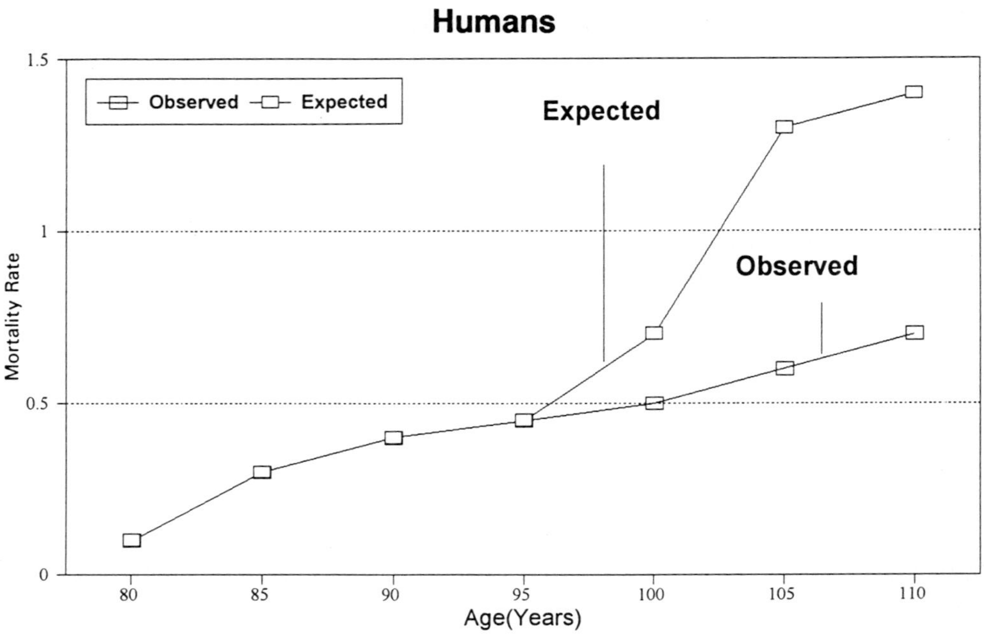

Figure 1. *Selective Survival. Abbreviation: Mortality Rate = Anual Death Divided by Number in Age Group. From: Thomas T. Perls. The Oldest Old. Scientific American, January 1995, pp 50-55.*

Although a complete chapter of this book could be devoted to speculations on the genetic background of these observations, this information would not simplify a proper pacemaker selection in an eighty years old patient suffering from a Stokes-Adams attack based on the sudden appearance of complete AV block. We, as clinical cardiologists, do better to accept these observations simply as facts and question its implications regarding the therapeutical approach of elderly patients who need pacemaker implantation.

For the moment, we may defer from these data, that there are two types of elderly people: Type I people, that has an improved life expectancy due to a change in life style, eating habits and all available tools of modern medical technology. These individuals have previous histories that include any or combinations of the following diseases: myocardial infarction, heart failure, hypertension, valvular heart disease, degenerative joint disease, cancer, cerebro-vascular disease and Altzheimer disease.

In contrast to these people, there are type II people. Type II people are elderly individuals that can be considered the fittest of the human race. They have no previous history of serious cardio-vascular disease, have very mild forms of diabetes, or dementia and have never had any tumor related disease. In addition, they never needed any tool of modern medical technology so far.

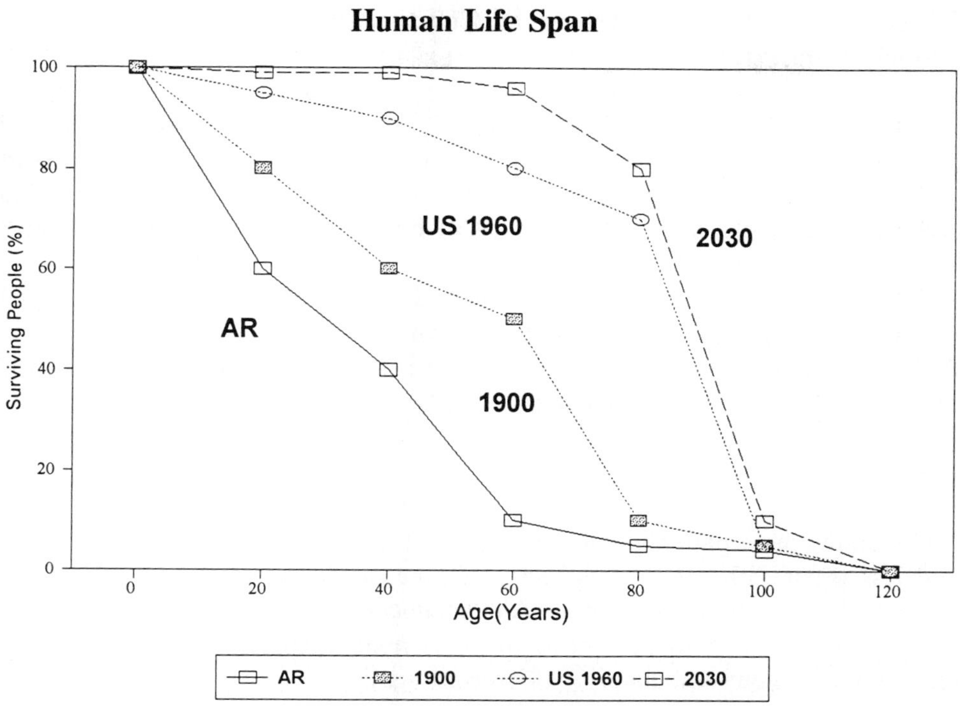

Figure 2. *Human Life Span. Abbreviations: AR= Ancient Rome; 1900 = developed countries around 1900; US 1960 = Population of the U.S.A. around 1960. From: Marvin Minsky. Will Robots Inherit the Earth? Scientific American. October 1994, pp 87-91.*

Admission to the Hospital

Based on the description of type I and type II patients in the previous section, life expectancy will greatly differ between a type I patient over 80 years of age is admitted to the hospital because of a Stokes-Adams attack or a type II patient.

When a type I patient is admitted, it is unlikely that his or her remaining life expectancy is greater than the battery life of the pacemaker to be implanted. However, when a type II patient is admitted with a Stokes-Adams seizure, battery life of the pacemaker to be implanted might be much shorter than the life expectancy of this new patient.

Thus on admission, even before one has established a diagnosis in a patient over 80 years of age, the previous history of the patient gives us important information on his or her remaining life expectancy independent of the permanent pacemaker to be inserted.

Diagnosis of Frequently Observed Conduction Disorders in the Elderly Population

A complete discussion on the work-up of syncope in the elderly population is beyond the scope of this article. A restriction is made to syncope related to the main conduction disorders observed in this subgroup of patients i.e., sick sinus syndrome, complete atrio-ventricular (AV) block and chronic atrial fibrillation with advanced or complete AV block.

Syncope based on complete AV block is more often observed in elderly patients than syncope based on sinus arrest due to sinus node dysfunction.[5,6] Patients with atrial fibrillation and slow ventricular response usually present with symptoms of fatigue and dizziness but seldom with fainting spells.[7,8]

Sick Sinus Syndrome

Generally, these patients visit the outpatient clinic because of dizziness, fatigue and less often with previous episodes of syncope.[5,6] The routine ECG displays normal sinus rhythm with intact AV conduction. Neurologic investigation is usually negative and the diagnosis of sinus node dysfunction is assessed after reading the 24-hour ambulatory ECG recording.

AV Block

Most of these patients are referred by the general physician to the emergency room of the hospital because of a serious fainting spell and the routine ECG on admission provides a diagnosis of complete AV block.[8] In a lesser degree, these patients are seen in the outpatient clinic because of symptoms of dizziness and fatigue. The routine ECG shows sinus rhythm with bifascicular or trifascicular AV block[9] and it is the value of the 24-hour ambulatory ECG recording that may show intermittent complete AV block to assess the correct diagnosis.[10,12]

Atrial Fibrillation with Advanced or Complete AV Block

Today, many new elderly patients are sent to the cardiology outpatient clinic with complaints of dizziness or fatigue and atrial fibrillation on the routine ECG. After a complete noninvasive work-up, a complete neurological investigation, and vital function laboratory examination, most of them are sent back to their general physician with a prescription of digoxin, ACE-inhibitor, a diuretic and anticoagulant therapy. Patients with atrial fibrillation showing a slow ventricular rate remain under supervision of a cardiologist. In this subgroup hard evidence lacks to delineate a cause-effect relationship between complaints and ECG or Holter recording findings. Since chronic atrial fibrillation and slowing of heart rates are age depending phenomena[11,12], there exists no golden ECG standard to decide whether to implant a pacemaker or not. Of course when syncope occurs and neurological and other non-cardiac causes are excluded, pacing has to be considered as therapy of choice.[13] However, when dizziness and fatigue are the main complaints, the indication for permanent pacing remains a gray area.[13,14]

Preoperative Evaluation

General Preoperative Investigation

When the diagnosis of a conduction disorder has been assessed and a decision has been made to implant a pacemaker, a general work-up has to be performed. Table 1 shows the general preoperative evaluation performed in every patient before the patient is taken to the operating room. Besides, depending on the established diagnosis additional measures needs to be made to select the proper pacing device.

Specific Measures in Sinus Node Dysfunction

The papers of Rosenquist[15,56] clearly proved that patients with sinus node dysfunction should not be treated by ventricular demand pacing. In terms of longevity, quality of life, cerebro-vascular accidents, hemodynamics and incidence of chronic atrial fibrillation, atrial pacing should be the preferred pacing mode. Based on this preference, one of the authors published the Dutch perspective on selection of the optimal pacing mode in 1992. We still follow the mode decision matrices presented in this report.[17] An adapted version of the decision matrices is depicted in figure 3.

However, in considering atrial pacing permanently, one has to assess additional aspects of the syndrome i.e., the quality of AV conduction, the occurrence of paroxysmal atrial fibrillation or flutter and chronotropic incompetence during exercise.

▸ *Assessment of AV conduction.* A proper evaluation of AV conduction includes a full disclosure 24-hour ambulatory ECG recording, an exercise test, an incremental atrial pacing test to assess the AV nodal Wenckebach point, the intravenous administration of atropin and isoproterenol to qualify sympathetic drive.[18,19]

Table 1.

General pre-operative evaluation	
History	Rationale: - provides information about mental and physical vitality of the patient. - use of drugs : aspirin, antirheumatic drugs, anti-coagualant drugs like warfarine and platelet aggregation-inhibiting drugs. All these drugs should at least be discontinued 5-7 days before surgery to avoid serious bleeding complications. - in patients with heart valve prosthesis, heparin should be administered i.v. Oral anticoagulant drugs must temporarily be discontinued.
Physical Examination	Rationale: - provides information on heart failure. Patients in overt heart failure have to be treated with ACE inhibitors, diuretics, digoxin or positive inotropic drugs to lower the risk during pacemaker implantation.
ECG	Rationale: - to assess the diagnosis of the conduction disorder.
Chest X-Ray	Rationale: - Lung cancer especially in the elderly population may initially produce very little symptoms or no symptoms at all. In patients with lung cancer in whom still pacemaker therapy is contemplated, an abdominal region for the pacemaker pocket avoids reoperation when radiotherapy is applied.
Laboratory Investigation	Rationale: - Hb, Ht, WBC, renal function and electrolytes thyroid function and blood sugar are mandatory in every patient undergoing pacemaker implantation.

In the past, electrophysiologic studies were also performed to establish HV intervals as a measure of infra-nodal conduction.[8] When these tests concluded that there is intact AV conduction a single chamber atrial pacemaker could be implanted because the likelihood to develop AV block was less than 1-2% in most of long-term studies.[20-25]

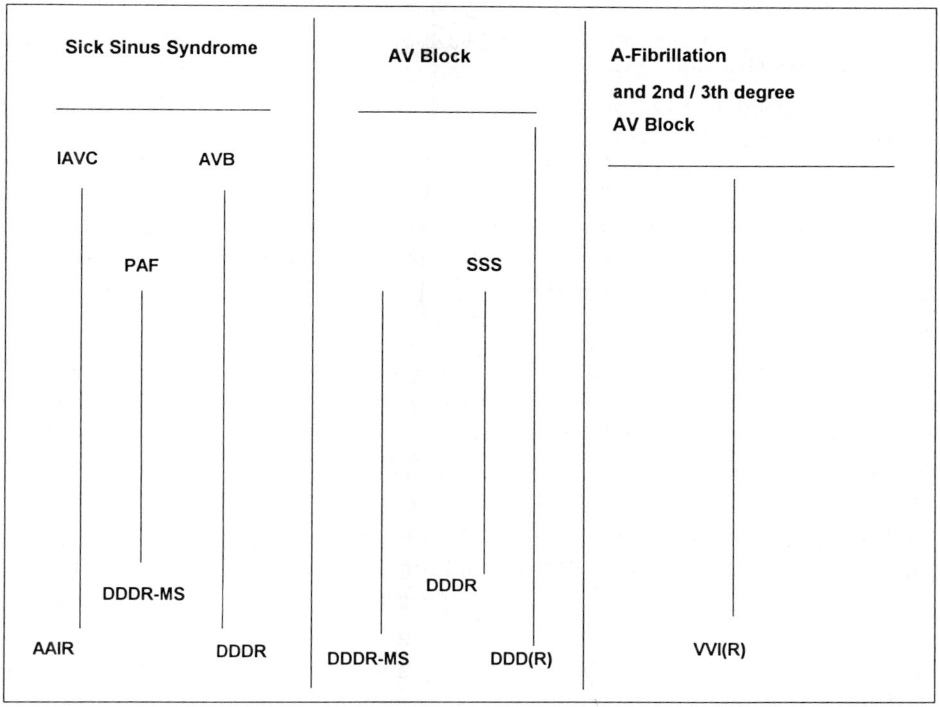

Figure 3. *Pacemaker Selection. Abbreviations: IAVC = intact atrio-ventricular conduction; PAF = paroxysmal atrial fibrillation; AVB = atrio-ventricular block; SSS = sick sinus syndrome; AAIR = single chamber atrial pacemaker rate modulation by sensor; DDD(R) = dual chamber pacemaker rate modulation by sensor; DDDR-MS = dual chamber pacemaker rate modulation by sensor and mode switch algorhythm implemented; VVI(R) = singel chamber ventricular pacemaker rate modulation by sensor.*

Although there still exists a place for these tests especially in the younger population with sinus node dysfunction in whom one considers to implant a singlechamber atrial pacemaker, a pre-operative evaluation as described is not attractive in patients over 80 years of age. This approach is time-consuming and burdening for elderly people. Besides, it definitely prolongs hospital stay with possible detrimental consequences. We therefore do not perform these tests.

▸ *Paroxysmal atrial fibrillation and atrial flutter.* To find out whether the atrium is suitable for an atrial based pacing system, it is mandatory in the elderly patient to obtain at least one 24-hour recording of the ambulatory ECG. If sinus rhythm is stable during this observation, the likelihood is great that an atrial electrode will adequately sense and pace the atrium, although the proof is in the peroperative testing phase.[26] If sinus rhythm is unstable and frequent episodes of atrial flutter or fibrillation occur as well during daily activity as during sleep, one could try to suppress the arrhythmia's by prescription of an antiarrhythmic drug that affects the effective refractory period of the atrial muscle. If such trial is ineffective, chronic atrial fibrillation waits around the corner, making the patient less suitable for an atrial based pacing device.[27]

▸ *Chronotropic Incompetence.* In young patients chronotropic incompetence can be tested by treadmill or bicycle ergometer exercise. In the elderly patient, this is seldom feasible, since most of these patients are hardly able to perform these tests because of knee or hip problems. Besides these tests are not representative for the normal daily activity these individuals are used to.[26]

Due to these limitations, it is impossible to perform a proper additional assessment and implant a single chamber atrial pacemaker. In these patients, one should implant a dual chamber pacemaker, whenever a stable sinus rhythm is observed. We program the pacing device after pacemaker implantation in the atrial demand sensor modulated mode when AV conduction is intact during a noninvasive incremental atrial pacing test and establish with Holter recordings during follow-up whether AV conduction remains intact. In patients with paroxysmal atrial fibrillation or flutter we program the AV synchronous sensor modulated pacing mode with the mode-switch algorithm programmed on. In patients with unstable sinus rhythm and frequent episodes of atrial fibrillation or atrial flutter despite antiarrhythmic treatment and in those were no acceptable atrial signals can be obtained to sense the atrium or the atrium cannot be paced by normal pacing energies, we implant a ventricular demand sensor modulated unit.

Specific Measures in AV Block

There is an overwhelming amount of literature that proves the hemodynamic benefit of AV synchronous pacing as compared to ventricular demand pacing in patients with symptomatic complete heart block.[28-33]

The majority of these studies were done at rest. However, during exercise the value of a properly timed atrial contraction seems to diminish as heart rate increases. Fananapazir *et al*[34] were the first to show that exercise tolerance during bicycle ergometer test were the same in patients during AV synchronous pacing and during sensor modulated ventricular asynchronous pacing.[33-35] Since elderly people lead a sedentary life, they have much more to expect in terms of quality of life from a dual pacing device than from a ventricular demand sensor modulated system. In contrast to patients with sinus node dysfunction, there is no hard data that proves that AV synchronous pacing prolongs life and improves quality of life. There are only two retrospective long term survival studies available in the literature on heart failure and pacing mode. Alpert *et al*[36,37] and Linde-Edelstam *et al*[38] showed that patients with AV block who presented with heart failure at time of pacemaker implantation had a worse outcome when a ventricular demand pacemaker was implanted than when a dual chamber pacing system was inserted. No statistically significant differences in prognosis were observed in patients with heart block but without congestive heart failure undergoing either a ventricular demand pacemaker or a dual chamber pacemaker. According to the literature, AV synchronous pacing in patients with complete AV block definitely improves the quality of life in comparison with ventricular demand sensor modulated pacing.[35,39,40] Yet we do not implant a dual chamber pacemaker in every patient over 80 years of age presenting with symptomatic complete heart block. There are several variables to be considered before a pacing device is selected: Concomitant sinus node dysfunction, the occurrence of paroxysmal atrial fibrillation or atrial flutter and left ventricular function as assessed by echocardiography.

▸ *Concomitant sinus node dysfunction.* Proper pre-operative assessment of concomitant sinus node dysfunction can hardly be done in elderly patients. Besides the necessity to do so, is also lacking. One only has to be aware of sinus bradycardia on the pre-operative ECG recording and pre-program the dual chamber pacemaker to be implanted at a lower rate of 70 ppm instead of a lower rate of 50 ppm as is usually done in patients with heart block but with a normal sinus rate.

▸ *Paroxysmal atrial fibrillation.* What has been stated about unstable sinus rhythm and the occurrence of atrial fibrillation in patients with sinus node dysfunction as the presenting conduction disorder, also holds true for patients with heart block as the presenting conduction problem. Therefore, it is desirable to obtain a 24-hour ambulatory ECG recording, which provides information on the stability of the sinus node and thus on the suitability of an atrial based pacing system.[41-43]

▸ *Echocardiography.* Earlier work done on the hemodynamic benefit of AV synchronous pacing performed in the seventies and eighties, showed the clear benefit of dual chamber pacing over single chamber ventricular pacing, especially in patients with normal left ventricular function as assessed by hemodynamic studies.[28-33]

The value of AV synchronous pacing in patients with poor left ventricular function was considered to be negligible since due atrial dilatation the atrial transport function was diminished and due to increased left ventricular enddiastolic pressure, atrial contribution to ventricular filling becomes insignificant. The ambiguity whether one should implant AV synchronous or ventricular demand pacemakers in patients with poor left ventricular function remained until papers appeared in the literature on systolic and diastolic left ventricular function performed by echo-doppler.[44-46] The majority of these studies clearly showed that atrial contribution to ventricular function is important. Especially in the elderly population a greater prevalence and severity of disease states has been observed that affect LV diastolic function.[47,48] Indeed, more than 30% to 40% of patients with systolic heart failure present with diastolic dysfunction as well.[47] This means that the optimal diastolic filling of the ventricles becomes more dependant of a properly timed atrial contraction than of the passive filling phase in early diastole.

Although, prospective randomized cross-over studies where patients with complete heart block and poor left ventricular function are either paced AV synchronously or ventricular on demand, are not available, these studies have to be performed to definitely find out the value of AV synchrony in terms of quality of life and prognosis in this particular subset of patients.

As a rule, we select a dual chamber pacemaker for elderly patients with symptomatic complete AV block. When the pre-operative ECG, or Holter recording shows signs of concomitant sinus node dysfunction, we pre-program the pacemaker to be implanted at a lower rate of 70 ppm. Is sinus rhythm unstable on these recordings and frequent episodes of atrial fibrillation are observed despite antiarrhythmic drug therapy, we refrain from a dual chamber pacing device and implant a ventricular on demand pacemaker. Patients with complete heart block and poor systolic and diastolic left ventricular function on the pre-operative echocardiogram are given the benefit of the scientific doubt. In these patients, dual chamber pacemakers are implanted.

Specific Measures in Atrial Fibrillation and Advanced or Complete AV Block

The decision to implant a pacemaker in this subgroup is limited to 3 types of ventricular demand devices i.e. single lead ventricular on demand unit without sensor implementation or sensor modulated single chamber devices that come with a single or a dual sensor. In terms of quality of life scores, patients prefer a rate modulated pacing device in comparison to a simple ventricular demand unit.[49,50] However, very little literature exits on the particular subject of patients with atrial fibrillation and advanced AV block. Although, there appeared reports on the hemodynamic benefit of dual sensor single chamber pacemakers as compared to single sensor devices, these studies were done in patients with all kind of conduction disorders but not specifically in the group with chronic atrial fibrillation and advanced AV block.[50] Selection of a pacing device in this subset is therefore based on common sense. Common sense tells us that a patient who leads a physically active life might benefit from a dual sensor system, whereas a patient who leads a sedentary life might not need such a sophisticated unit.

We usually implant ventricular sensor modulated on demand pacemakers. If the patient is still a sportsman or sportswoman, we first try to restore sinus rhythm with one or more trials of antiarrhythmic drugs and if not successful, perform electrical cardioversion. When the latter failures as well, only in this subset, we implant dual sensor driven ventricular demand pacemakers.

Preoperative Evaluation in the Future

Especially in the elderly, preoperative evaluation of pacemaker candidates can be cumbersome. In addition, no absolute guaranties can be given that after a complete work-up and a proper pacemaker selection at time of implantation, this specific selection remains optimal during follow-up. It would be desirable to minimize these imperfections even before the first implantation is performed.

One step in the direction to simplify the whole shebang and guarantee an optimal pacing mode during implantation also during follow-up, comes from the development of single lead pacing devices, which provide all desirable pace and sense modalities in the atrium as well as in the ventricle. With these units pacing modes can be noninvasively adjusted depending on the patient's needs.

Single Lead VDD Pacing Systems

These pacing systems provide AV synchronous pacing and single pacing lead implantation. The definite advantages have been published in the literature by several authors.[51-53] In summary, the procedure is fast, floating atrial sensing is, although not perfect, reliable enough to apply in patients with normal sinus function and AV block as the presenting conduction disorder. The disadvantages of these pacing systems are also clear: the inability to pace the atrium. When due to medication or due to degeneration the sinus node, or due to degenerative changes in the surrounding atrial tissue, the sinus rate drops below the programmed minimum rate of the pacemaker, asynchronous ventricular pacing results with the potentially undesirable consequences of retrograde AV conduction.

Single Lead DDD Pacing Systems

These pacing devices will offer the full functionality of a dual chamber pacing unit, packed in a single lead system. Recently, clinical investigation started in Europe[54] with these units (figure 4 and 5).

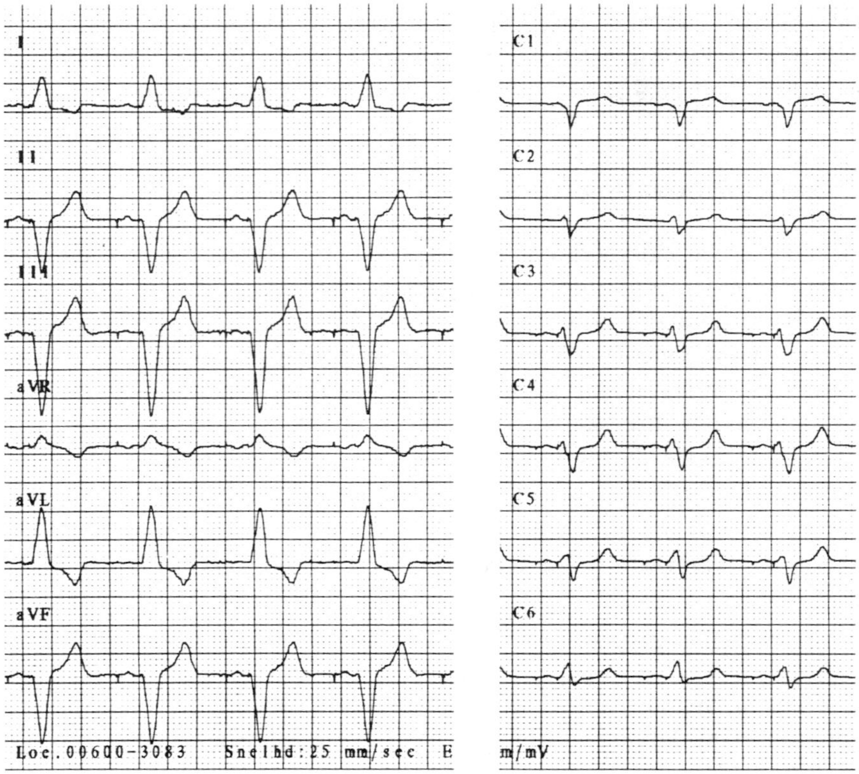

Figure 4. *Twelve-lead ECG of a patient with a single lead DDD pacemaker during AV sequential pacing. Note the positive P waves in I, II, III, and negative P wave in aVR. In the horizontal plane the P wave is positive in leads V4-V6. This P wave axis confirms an atrial activation sequence from superior to inferior and from right to left.*

At present, clinical results are not available, but it can be foreseen, that if implantation of these units becomes as simple as the implantation of a single lead ventricular demand pacemaker, the attraction to implant dual chamber pacemakers will gradually vanish among cardiologists and surgeons. Implantation of these units will take significantly less time and dislocation of the atrial leads will definitely belong to the past. In the future pre-operative evaluation concerning the specific conduction disorder will become superfluous. Patients will be

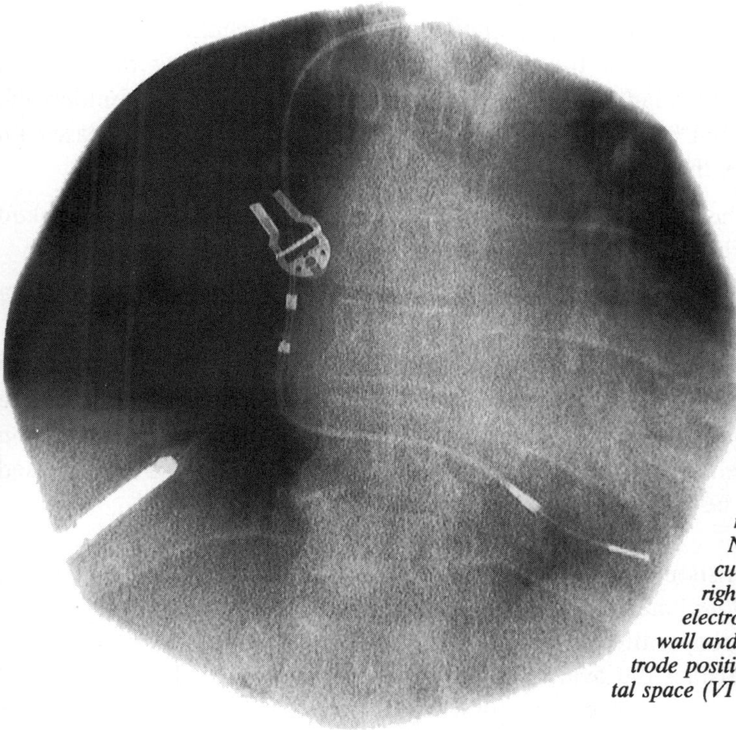

Figure 5. *Posterior-Anterior view during fluoroscopy after single lead DDDR pacemaker implantation. Note the bipolar ventricular electrode pair in the right ventricular apex, atrial electrode pair at the lateral wall and the surface ECG electrode positioned at the 4th intercostal space (VI lead).*

admitted to the hospital, a diagnosis of the conduction disorder will be established and a single lead pacemaker with dual lead functionality is subsequently implanted. Pacing modes will postoperatively and during follow-up be adjusted according to the patient's hemodynamic need.

Conclusions

After 30 years of permanent pacing experience, we will be back at where we started, although not only with much more intelligence implemented in the available pacing devices but also with a nearly quadrupled longevity of the pacemaker battery and an improved life expectancy of the elderly recipient of the pacemaker as compared to a patient of the same age that would have undergone a pacemaker implantation 30 years ago. We must realize however, that the improved longevity of the patient in the western world has more to do with a change in life style, eating habits and tools of modern medical technology over the last 30 years, than with the selected pacing system per se.[1-5] Nevertheless, it in the future it will become harder to deny that an improved pacing system contributes to the improved life expectancy of the recipient.

There is a growing realization that implantation of dual chamber pacemakers is an expensive technology in the older population.[55] In selecting the optimal pacemaker for a particular patient, a physician should always remember the importance of an atrial based pacing system and should resist decisions based on economic constraints that might not serve the patient's best interest.[27,56]

When choosing the type of pacemaker, three basic questions should be asked and a simple algorithm followed.[56]

The *first* question should be: *Is this a physically active individual who might benefit from a pacing system that closely mimics physiology of the normal heart?*
In the introduction of this paper, the importance of the patient's history was discussed to obtain information on the prognosis of the patient in relation to the longevity of the pacemaker battery. This item is important in any further decision making. If the patient is indeed a very active elderly individual, an atrial based pacing system must be the pacing device of first choice.

The *second* question should be: *What is the underlying conduction disorder and can the atrium be sensed and paced?*
In the session on preoperative evaluation, the importance of a proper diagnosis was discussed concerning the available literature on sinus node dysfunction, AV block and atrial fibrillation in combination with advanced AV block. In patients with sinus node dysfunction and reliable atrial function to sense and pace, at present there exists no controversy: these patients should receive an atrial based pacing system.
For patients with AV block the situation is less clear. Based on retrospective analysis, no statistically significant difference in prognosis was observed in patients when either a ventricular demand pacemaker or a dual chamber pacemaker was implanted when heart failure was absent.[36-38] On the otherhand, patients with overt heart failure at time of implantation, had a better prognosis when a dual chamber pacemaker was implanted than when a ventricular on demand pacemaker was inserted.[38] The explanation for these findings was given by echo-doppler studies.
For patients with AV block and heart failure, these observations mean that if the atrium is suitable for pacing and sensing, one should implant an atrial based pacing system. Uncertainty, remains whether one also should implant a dual chamber pacemaker in any patient with AV block, but without signs or symptoms of heart failure.
For patients with chronic atrial fibrillation and advanced AV block, the right ventricle is still the only place to implant a pacemaker lead. However, especially in the physically active patient one should try to restore sinus rhythm by anti-

arrhytmic drug treatment and if not successful, with electrical cardioversion.

The *third* question should be: *Is there atrial chronotropic incompetence?* Assessment of chronotropic incompetence in the elderly, is not an easy task to perform preoperatively as explained in the section of specific measures in sinus node dysfunction. The need for a sensor implementation can be at best be assessed after hospital discharge by a 24-hour ambulatory ECG recordings. Does this mean that in anticipation on eventual chronotropic incompetence one has to implant sensor modulated pacemakers in every elderly patient? The simple answer is yes. There is no reliable way to assess chronotropic incompetence pre-operatively, since standard exercise tests are not representative for the normal daily activity of the patient and walking around the ward while the ECG is monitored by telemetry, can only be performed in the subset of patients, who are not dependant of an isoproterenol drip, or temporary pacemaker.

With these three questions in mind, a tailored pacemaker prescription can be given. Patients with correctly programmed pacemakers, who are followed in the outpatients' clinic by a technician to assess pacemaker function and a cardiologist to assess the patient's cardiac function, rarely need to be readmitted to hospital because of pacemaker related problems.[56] A need exists for better physician education about the long-term consequences of the various pacing modes and their comparative cost effectiveness.

References

1. Fries JF. Aging, Natural death and the compresion of morbidity. NEJM 1980;303:3:130-5.
2. Suzman RM, Willis DC, Manton KG. The Oldest Old. Oxford University Press, 1992.
3. Manton KG, Corder S, and Stallard E. Estimates of change in chronic disability and institutional incidence and prevalence rates in the US elderly population from the 1982, 1984, and 1989 National Long Term Care Survey. Journal of Gerontology: Social sciences 1993;484;153-66.
4. Walford RL. Maximum Life Span. Norton and Company, New York, 1983.
5. Ferrer MI. The sick sinus syndrome in atrial disease. JAMA 1968;206:645-8.
6. Ferrer MI. The sick sinus syndrome. Circulation 1973;47:635-41.
7. Rubenstein JJ, Schulman CL, Yurchak PM, DeSanctis RW. Clinical spectrum of the sick-sinus syndrome. Circulation 1972;46:5-13.
8. Narula OS. Atrioventricular block. In: Narula OS (ed.), Cardiac Arrhytmias, Electrophysiology, Diagnosis, and Management. Williams & Wilkins, Baltimore London, 1979, pp 85-113.
9. Narula OS, Cohen LS, Scherlag BJ, Samet P, Lister JW, Hildner FJ. Localization of A-V conduction defects in man by recording of the His bundle and bundle branches. Am J Cardiol 1970;25:228-35.
10. Kennedy HL. Ambulatory electrocardiography. Ann Intern Med 1977;87:729-33.
11. Coumel P. Continuous electrocardiographic recording. Clinical, diagnostic and therapeutic value. Arch Mal Coeur 1975;68:941-5.

12. Harrison DC, Fitzgerald JW, Winkle RA. Ambulatory electrocardiography for diagnosis and treatment of cardiac arrhythmias. NEJM 1976;294:373-6.
13. Pitcher D, Papouchadou M, James MA, Russell Rees S. Twenty-four hour ambulatory electrocardiography in patients with chronic atrial fibrillation. Br Med J 1986;292:594.
14. Pollak A, Falk RH. Pacemaker therapy in patients with atrail fibrillation. Am Heart J 1993;125:824-30.
15. Rosenqvist M, Valin M, Edhag O. Atrial pacing for sick sinus syndrome. Clin Cardiol 1990;13:43-7.
16. Rosenqvist M, Brandt J, Schuller H. Long-term pacing in sinus node disease: Effects of stimulation mode on cardiovascular morbidity and mortality. Am Heart J 1988;116:16-22.
17. Den Dulk K, van Mechelen R, Cheriex EC, Wellens HJJ. Selection of optimal pacing mode. Neth J Cardiol 1992;5:214-25.
18. Rosen KM, Loeb HS, Ziad Sinno, Rahimtoola SH, Gunnar RM. Cardiac conduction in patients with symptomatic sinus node disease. Circulation 1971;43:836-42.
19. Narula OS. Atrioventricular conduction defects in patients with sinus bradycardia. Circulation 1971;44:1096-110.
20. Rosenqvist M, Obel I. Atrial pacing and the risk for AV block: Is there a time for change in attitude. PACE 1989;12:97-101.
21. Kerr CR, Tyres GFO, Vorderbrugge S. Atrial pacing: Efficacy, and safety. PACE 1989;12: 1049-54.
22. Ryden L. Atrial inhibited pacing: Un underused mode of cardiac stimulation. PACE 1988;11: 1353-79.
23. Van Mechelen R, Segers A, Hagemeijer F. Serial electrophysiologic studies after single chamber atrial pacemaker implantation in patients with symptomatic sinus node dysfunction. Eur Heart J 1984;5:628-36.
24. Mast EG, van Hemel NM, Bakema L, Derksen B, Defauw JAM. Is chronic atrial stimulation a reliable method for single chamber pacing in sick sinus syndrome. PACE 1986;9:1127-31.
25. Van Hemel NM. Why don't we pace the atrium more often in sinus node disease ? Neth J Cardiol 1990;6:176-7.
26 Holmes DR, Hayes DL, and Furman S. Permanent Pacemaker Implantation. In: Furman S, Hayes DL, Holmes Jr DR (eds), A practice of cardiac pacing. Futura Publishing Company, Mount Kisco NY, 2nd edition, 1989, pp 239-87.
27 Ruiter JH. Considerations in the selection and use of a cardiac pacing system. In Clinical Aspects of Cardiac Pacing for Bradyarrhythmias. Thesis, University of Rotterdam, 1992, pp 112-35.
28 Karlof I. Haemodynamic effect of atrial triggered versus fixed rate pacing at rest and during exercise in complete heart block. Acta Med Scand 1975;197:195-210.
29. Rediker DE, Eagle KA, Homma S, Gillarn LD, Harthorne JW. Clinical and hemodynamic comparison of VVI versus DDD pacing in patients with DDD pacemakers. Am J Cardiol 1988;61:323-9.
30. Samet P, Bernstein WH, Nathan DA, López A. Atrial contribution to cardiac output in complete heart block. Am J Cardiol 1965;16;1-10.
31. Samet P, Castillo C, Bernstein WH. Hemodynamic consequences of atrial and ventriuclar pacing in subjects with normal hearts. Am J Cardiol 1966;18:522-8.
32. Kruse I, Arnman K, Conradson TB, Rydén L. A comparison of acute and longterm hemodynamic effects of ventricular inhibited and atrial synchronous ventricular inhibited pacing. Circulation 1981;65:846-55.
33. Goldreyer BN. Physiologic Pacing: The role of AV synchrony. PACE 1982;5:613-5.
34. Fananapazir L, Brunett DH, Monks P. Atrial synchronized ventricular pacing: contribution of the chronotropic response to improve exercise performance. PACE 1983;6:601-8.

35. Linde-Edelstam C, Nordlander R, Pehrsson K, Rydén L. A double blind study of submaximal exercise tolerance and variation in paced rate in atrial synchronous compared to activity sensor modulated ventricular pacing. PACE 1992;15:905-15.
36. Alpert MA, Curtis JJ, Sanfelippo JF, Flaker GC, Walls ST, Mukerji V, Villareal D, Katti SK, Madigam NP, Krol RB. Comparitive survival after permanent ventricular adn dual chamber pacing for patients with chronic high degree atrioventricular block with and without preexisting congetive heart failure. J Am Coll Cardiol 1986;7:925-32.
37. Alpert MA, Curtis JJ, Sanfelippo JF, Flaker GC, Walls ST, Mukerji V, Villarreal D, Katti SK, Madigan NP, Morgan RS. Comparitive survival following permanent ventricular and dual chamber pacing for patients with chronic symptomatic sinus node dysfunction with and without heart failure. Am Heart J 1987;113:958-65.
38. Linde-Edelstam C, Gullberg B, Nordlander R, Pehrsson SK, Rosenquist M, Rydén L. Longevity in patient with high degree atrioventricular block paced in the atrial synchronous or fixed-rate ventricular-inhibited mode. PACE 1992;15;304-13.
39. Menozzi C, Brignole M, Morachinni PV, Lolli G, Bacchi M, Tesorieri MC, Tosoni GO, Bollini R. Intrapatient comparison between chronic VVIR and DDD pacing in patients affected by high degree AV block without heart failure. PACE 1990;13:1816-22.
40. Bubien RS, Kay GN. A randomized comparison of life and exercise capacity with DDD and VVIR pacing modes. PACE 1990;13:524-36.
41. Feuer JM, Shandling A, Messenger JC, Castellanet GD, Thomas LA. Influence of cardiac pacing mode on the long-term development of atrial fibrillation. Am J Cardiol 1989;64:1376-9.
42. Benditt D, Mianulli M, Buetikofer J. Prior arrhythmia history is the major determinant of post-implant atrial tachyarrhythmias in DDDR pacemaker patients. Rev Eur Tech Biomed 1990;12:95-9.
43. Gross J, Moser S, Benedek ZM, Andrews C, Furman S. Clinical predictors and natural history of atrial fibrillation in patients with DDD pacemakers. PACE 1990;13:1828-31.
44. Cheriex EC, Dulk K den, Pieters FAA, Wellens HJJ. Role of Doppler echocardiography in cardiac pacing. Neth J Cardiol 1992;5:208-13.
45. Pearson AC, Janosik DL, Redd RR, Buckingham TA, Blum RI, Labovitz AS, Mrosek D. Doppler echocardiographic assessment of the effect of varying atrioventricular delay and pacemaker mode on left ventricular filling. Am Heart J 1988;115:611-20.
46. Stewart WJ, Dicola VC, Harthorne JW, Gillam LD, Weyman AE. Doppler ultrasound measurement of cardiac output in patients with physiologic pacemakers. Am J Cardiol 1984; 54:308-12.
47. Aranow WS, Ahm C, Kronzon I. Prognosis of congestive heart failure in elderly patients with normal versus abnormal left ventricular systolic function associated with coronary artery disease. J Am Coll Cardiol 1990;66:1257-9.
48. Kupari M. Diastolic heart function and failure. J Intern Med 1991;229:479-81.
49. Wittkampf HF, Jongste MJ de. Rate stabilization by right ventricular pacing in patients with atrial fibrillation. PACE 1986;9;1147-53.
50. Kristensson BE, Arnman K, and Smedgard P. Physiological versus single-rate ventricular pacing: a double-blind cross-over study. PACE 1985;8;73-84.
51. Antonioli GE, Ansani L, Barbieri D, Guardigni G, Perloco GF, Toselli T. Italian multicenter study on a single lead VDD pacing system using a narrow atrial dipole spacing. PACE 1992;15:1890-983.
52. Crick JCP. European multicenter prospective follow-up study of 1002 implants of a single lead VDD pacing system. PACE 1991;14:1742-4.
53. Sutton R. The second coming of VDD. Eur J Cardiac Pacing Electrophysiol 1992;4:225-6.
54. Kruse IM, Mechelen R van, Bakels N, Lokhoff N. Early results with a new single-pass transvenous DDD-lead. PACE 1995: in print.

55. Clarke M, Sutton R, and Ward D. Recommendations for pacemaker prescription for symptomatic bradycardia. Report of the working party of the British Pacing and Electrophysiology Group. Br Heart J 1991;66:185-91.
56. Barold SS. The fourth decade of cardiac pacing: Hemodynamic, electrophysiological and clinical considerations in the selection of the optimal pacemaker. In: Zipes DP, Jalife J (eds), Cardiac Electrophysiology - from Cell to Bedside. W.B. Saunders Company, Philadelphia, Pennsylvania, 2nd edition, 1995, pp 1366-92.

2 CONSIDERATIONS BEFORE IMPLANT OF A PACEMAKER

Chapter 5

Single Lead Atrial Synchronized Ventricular (VDD) Pacing

Jonathan C. Pitts Crick

VDD Mode

The cause of symptomatic bradycardia in most patients is either sinus node disease or atrioventricular block. The aetiology is usually generalized disease of the conducting tissue and sensitive tests may reveal the coexistence of both defects in the same patient. In practice, however, it is uncommon to find this to a clinically significant degree: in sinus node disease it is not generally necessary to pace the ventricle and in heart block it is not generally necessary to pace the atrium. Therefore the logical choice of pacing mode to restore physiological rhythm is AAI or AAIR for sinus node disease and VDD for atrioventricular block.

Various reasons have been put forward for the widespread use of other pacing modes but these are mostly based on neither logic nor experience. In atrioventricular block the use of back-up VVI pacing may be justified on economic grounds where symptoms occur only occasionally while VVIR pacing may be appropriate in the presence of incessant or frequent atrial arrhythmias. In practice the major reason for use of VVIR pacemakers in heart block is the disinclination on behalf of the operator to insert a separate atrial electrode. The use of DDD pacing is appropriate where there is evidence of sinus node dysfunction, only at rest, (otherwise DDDR is required) but in the past majority of cases DDD mode is only employed as it is the default setting of dual-chamber pacemakers pre-programmed by the manufacturers.

Having established that VDD mode is correct for atrioventricular block with intact sinus node function is there any need to implant a device with wider capability? In the past very few specific VDD pacemakers have been manufactured and doubts have been raised about the use of such systems for three clinical reasons:

1. suspected unreliability in the diagnosis of sinus node dysfunction in the presence of heart block;
2. the possibility that sinus node disease might develop in the future;
3. the possibility that the patient may develop persistent drug refractory atrial fibrillation in the future.

The weight given to these considerations in the choice of pacing system should be based on actual documented experience in statistically adequate series of implants rather than just supposition or anecdote. Provided atrial pacing is not required a separate atrial lead may not be necessary.

Single Lead System

For many years attempts have been made to achieve reliable VDD pacing using a single lead with atrial ring electrodes in addition to the ventricular electrodes at the tip. A temporary system was developed over 20 years ago by Chamberlain, English and co-workers, and used successfully in the treatment of post-myocardial infarction patients.[1] Available technology at the time did not allow construction of an implantable device. Curry[2] and Antonioli[3] used leads with single atrial ring electrodes and connected them to standard implantable VAT pulse generators. These systems were troubled by atrial undersensing and myopotential triggering. Goldreyer[4] devised a lead with very close bipolar 'orthogonal' atrial sensing electrodes but atrial signals from this arrangement were not adequate for 1:1 triggering. Sowton[5] devised a lead with three atrial branches (on the basis that at least one would make contact with the atrial wall). This produced good signals for the use with standard pulse generators at the time but implantation of the leads was difficult and they proved mechanically unreliable in the long term. Ten years ago Morra[6] developed the first clinically successful implantable unit based on two atrial ring electrodes and a highly sensitive input amplifier appropriate to the signals produced. This device, the Medico Italia 'Phymos', was used extensively in Italy and in some other European centers. A rather similar device was developed in Italy and America and produced by LEM and CCS. In 1992 more sophisticated VDDR systems were introduced by Intermedics and Vitatron, and recently several other manufacturers, including Medtronic, Biotronik and Pacesetter, have developed single-lead VDD models.

Signals from Atrial Ring Electrodes

The amplitude and maximum slope of the unipolar signal diminishes rapidly with increasing distance of the electrode from the atrial wall.[7] The bipolar signal -the difference between two unipolar signals- diminishes even more rapidly, especially if the electrodes are close together. A mathematical analysis[8] suggests that in the worst case, where the lead passes through the center of the right atrium, the maximum bipolar signal is obtained with an electrode separation of around 3 cm. Far field signals, especially ventricular depolarization and repolarization are also greater with increasing electrode separation and this is an approximately linear relationship. The electrode distance for the optimal relation between atrial and far field signals (maximum signal to noise ratio) is 0.5-1.0 cm, though the worse case signal amplitude with this arrangement may be very low, 0.1-0.2 mV. The signal becomes poorer still if both electrodes move out of the right atrium into the superior vena cava, and may than become <0.1 mV.

In designing single lead VDD systems the choice lies between a widely spaced electrode system with a sensitivity of 0.2-0.3 mV, accepting a significant likelihood of far field signal oversensing, and a closely spaced electrode arrangement with a pacing sensitivity down to 0.1 mV, which will achieve more reliable sensing but at the expense of a probably higher battery consumption by the amplifier and difficulty in providing atrial pacing in the same (multipurpose) unit.

In many cases the lead, especially at implant, will be far from being in the worst-case position and if it is close to the lateral wall of the right atrium the signal amplitude may be several mV. This should not lead to false complacency as there is no fixation of the electrodes to the wall and so changes of posture and respiration may well lift the lead off the wall and towards the center of the atrium. Likewise, a low amplitude signal at implant does not predict sensing problems in the ambulant patient provided the ring electrodes do not move out of the atrium.

The atrial signals during atrial flutter and fibrillation are even smaller than those in sinus rhythm and so mode switching algorithms that depend on detection of a rapid atrial rate may fail unless the electrodes remain close to the wall. Signals may also become smaller in sinus rhythm if the right atrium enlarges both because of the Brody effect and also because of the lead moving further from the wall.

Implantation Technique

The implantation of a single lead VDD pacing system is only slightly different from that of a simple ventricular pacemaker.[9] It is somewhat preferable to insert the lead from the right because this gives greater positional stability to the atrial electrodes in terms of cranial-caudal movement (an approach from the left may bring the electrodes in closer to the right atrial wall, but this is not reliable). On the right side, the cephalic vein is usually of adequate size for any of the current multi-polar leads. A subclavian vein/introducer sheath technique may be used if necessary though this has a slightly increased potential for complications, especially damage to the complex lead by 'crush' between the clavicle and first rib.

Most manufacturers produce a choice of leads with different distances between the tip and atrial ring electrodes. The distance which is usually optimal for normal or slightly enlarged hearts is 13 cm, but for a very enlarged heart 15 cm may be necessary while for an unusually small heart 11 cm may be preferable.

The lead is inserted in the usual way using a stylet passed through the ventricular connector plug to the tip of the lead to guide it to the right ventricle. At this point fluoroscopy will show whether the atrial electrodes will lie comfortably at the mid right atrium. If they are rather high, then the tip should be positioned as close to the right ventricular apex as possible while if the electrodes are a little low and approaching the tricuspid valve, the tip should be moved back to a more proximal position on the inferior right ventricular wall. Once a stable position has been achieved, the stylet is gradually withdrawn and the lead advanced to produce a loop in the right atrium with a shape similar to the heel of a foot, with the atrial electrodes positioned approximately at the mid right atrium, close to the wall. There is considerable latitude in the position of the atrial electrodes and problems are only likely to arise if the electrodes are too high and liable to move out into the superior vena cava with changes in posture, or if the loop is af inadequate size to prevent dislodgement of the tip during deep inspiration on standing up.

With the lead in position routine checks of the ventricular electrode are made, including pacing threshold and signal. The signals from the atrial electrodes may then be checked though the results are of mainly academic interest as they will bear little, if any, relation to the long-term sensing threshold and the special sensing circuit should be able to cope with whatever signals are received provided adequate sensitivity is programmed.[10] Attempting to measure the signals using a standard pacing systems analyzer may cause unnecessary anxiety as the amplitude may well be too low for detection by the analyzer. If the position of the atrial electrodes is rather low, it is helpful to record the atrial bipolar signal to check that the far field R wave and especially the T wave are not too large. R wave oversensing can generally be prevented by programming the blanking period but T wave oversensing is more difficult. A large R wave (greater than 1 mV) in the atrial electrogram suggests that the lower atrial pole is close to or through the tricuspid valve and the lead should be repositioned.

Some current models use bipolar ventricular sensing and most use unipolar ventricular pacing so that it is important to make a pacemaker pocket with some tissue between the pulse generator and the pectoral muscle. It is conceivable that the system will not pace until the pulse generator is in the pocket.

Programming and Follow-Up

In the great majority of cases the atrial sensing should be programmed to the most sensitive setting as this will ensure reliable tracking as the patient mobilizes during the first few months. After about three months the lead becomes attached at points of contact with the endocardium and superior vena cava endothelium, and the mobility of the atrial electrodes is much reduced.[11] Associated with this, the atrial sensing threshold becomes more stable though there can still be quite large changes in the signal several years after lead implantation. The only problem with maximum sensitivity setting is the possibility of far field R wave and T wave sensing if the electrodes are near the tricuspid valve as mentioned above. R wave oversensing may produce no apparent change in the pacemaker rhythm but may result in a mode switch to asynchronous pacing (depending on the algorithm). The problem may usually be solved by extending the atrial blanking period. T wave oversensing may result in a pacemaker mediated tachycardia and, although extension of the post ventricular atrial refractory period (PVARP), where this is possible, may prevent it, this will result in a very limited maximum tracking rate. It is therefore best avoided by careful programming of the atrial sensitivity.

Basic pacing rate should be programmed sufficiently low that it is never reached other than with a post extrasystolic pause, as low-rate-limit pacing is not atrially synchronized and may even produce retrograde conduction and thus pacemaker syndrome especially at night. The correct rate may be determined by interrogating the pacemaker diagnostic data or, if necessary, by examining the trend plot of a 24 hour Holter recording. If the sinus rate at night is persistently below 45, there is either significant sinus node disease (in which case the wrong pacemaker had been chosen) or the patients has been put on a bradycardia inducing drug and alternatives to this should be considered. Similarly, the upper tracking rate limit should be sufficiently high that it is never reached in sinus rhythm. Provided there is no problem with atrial tachyarrhythmias it may be set five to ten beats per minute higher than the age predicted maximum heart rate or the highest rate achieved during an informal exercise test (e.g. stair climbing).

Atrial arrhythmias that cannot be satisfactorily controlled by drugs can pose a difficult programming problem. The most elegant solution is an automatic mode switch to VVIR immediately on the occurrence of the arrhythmia with a switch back to VDD mode when sinus rhythm returns. The facility is, of course, only available on VDDR systems and as mentioned above switching may be unreliable if the atrial signals are small. The other options are to program a very limited upper tracking rate or long PVARP, to reduce the atrial sensitivity so that only a proportion of the atrial signals are detected and to reprogram the pacing mode to VVI or VVIR with a basic pacing rate. If atrial fibrillation becomes established then the last option is best, and if rate responsive mode is not available consideration should be given to pulse generator replacement.

Clinical Experience

Follow-up studies of VDD pacemaker implants are especially important to answer the questions raised above concerning the incidence of atrial arrhythmias and sinus node dysfunction after implant. In an early prospective follow-up study[12] of over 1000 implants of the Medico Italia system conducted in 60 European centers, the mean follow-up period was over 14 months with a maximum up to five years. During that period no patient required pacemaker revision because of sinus node disease, and atrial fibrillation or flutter were seen in only 10 cases (1%).

Several smaller series have supported these findings. A study[13] of 73 patients followed up for up to 5 years (mean 27 months) after VDD implant (mainly LEM/CCS) showed only one case of AF and none of sinus node disease. In an American series[14] of 49 implants with mean follow-up of 16 months no case of sinus bradycardia and one of AF was found. A comparison of VDD and DDD pacing[15] showed no refractory AF in 62 patients over a mean follow-up of 21 months with paroxysmal atrial arrhythmias more frequent in the DDD group.

Longer term follow-up of these patients cohorts are required and some will be published in the near future. On the basis of these investigations the need for an included VVIR capability can be judged while in some cases there may be a haemodynamic benefit from the use of a rate adaptive sensor in addition to atrial tracking.[16]

As regards reliability of atrial sensing, this was already satisfactory with the early models[12,14] and is virtually faultless with the second generation of single lead systems.[10]

The evidence available from the studies published or presented so far suggests that there is a very low incidence of problems with single lead VDD/VDDR pacing and this should therefore become the standard treatment for atrioventricular block.

References

1. Fowler MB, Crick JCP, English MJ, Woollons DJ, Vencent R, Chamberlain DA. Haemodynamic advantages of synchronous (VDT/I) pacing after myocardial infarction using a single wire system. PACE 1980;3:370 (abstract).
2. Curry PVL, Raper DA. Single lead for permanent physiological cardiac pacing. Lancet 1978;2:757-9.
3. Antonioli GE, Grassi G, Baggiani GF, et al. New method for atrial triggered pacemaker. G Ital Cardiol 1980;10:679.
4. Goldreyer BN, Olive AL, Leslie J, Cannom DS, Wyman MG. A new orthogonal lead for P synchronous pacing. PACE 1981;4:638-44.
5. Sowton E, Wainwright RJ, Crick JCP. 'Crown of Thorns' single-pass lead – clinical results. PACE 1983;6:470-7.
6. Curzio G, Aquilina M, Morgagni W, Morra A, Travan M. In: Pérez Gómez F (ed.), Cardiac Pacing – Electrophysiology, Tachyarrhythmias. Editorial Grouz, Madrid, 1985, pp 865-73.
7. Crick JCP. Electrograms from the vicinity of the human heart in relation to artificial pacing. University of Sussex, thesis, D.Phil., 1984.
8. Pitts Crick. Unpublished (in preparation).
9. Pitts Crick JC, Papouchado M. Implantation technique for single-pass atrioventricular lead. Eur JCPE 1994;4:116.
10. Papouchado M, Goodfellow J, Burchard F, Pitts Crick JC. Single-pass lead VVD-R pacing: reliability of atrial sensing and atrial triggered ventricular pacing. PACE 1993;16:1929 (abstract).
11. Papouchado M, McConnell TJ, Freer T, Pitts Crick JC. Comparison of single-pass VDD pacing leads. Eur JCPE 1994;4:116.
12. Pitts Crick JC. European multicentre prospective follow-up study of 1002 implants of a single lead VDD pacing system. PACE 1991;14:1742-4.
13. Ansani L, Percoco GF, Guardigli G, Toselli T, Antonioli GE. Long-term reliability of single lead atrial synchronous pacing systems using closely spaced atrial dipoles: five year experience. PACE 1994;17:1865-9.
14. Gross JN, Andrews C, Ben-Zur UM, Ritacco R, Furman S. VDD pacing: chronic efficacy, incidence of atrial fibrillation and evolution of sinoatrial dysfunction. PACE 1993;16:881 (abstract).
15. Zanetta M, Parravicini U, Zenone F, Bielli M. Supraventricular arrhythmic events in advanced A-V block: single lead VDD versus DDD pacing. PACE 1993;16:1940 (abstract).
16. Lau CP, Tai YT, Leung SK, Li J, Won CP, Leung WH, Chung F, Au E. Improved aerobic capacity with single lead atrial synchronous pacing with a rate adaptive sensor. J Am Coll Cardiol 1993;21:383A (abstract).

3 PREVENTION OF PACEMAKER COMPLICATIONS

Chapter 6

Prevention and Treatment of Pacemaker Infection

Jo J.A.M.T. Defauw, Norbert M. van Hemel and Emile R. Jessurun

Introduction

For a number of reasons, infection of the pacemaker pocket is a serious complication.[1-3] The initial local infection may spread through one or more pacing leads and invade the bloodstream, which in turn can initiate septicemia or endocarditis. Secondly, treatment of the infection requires removal of the pacemaker to eliminate the infective process. This approach frequently requires long-term temporary pacing in pacemaker-dependent patients with inherent problems. Thirdly, removal of the permanent leads is frequently necessary, which constitutes a dangerous intervention.[4] It is very understandable that pacemaker pocket infection is associated with a high morbidity, lengthy hospitalization for careful surveillance of the infection and cardiac rhythm, and that this complication leads to high cost.

Fortunately, the rate of pacemaker infection after permanent pacemaker implantation is rather low, ranging from 1.7% to 5%, depending on the applied definitions.[1-3] Some authors also determine initial erosion of the skin of the pacemaker pocket as infection because this condition sometimes causes a late repeat surgical intervention for an infective process.[3] Culture tests most frequently identify Staphylococcus aureus and coagulase-negative staphylocci, but often the primary bacteria cannot be determined in pacemaker pocket infections late after implantation.

This study addresses measures to be taken for prevention of pacemaker infection, whereby emphasis will be laid on risky aspects of the implantation procedure, the value of antibiotic prophylaxis at implantation and replacement, and the identification of high risk patients. Guidelines for treatment of the infection and removal of the generator and leads will also be offered. Recent reports on infection rates of *temporary* electrodes are scarcely available, which hampers providing particular recommendations.

Implantation and Infection Risk

The Standard Implantation Procedure

The first principle of pacemaker implantation is a sterile approach, which is the responsibility of the operating team and the hospital facilities. The operation is performed in either the operating room or the catheterization laboratory. Prophylactic antibiotic against Staphylococcus aureus is administered thirty minutes to a maximum of two hours before the implantation procedure. The preferred antibiotic is flucloxacillin, or a first generation cephalo-sporin in selected cases.[5,6] When the procedure is performed in a catheterization laboratory, the room must have a positive air pressure installation to prevent external contamination. The skin of the patient must be thoroughly desinfected with either iodine or chlorhexidine and, when dry, sterile towels are placed around the pacemaker implantation area. Then the operative area is covered with surgical plastic.

The implantation area is infiltrated with a local anesthetic, e.g. 30 ml lidocain 1%, or the patient undergoes general anesthesia. The skin incision is made parallel to, and about 3 cm below the clavicle, extending medially about 4 cm from the deltopectoral groove. The next step is the formation of the pacemaker pocket by blunt dissection, which is either subcuteaneous, subfascial or subpectoral. Thereafter, careful hemostasis is performed by placing dry compresses or compresses soaked with 1% povidone iodine, in the pocket.

Depending on the operator's preference, a venous dissection of the cephalic vein or a pectoral vein is used. If no suitable veins are found, puncture of the subclavian vein is performed with a peel away introducer sheath. After positioning the electrode(s), one should carefully inspect the puncture site or the venous dissection for residual bleeding. The area should be absolutely dry and no hematoma may be present. When the electrode is connected to the pacemaker generator the compresses are removed and the pacemaker pocket is inspected for residual bleeding. The pocket should be absolutely dry and clots must be carefully removed. With the excess parts of the electrode(s) curled behind the pacemaker generator, it is positioned in the pocket. The wound is closed in layers with resorbable sutures for the subcutaneous layers and non resorbable sutures for the skin closure.

It should be emphasized that sterility must be maintained at all times. Only authorized personnel necessary for performing the implantation are permitted to enter the operating room.

Operative Risk Factors for Pacemaker Infection

a. Operation room or cardiac catheterization

With the advent of the transvenous approach of pacemakers in the mid 70's, the implantation procedure appears to be no longer restricted to the operation room. Advantage of the catheterization laboratory is the availability of high resolution fluoroscopy favouring lead positioning and insertion, but this location might compromise sterility. Despite these differences, Miller *et al*[7] could not observe in a retrospective study any infection in a small population of patients (N=80) in whom implantation was done in either the catheterization laboratory or operating room.

b. Clinical characteristics[8]

Predisposing factors favouring infection include diabetes mellitus, use of corticosteroids, immuno-compromised patients and cancer. Administration of coumarins or platelet aggregation inhibitors may cause excessive bleeding and the development of hematoma in the pacemaker pocket despite all surgical precautions.

c. Local depressed resistance

Skin erosion may be caused by defibrillation burns, tape, telemetry, monitor skin electrodes, diaper rash, tight clothes, trauma and sunburn. An increased risk for infection can be expected after prior multiple pulse generator replacements and early manipulation of leads after implantation e.g. for early dislodgement of the lead. When shaving of the operative area is required, it should be done as shortly as possible prior to surgery to prevent infection.

d. Pacemaker techniques

Temporary pacing with a lead adjacent to the side of the scheduled pacemaker implantation can facilitate pacemaker infection and venous thrombosis, causing an obstacle for the implantation. Prolonged placement of an external pacemaker can be a source of infection. The duration of the surgical procedure and the length of the incised skin are well-established risk factors for surgical site infection.[8] Finally, needle aspiration of pocket fluid or hematoma, and drainage of the pacemaker site after implantation also constitute increased risk for infection.

However, this survey of assumed predisposing factors favouring pacemaker infection cannot assign any clinical or methodological variable as a statistically valid risk factor. To establish a certain risk factor, the currently very low infection rate of less than 5% requires a very large number of patients to include in a prospective study. In addition, many studies suggesting a risk factor, are based on surgical methods and pacemakers in the years of infancy of pacemaker implantation. With the presence of thin and small sized pacemakers, skin erosion, one of the most important risk factors, has become a rare event. We conclude, that although above-mentioned conditions are not proven risk factors for pacemaker infection, they will affect the decision on when and where to place the temporary and definitive lead(s) and pocket.

Antibiotic Prophylaxis

Antibiotic prophylaxis intends to minimize pacemaker infection by administration of antibiotics. An establishment of the practical value of antibiotic prophylaxis requires randomized studies based on comparable patient groups, timing of treatment, surgical methods and implantable devices. In view of the low infection rates, the number of included patients should be very large. Because unheralded and delayed infection of a pacemaker may occur, surveillance of the studied patients should be extended to at least two years after surgery.[8] These considerations were applied in the literature review on this subject.

To compare the outcome of prophylactic systemic flucloxacillin (2 gm i.v. one hour before surgery, followed by 3 gm orally in the next five days) versus local administration of 500 mg cloxacillin in a dextran emulsion, Bluhm *et al* included 105 patients who underwent replacement of the pacemaker using an abdominal pacemaker pocket.[9] This study, carried out between 1980 to 1982, does not show any difference because no infection occurred in the systemic approach (0/53 patients), and in only 2/52 patients in the locally administered regimen after a follow-up ranging from 7 to 38 months. These results, however, are of less practical value due to the fact that both the abdominal pacemaker pocket and local administration of antibiotics are today outdated. In addition, generator replacement is a smaller operation, and therefore the risk of contamination is less than during the first implant. In a following study, Bluhm *et al* also could not demonstrate any difference in infection rate between antibiotic prophylaxis with flucloxacillin during the same above-mentioned administration scheme versus placebo.[10] In this study, 106 patients were included with first implantation routinely using the right cephalic vein and placement of the pacemaker in the upper right thoracic region in a subcutaneous pocket or, in a few cases, beneath the pectoralis muscle fascia. Infection was never observed during a mean follow-up of 14, range 7 to 35 months after implantation. Absence of wound contamination was ascribed by the authors to modified surgical technique consisting of a different anatomical pocket position and/or improved surgical methods. Although the authors concluded that antibiotic prophylaxis was meaningless, we believe that the number of included patients was too small to justify this opinion.

This was not the case with the randomized study comparing prophylactic flucloxacillin versus placebo carried out by Mounsey *et al* in 473 patients who underwent first implantation.[11] In nine cases pacemaker infection, defined as a infective process requiring repeat surgery, emerged in patients not receiving flucloxacillin, showing a significant difference and benefit from antibiotic prophylaxis ($p=0.003$). Furthermore, the total population screened between 1991 to 1993 for inclusion in this study, was 715 consecutive patients allowing for identification of risk factors for infective pacemaker problems. Infections increased significantly in the hands of unexperienced surgeons, when the operation was prolonged (>55 minutes) or after a repeat operation for noninfective complications, such as lead dislodgement. Finally, the infection rate with or without antibiotic prophylaxis in patients with *temporary* electrodes did not show any difference.

A large number of patients was also included by Ramsdale *et al* in a randomized study comparing 1 gm cloxacillin and 1 gm amoxicillin intravenously administered one hour before surgery, and 2 gm ampicillin/flucoxacillin for two days after surgery versus placebo.[12] Five hundred patients were included in the study, and underwent first implantation or pacemaker replacement. In all patients antibiotics were sprayed into the pocket before insertion of the pacemaker. The number of patients showing wound infection and pocket infection (0.6%) or superficial inflammation (3.6%) did not show any difference in both arms during a follow-up of at least three months. The authors concluded that prophylactic antibiotic treatment has no practical value.

These results show a conflicting opinion on the validity of antibiotic prophylaxis for pacemaker implantation or replacement. Absence of a clear consensus is due to the low infection rate requiring large groups patients for randomization, improving surgical techniques, smaller pacemakers, and better identification of unfavourable conditions as well as patients at risk. Based on these results and on our own experience we advise the following scheme:

1. Antibiotic prophylaxis is recommended:[5,6,13]
    a. in high risk patients: use of corticosteroids, immuno-suppressive agents, treatment with cytostatics, insulin-dependent diabetes mellitus;
    b. in carriers of heart valves or artificial cardiovascular prostheses;
    c. in early repeat pacemaker surgery (<3-36 days after first surgery), e.g. correction of pacemaker dislodgement;

d. in case of prolonged implantation procedure (>30 minutes opened skin).

Drug of choice, dosage and timing: administration of 1 g cephazolin or 1 g flucloxacillin intravenously at induction of anesthesia (figure 1). When penicillin allergy is established, 600 mg clindamycin intraveneously offers an alternative. Continuation of antibiotic prophylaxis is not warranted.

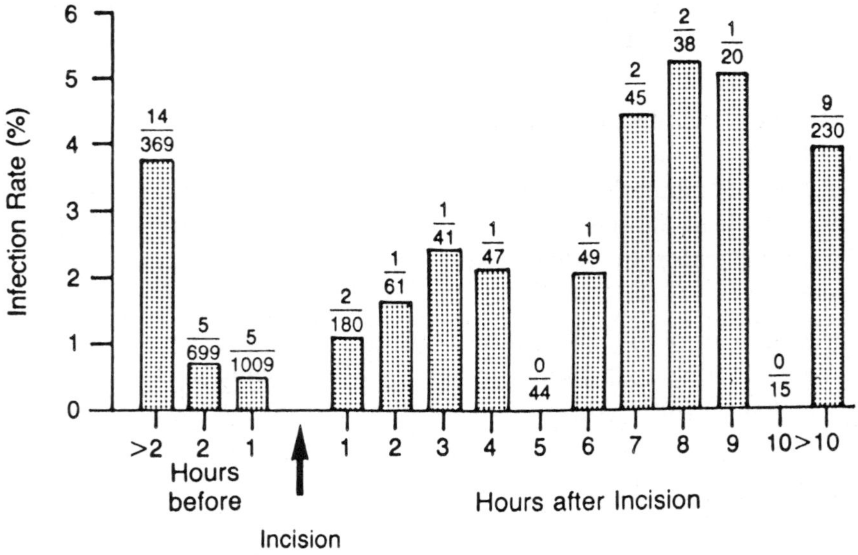

Figure 1. *Rates of surgical-wound infection corresponding to the temporal relation between antibiotic administration and the start of surgery.*
The number of infections and the number of patients for each hourly interval appears as the numerator and denominator, respectively, of the fraction for that interval. The trend toward higher rates of infection for each hour that antibiotic administration was delayed after the surgical incision was significant (z score, = 2.00; $P<0.05$ by the Wilcoxon test).[5] (With permission of the N Eng J Med).

2. Antibiotic prophylaxis is *not* recommended:

   in all routine cases without predictable risk in order to avoid the occurrence of drug resistance.

Treatment of Pacemaker Infection

Pacemaker infection might become manifest by several aspects, such as skin erosion or decubitus of the pocket or lead, pocket abscess, lead infection, septicemia and endocarditis.[3] Pacemaker infection almost always starts during surgery with bacterial contamination of the incised skin or deeper tissue layers composing the pacemaker pocket. Dependent on the type of causative micro-organisms, local (e.g. the degree of scarring) and systemic resistance of the patient, the infection will become manifest early or late after the surgical procedure. These factors also determine whether the infection will be limited to the pocket or spread out. The successive phases of pocket infection, lead infection, septicemia and endocarditis, and the corresponding therapeutical management will be discussed together.

Decubitus and Abscess of the Pocket

Decubitus results from a disproportion between pacemaker volume or shape and the initial or late dimension of the subcutaneous or subfascial pacemaker pocket. Due to continuous pressure, tissue layers above the pacemaker and/or lead weaken until finally the pacemaker migrates through necrotic tissue. Infection with micro-organism is a logical consequence of pacemaker protrusion. It often remains untraceable whether infection preceeds the decubitus or the opposite happens. Infection of the pocket *without* decubitus is suspected when redness, swelling or tenderness of the pocket develops, and sometimes fever accompanies the symptoms. When pacemaker pocket infection is diagnosed, two approaches are applicable:

1. Local wound care, continuous irrigation of the pocket and systemic antibiotic treatment

This conservative management is attractive because the same pacemaker can be used and temporary pacing can be avoided. Careful debridement of the infected pocket and vigorous enlargement of the pocket to guarantee adequate closure without tension is required.[14] Then a closed irrigation system (figure 2), containing a solution of tyloxapol and tobramycin is used for at least five days. It is very important that this system flows continuously, without any obstruction from clots or other particles. Successful examples of local therapy with a favourable long-term result have been reported.[14] However, a high recurrence rate of infection can be expected, probably by migration of the infection into the leads or adjacent tissue, particularly in cases with infection months after implantation and caused by coagulase-negative staphylococci.[2,3]

We emphasize that when this method is used, irrigation of the pocket should be done with NaCl 0.9% to achieve mechanical cleaning of the infected pocket because the advantage of irrigation with antibiotics has never been proven. In addition, administration of an aminoglycoside is not warranted, because these antibiotics are not the drugs of first choice against staphylococci.

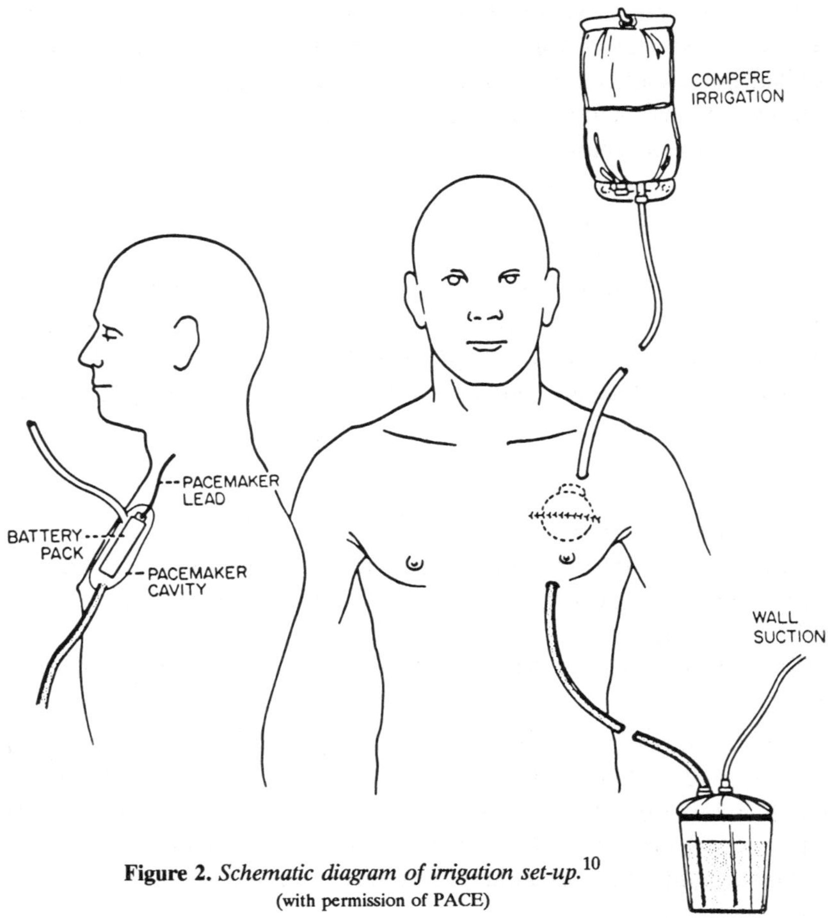

Figure 2. *Schematic diagram of irrigation set-up.*[10]
(with permission of PACE)

2. *Complete removal of the pacemaker and leads, local spraying with povidone-iodine solution and implantation of a new pacemaker on the opposite side*

This aggressive approach is based on the concept that removal of foreign material located in an avascular fibrocollagenous pouch, is the only appropriate method to eliminate the infection.[15-17] It also prevents the spread-out of the infective process into the leads and reduces the chance for septicemia and endocarditis. The therapy includes complete removal of the leads because this hardware may become a new focus of infection.[18] To stimulate secondary wound healing, wound debridement and drainage of the pocket will be done afterwards. Culture tests of the removed hardware and infective material will guide the administration of antibiotic therapy afterwards and during the next implantation at the opposite thoracic side.

We prefer radical removal of all hardware in proven or suspected pacemaker infections, emerging early or late after pacemaker implantation or replacement, followed by reimplantation at the opposite side.[17] Limitation of the infective process to the pocket area and prevention of secondary infections through an irrigation system, e.g. low grade infections with coagulase-negative staphylococci, are in favour for this concept, which eventually results in shorter hospitalization and better cost-effectiveness. An exception constitutes threatening decubitus without skin perforation. Under these circumstances, local skin excision and pocket replacement can be considered. This approach is based on assumed absence of necrosis of superficial tissue layers and hence a still existing barrier against infection from outside. Absence of infection has to be established with culture test during surgery.

Infected Leads

Lead infection can only be indirectly suspected by signs of infection of the pacemaker pocket and/or by septicemia. On occasion, transoesophageal echocardiography can show vegetations attached to the lead. For percutaneous removal of implanted leads, several approaches are available to date.[4] Their success rate depends on shape and size of the distal electrode. For example, tined and flange-tipped leads may interfere with extraction, can provoke myocardial perforation and injury of the tricuspid valve and the venous system. Secondly, endothelialization of leads by fibrocollagenous material may complicate extraction because leads are frequently firmly attached to the venous system. Finally, the force necessary to extract, sometimes causes desintegration and rupture of the lead. Currently available percutaneous methods for removal can be summarized as follows:

a. Direct traction of the lead after disconnection of the generator, a frequently time-consuming method with a low success rate, and often complicated by lead fracture instead of complete removal of the lead.
b. Grasping and withdrawal of the lead when the proximal end is intravascular or has migrated, using a rigid grasping forceps, a snare catheter or a Dotter helical basket with the help of a pigtail or right Amplatz catheter. All methods require traction and are characterized by the risk for vascular or myocardial injury.[19]

c. Introduction of a locking stylet into the lead for permitting direct traction followed by passing dilating coaxial sheets over the electrode, to disrupt the endothelialization of the lead, and to permit countertraction to the myocardium. Advantages of this approach are more support for extraction and prevention of vascular injury.[19,20]
d. Not the use of a locking stylet but tying of a 26 gauge surgical wire around the proximal end of the lead, for direct traction on the lead followed by a coaxial extraction approach with a 12 French billiary dilator (see further c).[21]

Leads that recently have been inserted and therefore have few fibrous adhesions to the venous system, or leads without active fixation are most suitable for percutaneous extraction.[15] When excessive force is needed or when the lead is implanted in the atrium, the risk for complications increases.

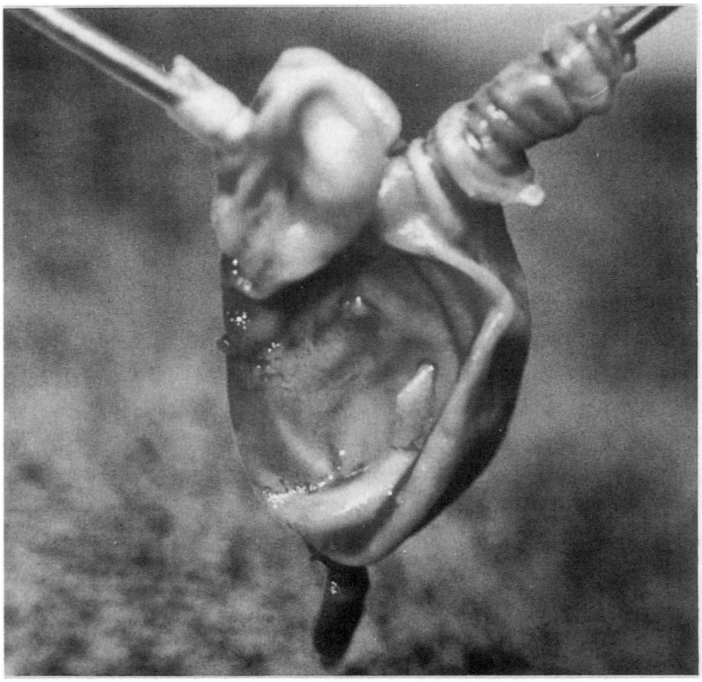

Figure 3. *Pacemaker lead with vegetations.*

Infected leads or remnants should always be removed because their presence maintains the infection process due to insufficient efficacy of antibiotic therapy in this foreign body. There are reports documenting a morbidity of up to 66% for infected retained electrodes.[4,19-21] Training and experience with percutaneous methods are required, and it is advocated to refer patients with infected leads to specialized centers, preferably with full facilities for cardiac surgery back-up.[22]

Presence of vegetations (figure 3) attached to a lead as demonstrated by trans-oesophageal echocardiography, is an undisputable reason for surgical removal, using thoracotomy and cardiotomy to avoid the risk of septic pulmonary embolism.[21]

Septicemia and Endocarditis

In this serious and life-threatening systemic infection, removal of all hardware combined with antibiotic chemotherapy is required. Prior to surgery, the difficult decision of whether percutaneous extraction of the lead can be done, or open intracardiac removal is necessary. Percutaneous extraction of the lead appears justified when lead vegetations and signs of tricuspid endocarditis can be fully excluded with echocardiographic studies. Presence of multiple leads whether abandoned or not, age and physical condition are also important determinants. In view of the above-mentioned complications of percutaneous extraction, experience with this approach is another requirement to make a correct decision on lead extraction after opening the pacemaker pocket or surgical removal. Conceivably, culture tests of all removed hardware should be performed.

When the nonthoracic approach is excluded, open intracardiac removal through a right-sided atriotomy with the use of cardiopulmonary bypass will be done, allowing controlled explantation of the lead under direct vision.[23-25] The semi-open method through a purse string suture on the beating heart without bypass constitutes an alternative approach, contributing to a shorter recovery period and hospital stay.[22] Simultaneous implantation of a new pacemaker and epicardial leads can be considered, but we prefer temporary epicardial pacing for five to seven days to evaluate the results of the infective treatment. When fever abates and wound healing is complete, replacement of the pacemaker at the opposite side can be done in a second procedure, with antibiotic prophylaxis.

Conclusions

Many measures, consisting of small-sized pacemaker generators, high quality fluoroscopy, improved experience and better training in implantation techniques have strongly contributed to a very low infection rate of pacemakers in the 90's. This observation can diminish alertness on infection in the pacemaker clinic. Pacemaker infection remains to date a serious, time consuming and expensive complication of pacing therapy, and deserves continuous attention for prevention and early detection with all available tools. Because pacemaker infection can deteriorate into a systemic, life-threatening disease, an aggressive therapeutical approach is justified. Finally, in view of the currently diminishing efficacy of antibiotic prophylaxis, the surgical technique is more important than ever.

The authors wish to thank B.M. de Jongh, MD, PhD, and B.P. Overbeek, MD, PhD, Department of Medical Microbiology and Immunology, Sint Antonius Hospital, Nieuwegein, The Netherlands, for review of this report.

References

1. Brodman R, Frame R, Andrews C, Furman S. Removal of infected transvenous leads requiring cardiopulmonary bypass or inflow occlusion. J Thorac Cardiovasc Surg 1992;103:649-54.
2. Berge PG, Winter UJ, Dünnebacke M, Deutsch HJ. Pacemaker infections from the clinical point of view: Review and own experiences. In: Winter UJ, Zegelman M (eds), Herzschrittmacher- und Defibrillator-Infektionen, 1994, Thieme Verlag, Stuttgart, pp 20-26.
3. Choo MH, Holmes Jr DR, Gersh BJ, Maloney JD, Merideth J, Pluth JR, Trusty J. Permanent pacemaker infections: characterization and management. Am J Cardiol 1981;48:559-64.
4. Myers MR, Parsonnet V, Bernstein AD. Extraction of implanted transvenous pacing leads: A review of a persitent clinical problem. Am Heart J 1991;121:881-8.
5. Classen DC, Evans RS, Pestotnik SL, Horn SD, Menlove RL, Burke JP. The timing of prophylactic administration of antibiotics and the risk of surgical-wound infection. N Engl J Med 1992;326:281-6.
6. Page CP, Bohnen JMA, Fletcher JR, McManus AT, Solomkin JS, Wittmann DH. Antimicrobial prophylaxis for surgical wounds. Arch Surg 1993;128:79-88.
7. Miller GB, Lemna RB, Kratz JM, Gillette PC. Comparison or lead dislodgement and pocket infection rates after pacemaker implantation in the operating room versus the catheterization laboratory. Am Heart J 1988;115:1048-51.
8. Consensus paper on the surveillance of surgical wound infections. Infect Control Hosp Epidemiol 1992;13:599-605.
9. Bluhm G, Jacobson B, Ransjö U. Antibiotic prophylaxis in pacemaker surger: a prospective trial with local or systemic administration of antibiotics at generator replacements. PACE 1985;8:661-70.
10. Bluhm G, Norlander R, Ransjo U. Antibiotic prophylaxis in pacemaker surgery: a prospective double blind trial with systemic administration of antibiotic versus placebo at implantation of cardiac pacemakers. Pace Clin Electrophysiol 1986;9:720-6.
11. Mounsey JP, Griffith MJ, Tynan M, Gould FK, MacDermott AFN, Gold RG, Bexton RS. Antibiotic prophylaxis in permanent pacemaker implantation: a prospective randomized trial. Br Heart J 1994;72:339-43.
12. Ramsdale DR, Charles RG, Rowlands DB, Singh SS, Gautam PC, Faragher EB. Antibiotic prophylaxis for pacemaker implantation: a prospective randomized trial. PACE 1984;7:844-9.
13. Dellinger EP, Gross PA, Barrett TL, Krause PJ, Martone WJ, McGowan Jr JE, Sweet RL, Wenzel RP. Quality standard for antimicrobial prophylaxis in surgical procedures. Clinical Infectious Diseases 1994;18:422-7.
14. Hurst LN, Evans HB, Windle B, Klein GJ. The salvage of infected cardiac pacemaker pockets using a closed irrigation system. PACE 1986;9:785-92.

15. Goldman BS. Commentary for 'Salvage of infected cardiac pacemaker pockets using a closed irrgation system'. PACE 1986;9:915-6.
16. Ruiter JH, Degener JE, Mechelen R van, Bos R. Late purulent pacemaker pocket infection caused by Staphylococcus epidermidis: Serious complications of in situ management. PACE 1985;8:903-7.
17. Byrd CL, Schwartz SJ, Hedin NB, Saunkeah B. Experience with 234 pocket infections: what works? PACE 1992;15(II):510.
18. Praeger PI, Kay RH, Somberg E, Herman MV, Reed GE. Pacemaker remnants - another source of infections. PACE 1984;7:763-4.
19. Fearnot NE, Smith HJ, Goode LB, Byrd CL, Wilkoff BL, Sellers TD. Intravascular lead extraction using locking stylets, sheats, and other techniques. PACE 1990;13:1864-70.
20. Byrd CL, Schwartz SJ, Hedin NB, Goode LB, Fearnot NE, Smith HJ. Intravascular lead extraction using locking stylets and sheats. PACE 1990;13:1871-5.
21. Hager WD, Brown L, Ramsby G. Percutaneous removal of infected permanent pacemaker leads using a simple coaxial dilating system. PACE 1994; 17:2345-8.
22. Sloman G, Strathmore N. Permanent pacemaker lead extraction. PACE 1993;16:2331-2.
23. Niederhäuser U, Segesser LK von, Carrel TP, Laske A, Bauer E, Schönbeck M, Turina M. Infected endocardial pacemaker electrodes: Successful open intracardiac removal. PACE 1993;16:303-8.
24. Dubernet J, Irarrázaval MJ, Lema G, Maturana G, Urzua J, Morán S, Navarro M, Fajuri A. Surgical removal of entrapped endocardial leads without using extracorporeal circulation. PACE 1985;8:175-80.
25. DeLeon SY, Bojar R, Koster NK, Ilbawi MN, Munez H, Idriss FS. Recurrent sepsis from retained endocardial electrode in children: Successful removal with cardiopulmonary bypass. PACE 1984;7:166-8.

3 PREVENTION OF PACEMAKER COMPLICATIONS

Chapter 7

Technical Follow-up of Implanted Pacemakers

Peter van der Kemp and Lex Bakema

Introduction

A patient with a cardiac pacemaker is condemned for life to attend a pacemaker clinic for follow-up. One of the main objectives for follow-up is to anticipate impending pacemaker system failure before there is risk to the patient. Battery depletion impairs pacemaker function and is still the main reason for surgical intervention.[1] Beginning or actual failure of systems must be ascertained in the clinic and the necessary steps taken to remedy the situation.

Historically, pacemaker follow-up became necessary because of the short battery life, the poor performance of pacemaker leads and the unpredictability of pulse generator components.[2] Surveillance of pacemaker function was mostly carried out by electronic engineers, some having a background in medical physics. The current widespread use and complexities of pacemaker therapy has led to a need for specially trained associated professionals in follow-up. Despite the enormous technological improvements and widespread application of pacemaker therapy there is, however, still no consensus about the method, intervals and organization of pacemaker follow-up. The equipment required and the schedules used will depend to some extent on the nature of the pacemaker system employed. There are also remarkable differences between the procedures, schedules, degree of physician involvement and the administration of collected data between various hospitals. Recently, more than 35 years after the first pacemaker implantation, the North American Society of Cardiac Pacing (NASPE) issued a policy statement about antibradycardia pacemaker follow-up.[3] This policy statement initiated a broad consciousness about the necessity to thorough organize follow-up of implanted pacemakers.

Rationale of Follow-up

The development of new symptoms and changes of cardiac function in patients require a dynamic adjustment of implanted pacemaker systems. Present pulse generators are becoming more adaptable to changing cardiac demands. It is therefore that the periodic check-up provides an excellent opportunity to optimize cardiac therapy.

With most modern programmable pulse generators, energy consumption, and therefore longevity, can be influenced by programmed parameter setting. Safe optimization of energy consumption requires careful planning. Pulse generators and pacemaker leads are, like other technical devices, vulnerable to unpredictable malfunction. A periodic assessment of a pacemaker system may prevent clinically important incidents resulting from further technical deterioration of the system. Malfunction may originate not only from failing pulse generator components but also from changes in the lead system or from changes in the heart itself. More frequent monitoring in the early stages after implant is advisable since early malfunction due to lead dislodgement or to pacing threshold changes as well as changes in the native heart rhythm can occur. Malfunctioning pacemaker systems will not always lead to dramatic events and the patient may not be aware of a faulty system. In some cases, however, it can lead to serious and even fatal complications.

Pacemaker Technology

▸ *Battery characteristics.* The projected period of time that the pulse generator battery and with that the pulse generator itself will function within manufacturers specifications, is expressed as longevity. Longevity depends on several predictable and unpredictable factors. Information about battery capacity, internal circuit drain and the efficiency of battery voltage transformation are provided by the manufacturer of the generator. Others parameters, such as pacing voltage and pulse width, are user-programmable and have a major influence on longevity (figure 1). Average pacing impedance varies with lead design and tissue interface intimacy while the pacing percentage depends on the interaction between programmed rate and the patient's intrinsic rhythm. The relation between pulse width, pacing amplitude and pacing percentage on longevity is explained in Appendix I. The above mentioned factors makes it impossible to predict the exact time of battery depletion.

To anticipate the generator's end of life one has to monitor cell usage. In conventional generators this is done by monitoring battery voltage. The voltage of a battery drops during its lifetime in a fairly predictable but non-linear manner.

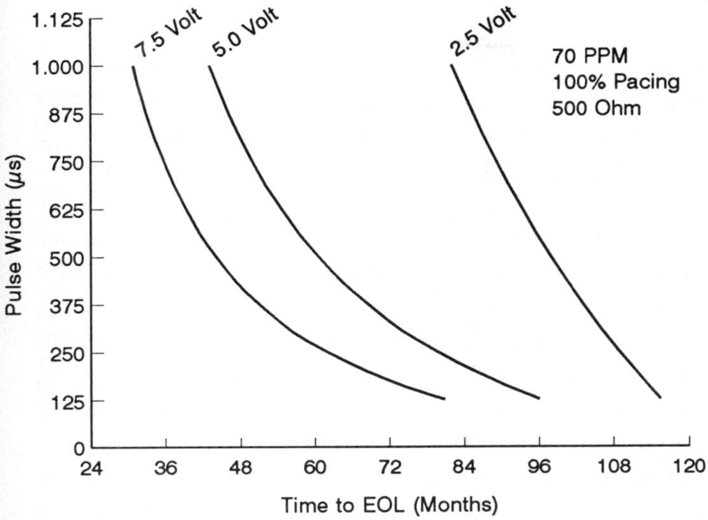

Figure 1. *Theoretical longevity of a Pulse Generator. Pulse width is plotted against longevity for a standby rate of 70 ppm. Three pacing voltage amplitudes are shown with lines representing 100% pacing against a nominal 500 Ω load.*

The very first pulse generators used simple electronic oscillators. The rate of these oscillators was (unintentionally) dependent on battery voltage[4], so that the pulse stimulation rate was a measure of the battery function. By counting the pulse rate, the patient could monitor the battery status and report abnormalities to the follow-up clinic. This practice was of limited use for patients with spontaneous rhythm or patients incapable of self monitoring. Hence, a periodic technical evaluation of pulse generator function became an essential safeguard to prevent sudden loss of pulse generator function due to battery exhaustion.

With present pulse generators, which have voltage independent crystal oscillators, design engineers had to develop other ways to indicate battery status. The simplest indicator chosen to show end-of-life behaviour is a distinct and abrupt fall in the pulse generators stimulation rate when the battery voltage falls below a certain level. With most modern generators, however, one can assess battery status very simply by placing a magnet over the pulse generator. The *magnet mode* usually is a fixed rate pacing mode that continues as long as the magnet is placed over the pulse generator. The stimulation rate during application of a magnet, the *magnet rate*, reflects the battery voltage and the remaining battery capacity. A typical decrease of magnet rate during battery depletion is given in figure 2. Comparing the magnet rate with the battery depletion data provided by the manufacturer or pulse generator databooks[5,6] gives an indication of the actual battery status. The magnet rate, measured when battery and circuitry are assembled, is called the magnet rate at Begin Of Life (BOL). The Elective Replace-

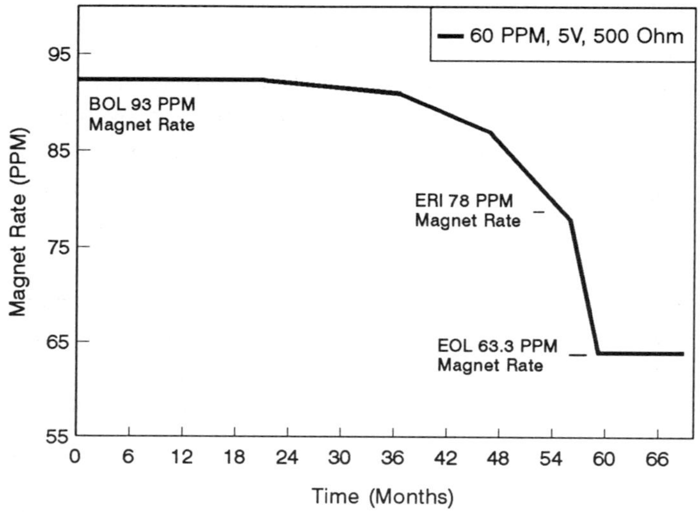

Figure 2. *Theoretical model of magnet rate versus time in a dual-chamber pacemaker at 100% pacing with 0.5 ms pulse width and pacing rate, pulse amplitude and average pacing impedance. By its nature, the voltage of a lithium-iodine battery decreases more sharply at the end than at the beginning of its life. Therefore the resulting magnet rate remains rather constant in the first part of the pulse generators life.*

ment Indicator (ERI) is a distinct magnet rate at which elective replacement of the implanted pulse generator is recommended. Some manufacturers designate the point of advised pulse generator exchange as Recommended Replacement Time (RRT). If the ERI/RRT point has passed, the function of the pulse generator will be unaffected for several months. Eventually, if the pulse generator is not exchanged, the End Of Life (EOL) point will be reached. At EOL most of the presently available pulse generators switch to a low energy program. As current consumption continues, the pulse generator will inevitably cease function within weeks. This point is called End Of Service (EOS) and the moment it is reached is not defined. The relation between magnet rate, battery (cell) impedance and the defined points is plotted in figure 3.

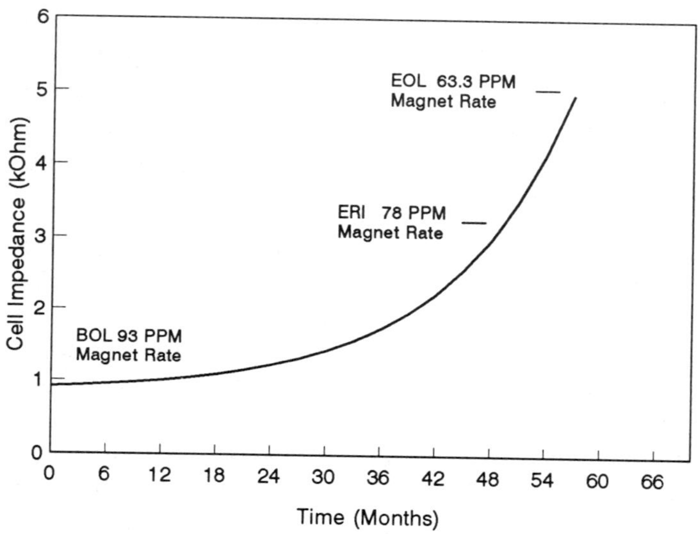

Figure 3. *Typical change in battery (cell) impedance over time during constant current drain.*

There are, however, more sophisticated approaches to predict remaining battery longevity. With some pulse generators, the battery impedance can be obtained from the telemetry data and this provides a useful estimate of the remaining energy and possible longevity. It is also possible to make an estimation of future energy consumption based on the current pacing data and therefore to predict how long the energy remaining in the cell may last. This calculation can be made manually or by the pulse generator itself in conjunction with the programmer.

In conclusion, the follow-up program must aim at prevention of acute interventions caused by battery exhaustion. Monitoring of the battery discharge at regular intervals in conjunction with information about the properties of the battery and the actual energy consumption of the system, determines the optimal moment for pulse generator exchange.

▸ *Detection characteristics.* Detection of signals from the heart muscle or 'sensing', is necessary for synchronization of the pulse generator to the patients native heart rhythm. The detection circuit of the pulse generator must differentiate between spontaneous heart beats and electrical signals of extra-cardiac origin as well as repolarization potentials.[7] The detection circuitry of the pulse generator therefore requires special filters. Such filters may differ slightly for the atrial and ventricular signal amplifiers.[8]

After a stimulation impulse, or detection of a spontaneous depolarization, there will be a period in which the pacemaker electrode senses depolarization and repolarization potentials. This can potentially mislead the pulse generators timing circuit since the incoming signals may be interpreted as new spontaneous heart activity resulting in premature reset of the timing circuit. To prevent such malsensing, a period of time in which the pulse generator signal amplifier is made insensitive to incoming signals is built into the circuitry: the refractory period. Refractory periods may be initiated by both paced beats and by sensed spontaneous depolarization. To adapt to specific needs the programmable pulse generator has several sensitivity and refractory period settings.

By programming decreasing levels of sensitivities the 'sensitivity threshold' can be defined. This sensitivity threshold is the lowest sensitivity setting at which correct sensing of the relevant intrinsic heart activity occurs.[9] Failure of correct sensing is generally called malsensing. It can be classified as oversensing, when unwanted signals are sensed or as undersensing when relevant cardiac activity is not detected. Malsensing may be intermittent and transient. It can lead to either competition with spontaneous rhythm or to unwanted inhibition. The electrocardiogram during follow-up, possibly in addition to ambulatory ECG (Holter) monitoring, is best suited to reveal malsensing. With correct pacing lead performance, malsensing can often be corrected by careful programming of sensitivity and/or refractory periods.

Even with optimal filtering and amplification techniques, the cardiac signals must be of a minimal amplitude and of a suitable frequency content to guarantee proper sensing.

▸ *Communication features.* Modern pulse generators are equipped with bidirectional telemetry. This means that the operator can not only send data to the pulse generator, but also receive data from the pulse generator by non-invasive electronic transcutaneous interrogation. This makes it possible to retrieve the actual settings of programmable parameters and in addition, much useful supplementary diagnostic data may be available. This diagnostic data may include technical data about the performance of the pulse generator such as battery impedance and cell voltage, and data on lead function such as the pacing impedance. It may also provide long-term information about the patient's heart rhythms by disclosure of the stimulation incidence. The availability of endocardial electrograms and timing event markers may help considerably with problem solving in follow-up (figure 4).[10] With telemetric diagnostic data, the consequence of changing pulse generator settings can be immediately observed, which reduces the need for other diagnostic procedures. However, pulse generators are becoming increasingly equipped with such diagnostic tools, and some caution is needed before they become incorporated in routine follow-up programs. For example, the information provided by event counters needs careful evaluation. Events can only be counted accurately if they can be detected reliably. Until the pulse generator contains a full disclosure Holter monitor, interpretation of compressed data as provided by event counters can be misleading. Validation of the data logging process is obligatory before any therapy, based on compressed pacemaker data, is established.[11]

▸ *Interference with other devices.* Pacemakers are vulnerable to interference. Endogenous interference can originate from electrical sources such as muscle potentials. Most common interference from exogenous sources is caused by ElectroMagnetic Interference (EMI) from other electrical devices.[12] The pulse generator's response to EMI is dependent on the characteristics of the EMI, proximity to the source of interference, available shielding, the sensing characteristics and polarity of the implanted pulse generator. EMI can alter pulse generator function both temporarily or permanently. If a persistent change in programming occurs, it may be corrected by re-programming. But EMI may also cause irreversible damage to the pulse generator circuitry. In the latter case explantation of the pulse generator may be required.

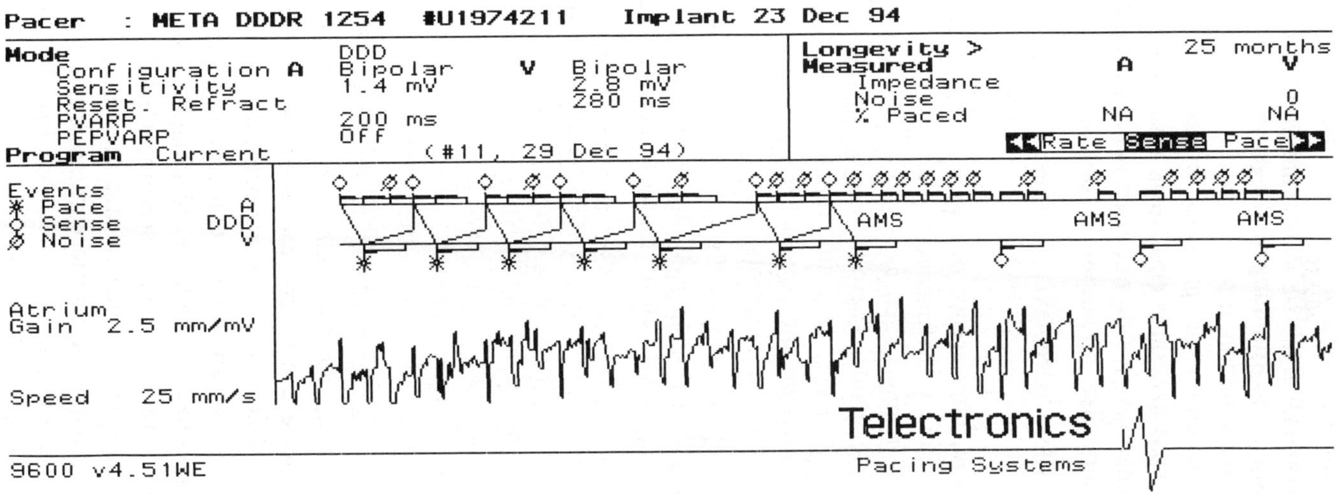

Figure 4. *Endocardial atrial electrograms in combination with Main Timing Events are very valuable during follow-up to analyze complex timing operations such as Automatic Mode Switching (AMS).*

If the EMI mimics intrinsic heart activity, the most common type of response of pulse generators is false inhibition or asynchronous stimulation.[13] Normal pulse generator function will resume immediately if the source of the interference is removed. Interference causing reprogramming of the pulse generator, is called as *phantom programming*.[14] In this situation, a persistent change of the programming occurs without any documentation of previous intentional reprogramming. Permanent damage to the pulse generator circuit can result from EMI exposure and may lead to minor anomalies which do not affect function but can rarely also induce potentially lethal failures like 'no output' or 'runaway'.[15]

There are four situations where pacemaker patients may become exposed to EMI:

In the *domestic environment*, interference due to electrical equipment is rare and mostly restricted to temporary dysfunction.[16] Very near approach of some devices equipped with heavy magnets such as audio speakers, may temporarily engage pulse generators magnet mode. There is an ongoing discussion about the possible effects of microwave ovens, induction heaters and (digital) cellular telephones.[17,18] In *public environments* the pacemaker patient can be exposed to EMI by installations such as metal detectors used at airports and anti-theft devices in shops and libraries. Interference from these devices is generally limited to short and transient periods of malfunction during the patient's passage through the installation. Other sources of EMI can be found in the *industrial sector*. Arc welders, degaussing installations and power plants may produces high levels of electromagnetic radiation. Several publications however, suggest that these high levels do not always lead to malfunction, and many patients have safely worked in these environments without any problem.[19-21] Not only temporary reversion of function but also permanent damage of the pulse generator circuit may occur during *medical procedures* such as radiotherapy[15,22], electrocautery[23], transthoracic defibrillation, magnetic resonance imaging, catheter ablation[24], transcutaneous electrical nerve stimulation, and extracorporeal shock-wave lithotripsy.[12]

If appropriate precautionary measures are taken, significant clinical incidents from electromagnetic interference can be avoided. Such measures can consist of comprehensive advice to the patient and field research for work environments. During field research, 'safe zones' can be delineated and other specific recommendations can be given. Recurring symptoms in specific situations, for instance during the use of heavy machines, can raise suspicion of EMI and need to be carefully evaluated. If confronted with permanent damage to the pulse generator, it is crucial to discover the source of interference in order to avoid similar damage to the replacement generator.

Lead Technology

The mechanical construction and design of pacing leads might appear to be relatively simple. Historically pacing leads have been a source of major problems and failures still occur despite much research and precise engineering. In the past, failure rates of almost 70% were reported.[25] The lead dimensions, flexibility, fixation mechanism, threshold behaviour, sensing characteristics, surface roughness and bio-compatibility all affect performance. At patient follow-up, full details of the lead specifications are required as well as updated information about it's performance in practice. The description of the several parts of a lead system is given in figure 5.

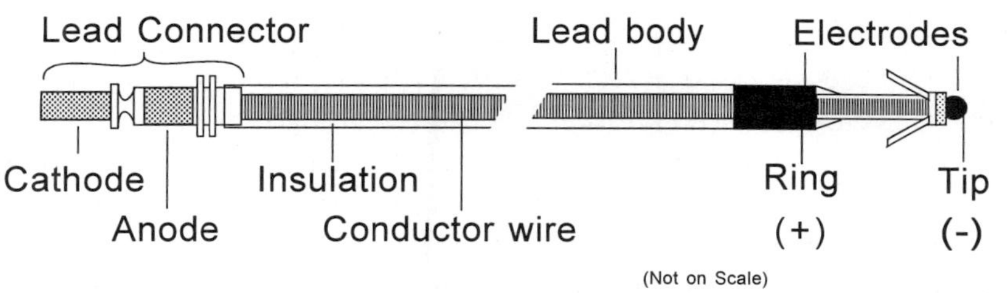

Figure 5. *The definition of the several parts of a cardiac pacing lead.*

▸ *Lead fixation.* To facilitate fixation during the first hours and days after implantation, an implantable pacemaker lead is equipped with an anchoring mechanism. Passive, *atraumatic*, leads use mechanisms such as tines, fins, flanges or conical constructions to stabilise their position. The tissue growth around the anchoring mechanism provides chronic fixation. Active, *traumatic*, fixation leads prevent the electrode in the acute and chronic phase from dislodgement (displacement) by the use of screws, springs, needles, pins and claws.[26]

Dislodgement can be classified into macrodislodgement and microdislodgement; the former being, by definition, radiologically visible. For example, a ventricular lead may have been withdrawn back to the atrium. Macrodislodgement is also referred to as 'dislocation'. It happens mostly in the early stage after implantation. It may be a result of poor implantation technique or due to some manoeuvres in the early post implant phase such as stretching or raising the arms above the head. Poor design of the electrode anchoring mechanism may sometimes lead to electrode dislodgement at a later stage.[27] Dislodgement often leads to loss of sensing, loss of capture or stimulation of extracardiac tissues. Analysis and comparison with previous ECG recordings of the ventricular-paced evoked response is valuable for evaluation of dislodgement (figure 6).

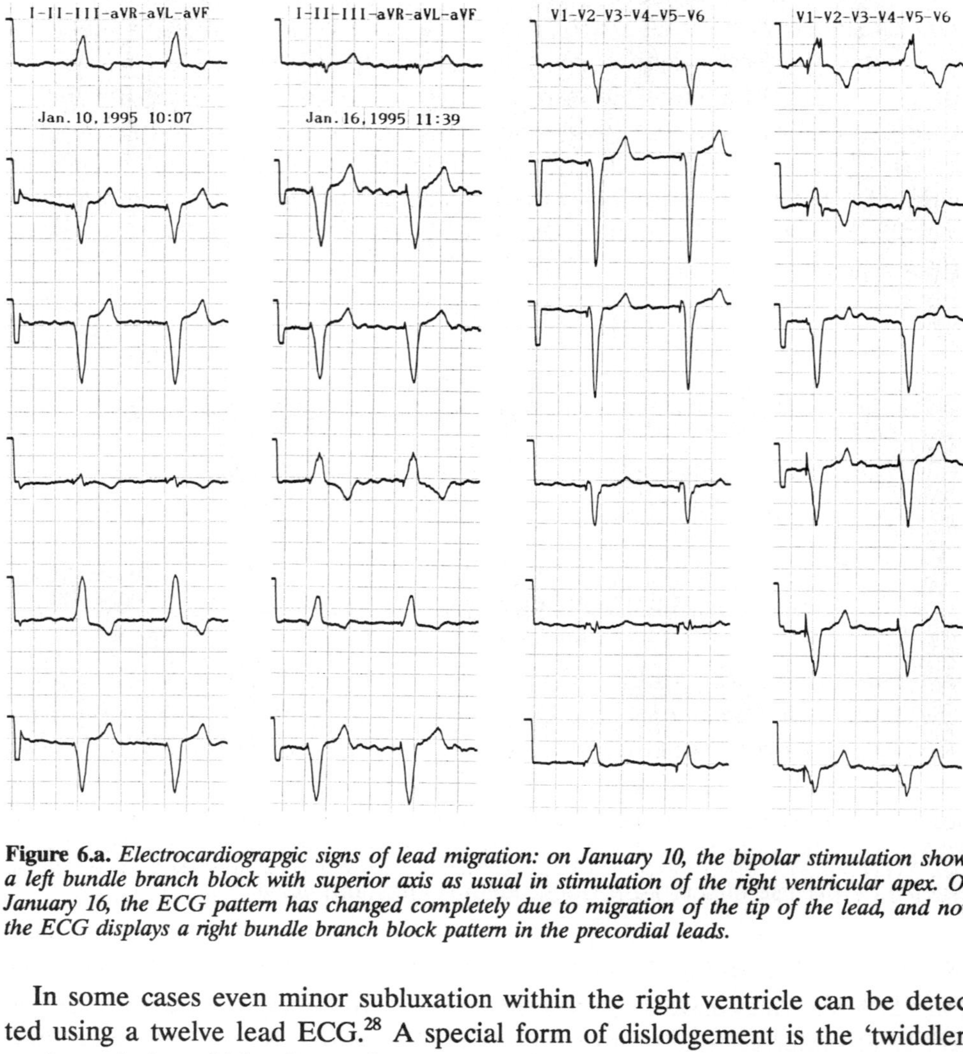

Figure 6.a. *Electrocardiograpgic signs of lead migration: on January 10, the bipolar stimulation shows a left bundle branch block with superior axis as usual in stimulation of the right ventricular apex. On January 16, the ECG pattern has changed completely due to migration of the tip of the lead, and now the ECG displays a right bundle branch block pattern in the precordial leads.*

In some cases even minor subluxation within the right ventricle can be detected using a twelve lead ECG.[28] A special form of dislodgement is the 'twiddlers syndrome', in which the patient constantly twists or fiddles with the pulse generator which winds up the lead, thus pulling it out of the heart (figure 7).

Perforation is the other important form of electrode displacement where the tip penetrates through the right ventricular or thin atrial wall. Usually, perforation occurs during the implant procedure but sometimes late perforation occurs. Low amplitude intra-cardiac signals, high pacing threshold, chest discomfort,

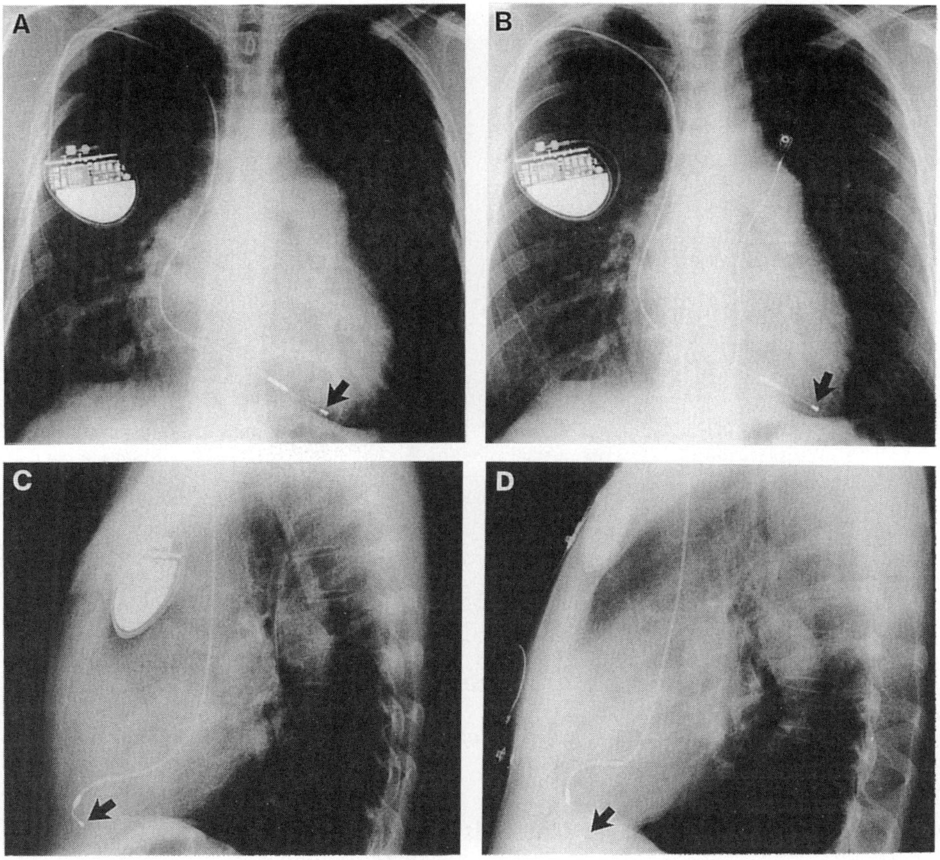

Figure 6.b. *Radiological signs of lead migration. Same patient as in figure 6.a. The anterior (panel A) and lateral (panel C) X-rays view at January 10 show placement of the lead into the right ventricular apex. X-rays made on January 16 (panels B and D) show a change in position of the tip of the lead to a more left lateral diaphragmatic position, suggestive for perforation of the apex or distal septum.*

hiccup from diaphragmatic stimulation and the fluoroscopic appearance of the lead tip in abnormal position may result from perforation. Some degree of partial perforation is probably not uncommon and may go unrecognized but occasionally serious problems such as cardiac tamponade, do occur. During follow-up, changes in pacing impedance, sensing threshold, pacing threshold and morphology of the paced ventricular complex may suggest lead dislodgement.

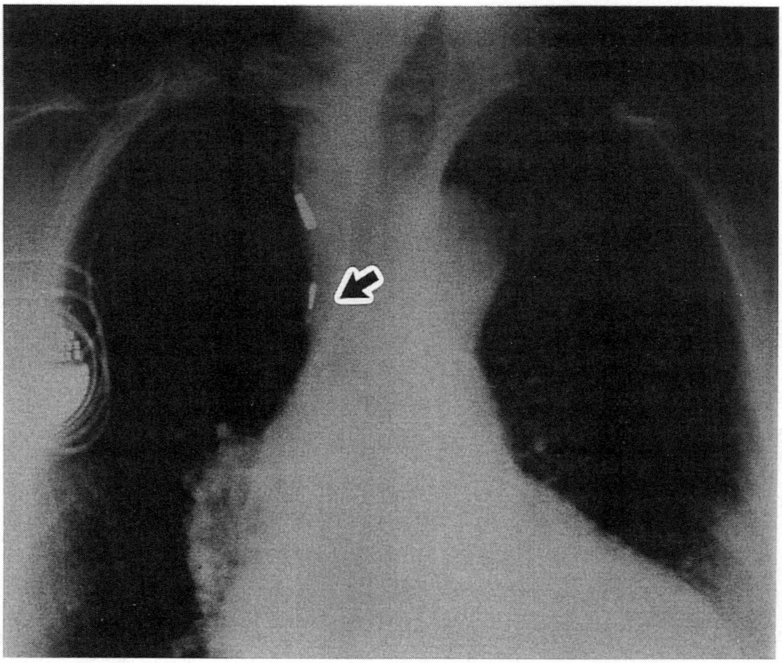

Figure 7. *The pacing lead is pulled out of the heart as a result of twisting with the pulse generator. (Twiddlers syndrome.)*

▸ *Lead integrity.* Implantable materials have to function reliably for years in a very hostile environment and are exposed to severe mechanical loads during their lifetime.[29] A pacemaker lead consists of one or two electrically insulated conductors. Commonly used insulation materials are silicone elastomer and polyurethane polymers. The electrical integrity of a lead can be affected by mechanical or chemical processes. Mechanical damage can be a result of the implant procedure.[30] A fracture of the lead by subclavian crush[31] is a result of the electrode becoming repeatedly compressed between the clavicle and the first rib (figure 8). Subclavian crush can be avoided by inserting the lead by cephalic cut down or by using a safe introducer technique.[32] Extreme mechanical stress as a result of excessive activity of the patient is

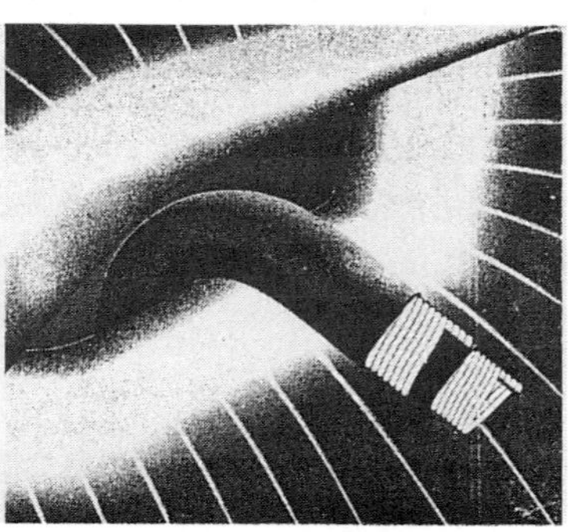

Figure 8. *Clamping of the lead between the clavicle and first rib (subclavian crush) has been related to high failure rates for some leads.*

rare but has been reported.[33] Chemical failure mechanisms such as Environmental Stress Cracking (ESC) result in surface crazing or cracking of the insulation material which can deepen and lead eventually to insulation failure.[34] Tests on the different types of polyurethane have shown that the harder 55D polyurethane is far more resistant to ESC than other types.[35] Another degradation process of the insulation material is Metal Ion Catalyzed Oxidation (MIO). MIO is caused by oxidation of the highly fatigue resistant Elgiloy or MP35N conductor material. MIO in the presently marketed electrodes is uncommon since conductors have been platinum coated.[36] Insulation failure can lead to intermittent oversensing and undersensing, loss of capture, extracardiac stimulation and sudden changes in pacing impedance. Pacing impedance measurements during follow-up have been proven to be useful in the detection of insulation failure.[37] A complete fracture of the conductor wire, with unimpaired insulation causes a very high pacing impedance. However, if the fractured wire protrudes through the insulation, the pacing impedance still can be within normal range. If the pulse generator is not capable of measuring pacing impedance, *pulse analysis* may be useful to detect lead anomalies. Pulse analysis studies the voltage across the Einthoven (surface) leads associated with the stimulus current through the body.[38] With this method and knowledge of the output specifications of the utilized pulse generator, an estimation of the unipolar pacing impedance can be made (figure 9).[4] Insulation defects can be localized by the construction of equipotential lines of the pulse generator artefact on the thoracic wall.[25]

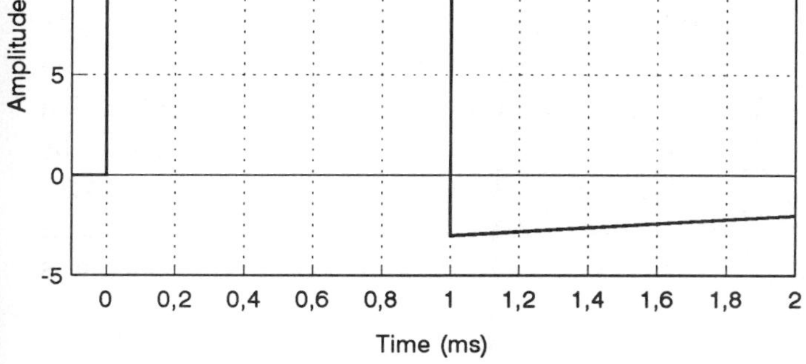

Figure 9. *With the use of pulse analysis by measuring the resultant voltage of the stimulus across the Einthoven leads an estimation of the unipolar lead impedance can be made. Specific properties of the utilized pulse generator must be known, such as the capacity of the output capacitor and the output impedance of the pulse generator circuitry.*

In conclusion, loss of integrity of a pacemaker lead may induce malsensing, alterations in pacing impedance and threshold increases. Intervention is indicated if the integrity of the lead is damaged. In the long term, a compromised lead will ultimately result in a failing pacemaker system.

The Interface Between the Implanted Pulse Generator and Cardiac Tissue

▸ *Stimulation threshold.* By measuring the voltage stimulation threshold at various pulse duration settings it is possible to compose a strength-duration curve. From the curve, the minimum output voltage required to provoke a depolarization at any given pulse width can be obtained. Stimulating the heart using an infinite pulse duration results in a minimum voltage threshold called the *rheobase*. The pulse duration of a threshold stimulus which has a voltage value of twice the rheobase, is called the *chronaxie*. From the curve in figure 10, it can be seen that the stimulus required for a threshold depolarization of the heart, which uses up the least energy, is one where the voltage and pulse width values are similar to those at the chronaxie.[39] A parabolic energy curve can be constructed from the strength-duration curve. It is useful to bear this energy curve in mind when a pulse generator has to be programmed to its final output setting. It should be

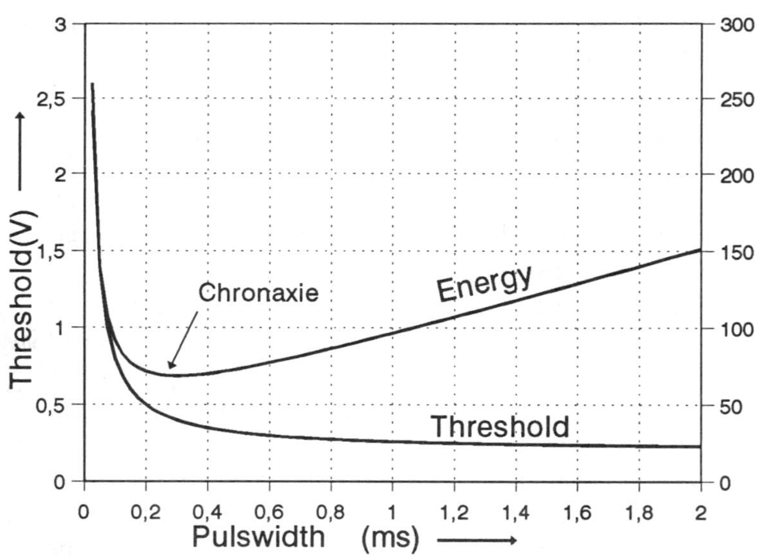

Figure 10. *The voltage threshold and the energy consumption for stimulation as a function of pulse duration. At the chronaxie pulse duration the voltage threshold is by definition twice the rheobase. The required energy for threshold stimulation is minimal in the vicinity of the chronaxie.*

pointed out from this curve that, above chronaxie, an increase of pulse duration is more effective in terms of energy consumption and safety margin than an increase in output voltage. To program a margin of safety above the threshold values shown by the strength-duration curve, pulse duration should be increased by a factor higher to that of a voltage increase. This will provide some protection against any further threshold rise while maintaining a balance between the two where energy usage is at it's minimum.

The pacing threshold, like the sensing threshold, will depend on the structure and surface area of the electrode tip and very much on the tissue interface at the electrode tip, which can change unpredictably. Occasionally other factors may also affect the pacing threshold by influencing the electrical properties of the underlying myocardium, such as ischemia and antiarrhythmic drugs. Therefore, the output parameters setting of a pulse generator has to be a compromise between safety and energy consumption. There is general consensus, that when the electrode has settled and reached a stable chronic threshold, the pacing output setting can be safely decreased to a minimum of twice the voltage threshold.[40] Output reduction with a balance between voltage and pulse duration will significantly prolong the life of the pulse generator battery.

▸ *Sensing cardiac signals.* Excitation of the muscle fibres initiates a propagating depolarization wavefront. As such a wavefront travels toward an implanted electrode a positive deflection is recorded. During the passage of the wavefront under the electrode, the electrode develops a negative polarity as the adjacent cells become negatively charged. This abrupt change of polarity is called the *intrinsic negative deflection*.[41] The sensing of cardiac signals by the pulse generator will depend largely on the amplitude (voltage) and the frequency content of that signal. The change in voltage divided by the period of time over which the voltage change occurs is called the *slew rate.* Higher slew rates suggest that higher frequencies are present which facilitate sensing. The geometry and surface area of the electrode tip will affect the amplitude of the cardiac signal as sensed by the pulse generator. Intracardiac factors which profoundly influence both the voltage and frequency of the sensed signal include the nature of the tissue interface, the position in the heart and the integrity of underlying heart muscle (myocardium). Myocardial function can be impaired by myocardial infarction or ischaemia as well as by cardiomyopathy and intraventricular conduction disturbances.[7] At the time of pacemaker implantation these problems can be avoided if a good electrode position can be selected such that the amplitude of the sensed signal and it's slew rate are sufficiently high. In the course of time, however, changes in the condition of the underlying myocardium and in the tissue interface may occur. This may cause a decrease of amplitude and slew rate of the electrogram and undersensing may result.

During follow-up, failure of sensing may be evident from a standard ECG or Holter monitoring. Quite commonly however, a false impression may be given that undersensing has occurred. An electrode will only sense the passage of a depolarization wave when this is passing directly underneath it. When a wavefront approaches an electrode from a distance, a substantial part of the myocardium may have been depolarized before the signal reaches the electrode and is sensed by the pulse generator. If the timing circuit of the pulse generator causes a paced beat, just before spontaneous local depolarization, there will be a second depolarization wavefront spreading out from the pacing electrode. The merging of the spontaneous and evoked depolarization wave fronts is called *fusion* and the resulting QRS complex seen on the surface ECG during this fusion beat will be a mixture of the morphologies of a spontaneous and a paced beat. Fusion beats are easily distinguished from malsensing and are a normal phenomenon in paced patients. If the pulse generator stimulus occurs at the very moment that heart cells in the vicinity of the pacemaker electrode are already depolarized (but just too early to permit sensing and inhibition), the pacing stimulus will be too late to initiate a wavefront and will not contribute to any further depolarization. The ECG appearance of the native P wave or QRS complex is not altered by the pulse generator stimulus. A pulse generator stimulus superimposed upon the beginning of a spontaneous beat without altering its morphology is defined as a *pseudofusion* beat.

The choice of unipolar as opposed to bipolar electrodes, has important implications for the way in which signals localized within the heart and those arising at a distance are sensed. A bipolar electrode will only sense signals that are close enough to cause a potential difference between the two poles and its sensing is therefore much more specific to signals arising near to the two electrodes. With a unipolar system, a potential difference between the heart electrode tip and the second pole which is the pulse generator housing (can) may be caused by signal sources near to either pole such as the musculus pectoralis in contact with the can or other extracardiac sources, such as electromagnetic interference external to the patient. With unipolar electrode configurations, oversensing is quite frequently observed. Fortunately, in the case of oversensing from skeletal muscle potentials, it is often self-limiting, since if the patient becomes unwell, while performing a certain activity he is likely to stop this activity. If certain activities are causing a real clinical problem, for example lifting heavy objects as part of daily work, then provocative testing with continuous ECG recording may confirm the situation. In some cases, reprogramming the sensitivity to a higher value may help.

Since, the amplitude of the ventricular intracardiac signal is usually well in excess of the programmed ventricular sensitivity, a precise determination of the sensing threshold is unnecessary if ventricular sensing appears to be adequate. In contrast, the atrial electrogram is of much lower amplitude than the ventricular and is more suspectable to change after implantation. Atrial undersensing is a well known problem and if it results in inappropriate atrial stimulation, atrial fibrillation may be induced.[42] Therefore, in contrast with the ventricular electrogram, routine assessment of the P wave amplitude is recommended. Assessment of the amplitude and character of the P wave electrogram is achieved by using the intra cardiac electrogram (ICEG) facilities of the pulse generator or by measuring P wave sensing threshold by successively decreasing the P wave sensitivity of the pulse generator until sensing ceases.

▸ *Tissue reaction, intracardiac.* After implantation of foreign material, heart tissues reacts with a sterile inflammation around the tip of the electrode. This inflammation elevates the pacing threshold up to about three times acute threshold. Threshold rise may be explained by the increase in effective stimulation surface area as non-excitable connective tissue grows around the electrode. The current density is the amount of current per unit of a cross sectional area. An increase of surface area leads to an decrease of current density. Local current density is the parameter which evokes cell depolarization. It is clear that threshold increases with decreasing current density.[43] When the formation of connective tissue is completed, pacing threshold stabilizes. This threshold is called the chronic pacing threshold. The tips of some pacing electrodes are a source of the steroid dexamethasone which leaches out slowly and minimises the tissue reaction after implantation. It has been confirmed that the use of this steroid reduces the usual rise of pacing threshold after implantation.[44] After several months the dexamethasone supply will be depleted but the threshold does not rise further.

In some cases the excessive inflammatory response at the electrode/tissue interface leads to an extreme increase of threshold. When the threshold exceeds the output of the pulse generator there will be failure to capture by the stimulation impulse. This situation is defined as *exit block*. Rarely, exit block may arise from other causes of threshold increase (see above), such as myocardial infarction and antiarrhythmic drugs, and transiently after cardiac defibrillation. Follow-up in the post-operative phase must include threshold measurements to anticipate exit block due to excessive inflammatory response. The intervals between threshold measurements might follow the scheme suggested in the section concerning follow-up organization. An exception should be made for patients which have had an abnormal threshold response in the past, or whose threshold is rising rapidly in the first days after implantation (for example, where the threshold has risen above 1.5 Volt within 10 days following implantation). Such patients should be seen weekly until the threshold has stabilized at an acceptable value. If pacing threshold in the chronic phase increases abruptly, lead integrity, catheter position and the connection to the pulse generator should be investigated rather than suspecting abnormalities in the electrode/tissue interface.

▸ *Extracardiac stimulation.* The delivery of a pacing impulse may not only lead to spontaneous propagated depolarization of the heart muscle but also to the stimulation of other structures in proximity to the positive or negative poles of the pacing system. With any ventricular pacing system, an occasional problem can occur with contractions of the diaphragm. The muscle of the diaphragm may be stimulated either directly from the pacing impulse or indirectly when the phrenic nerve (which innervates the diaphragm and lies over the surface of the heart) is stimulated.[45,46] In some cases diaphragmatic stimulation is caused by perforation of the lead tip through the ventricle and this is especially suggested when the symptoms appear suddenly after implantation. Pectoralis muscle stimulation in the shoulder sometimes occurs due to stimulation by the can of the pulse generator (the positive pole) but cannot occur if bipolar electrodes are used. Rarely, if the insulation of a pacemaker lead is damaged, stimulation of other muscular structures in the neighbourhood of the exposed metal conductor can occur. Any muscle stimulation appearing for the first time late after implantation may suggest such insulation defects or perforation or dislodgement of the electrode.

Organizational Aspects of Follow-Up

To fulfil the objectives for a rational follow-up program there has to be a well defined follow-up schedule. A follow-up visit must be cost effective and there must be assurance that the patient is unlikely to be at any risk from pacemaker system failures at least until the next follow-up. Although a periodic check is only a snapshot and some intermittent failures may be missed, the systematic collection and interpretation of data can bring to light many failures before becoming clinically important. Ideally there should be a protocol to determine the intervals between follow-up visits and for the minimal assessments required at each visit. Some kind of certification for the associated professionals performing pacemaker follow-up appears to be justified. In some hospitals, clinical follow-up by the cardiologist is combined with technical pacemaker follow-up and this is probably most ideal since the clinical needs and problems of the patients are often inseparable from technical aspects.

▸ *Interval of follow-up.* There should be a schedule for the minimum intervals between follow-up visits and this routine should not be allowed to lapse even without clinical symptoms. To determine the interval between follow-up visits, several aspects should be considered:

The *indication for cardiac pacemaker implantation* can affect the follow-up interval, particularly where more complex clinical problems than the usual pacemaker indications of straightforward heart block, atrial fibrillation and sick sinus syndrome are present. For example in patients with additional tachycardias, heart failure and cardiomyopathy, congenital heart disease, and after ablation therapy, more frequent clinical and technical reassessment is required. There is, unfortunately, no distinct definition of *pacemaker dependency.* However, in patients who do not appear to be dependent on their pacemakers, it may be possible to extend the interval between visits. The use of other therapeutic measures which may affect pacemaker function, such as radiotherapy and some forms of physiotherapy, and the exposure to powerful sources of electromagnetic radiation may initiate earlier reassessment. *The type of pacemaker* may also influence the decision about the follow-up frequency. For example, in patients with rate responsive systems and dual-chamber systems, it may be advisable to review the patient more often than the basic minimum in the first months after implantation since it may require more effort to adjust the programming correctly. *Threshold behaviour of the pacemaker electrode in use* may suggest a need for more frequent threshold assessments. Some older *battery systems* such as Lithium Copper Sulphide have depletion characteristics which give warning of approaching exhaustion only a few months before the pulse generator ceases to function. This makes frequent observations necessary as the pulse generator ages. Manufacturers frequently issue product performance reports. For some identified pulse generators or pacing leads *disposition to malfunction* may indicate intensified follow-up. *Integration of follow-up with other medical care* may change the arranged protocol.

In scheduling pacemaker follow-up visits, the requirements of the individual patient should be taken into account. The following proposed scheme may be adequate for the majority of patients.[28]

- Pre-hospital discharge.
- Ten days post implant, for removing stitches and inspection of the pulse generator site.
- Six weeks post implant, for the definitive programming of parameters.
- Further follow-up once every six months.

If the minimum period which can elapse between activation of the Elective Replacement Indicator (ERI) and activation of the End of Life Indicator (EOL) (at the current setting) is known, it can theoretically be used to determine the safe maximum interval between follow-up visits. As this interval depends on the actual current drain of the pulse generator, no general rules can be given. Usually the pulse generator manufacturers predict the minimum interval between ERI and EOL under certain conditions. With the aid of the formulas in Appendix I it is possible to predict the maximum follow-up interval for any actual setting.

Unexpected change in battery impedance, pacing threshold or lead impedance may initiate reduction of the routine follow-up interval to make observation of progression possible. Intervals which has to be reduced to a period as short as two weeks usually indicate surgical intervention.

▸ *Measurements.* The minimal requirement for measurements during a follow-up visit are:[28,47-49]

- Visual inspection of the pulse generator site.[50]
- An ECG Rhythm strip with preferably twelve leads, but a minimum of three leads.[12]
- Pulse interval or pulse rate of the pulse generator.
- Pulse interval or pulse rate of the pulse generator in magnet mode.
- Pulse duration.

If the pulse generator is programmable, one should acquire:

- The stimulation threshold.[51]

If the pulse generator is equipped with bidirectional telemetry, interrogate the pulse generator and record:

- The current programmed parameter setting.
- Pacing impedance.
- Cell (battery) impedance.

Should there be a clinical indication of suboptimal pacemaker performance or if malfunctioning is suspected additional tests should be performed:

- Evaluation for pacemaker dependency.[52]
- Pacing impedance using pulse analysis for pulse generators not equipped with impedance measurement facilities.[53]
- The sensing threshold.[16]

- ▹ Oversensing of myopotentials (provocation test).
- ▹ Retrograde conduction, by observation of the intracardiac atrial electrograms during asynchronous ventricular stimulation.[54]
- ▹ AV cross talk provocation test.[13]
- ▹ Position of pulse generator and leads, by the cardiologist using fluoroscopy.

Sometimes built-in features of the pulse generator can assist in Trouble Shooting:

- ▹ Built in Holter.[10]
- ▹ Intra-cardiac electrogram (ICEG).
- ▹ Main timing events (MTE).[55]

To investigate possible malfunction outside the pacemaker clinic, a 24 hours ambulatory (Holter) monitoring may supply additional information. If there is doubt about the setting of the rate response during exercise in a rate-responsive pulse generator (or the adequacy of patient's own sinus node response), an exercise test can be performed as part of the follow-up program.[48] Interpretation of the chronotropic response of the sensor during exercise is however complex, and often subjective assessment by the patient himself has to be translated into specific rate response parameters.[56]

Although it is not possible to detect every possible deficiency in the pacemaker system and the way it has been programmed during a routine follow-up visit, systematic collection of specific data increases the chance of bringing any important abnormality to light.

▸ *Associated professionals.* The basis of a successful pacemaker clinic is a well educated and motivated staff. Special effort is required to motivate personnel in order to maintain at a high quality level. Follow-up clinics are at present manned by:

- ▹ a cardiologist alone;
- ▹ an associated professional, who refers to the cardiologist if necessary;
- ▹ an associated professional in conjunction with the follow-up cardiologist.

Technical follow-up of pacemakers is not complete without simultaneous clinical assessment. Liaison between the associated professional and the clinician cardiologist responsible for the patient is indispensable. Only recently have educational guidelines for structured training programmes and independent examination been published for associated professionals.[57] Personnel may be recruited from miscellaneous departments of the hospital. As a result, the education and skill of the associated professionals in the pacemaker clinic varies widely. Education in pacemaker technology for those involved with follow-up is often offered by pacemaker companies as part of their continuing education program. The Educational Guidelines for Pacing and Electrophysiology published by the North American Society of Cardiac Pacing(NASPE) can be used as a reference for further training programs.[57]

▸ *Equipment requirements.* The main tool during pacemaker follow-up is a three channel, or better, a twelve lead, electrocardiograph. This ECG machine needs to provide linear amplification of input signals and must have a high dynamic response to cope with the high amplitude pacing signals. It must write three channels simultaneously, on line and without delay. Signal processing and low pass filters may distort the pacing artefact making interpretation of the amplitude and vector of the stimulus almost impossible. Many digital cardiographs are not suitable for pacemaker follow-up. The sampling rate of the input signal is often to low for the very short lasting pulse generator stimulus, which can lead to misinterpretation of pulse generator output amplitude and vector. In some electrographs the poor performance of the writing mechanism, for instance a thermal stylus, is compensated by the synthetic generation of a pulse generator artefact. This mechanism will generate a uniform spike with constant amplitude and vector if it detects a stimulus at the input circuit. Consequently, variations of spike amplitude due, for example, to insulation failure will be masked and the diagnosis will be missed. Sometimes artifacts on the input circuit of the cardiograph are presented as pacemaker spikes which mislead interpretation.

To analyze the native heart rhythm as well as the paced evoked response the cardiograph must be capable of recording the precordial leads.
Programmers for pulse generators are generally supplied to hospitals by the pacemaker manufacturers. It is preferable for pacemaker programmers to be battery operated. Battery operation avoids injection of 50 Hz interference in other sensitive follow-up equipment, survives mains supply interruptions at critical moments and battery operation enables field survey. Most pacemaker programmers are software operated, which means that different software and different methods of administrating the data have to be available for the different models in use. This software is supplied on floppy disks, tape cartridges or chip-modules. Keeping track of the required software and programmers for the different pulse generator models is essential. If the programmer needs to be connected to the patient by means of ECG electrodes, internal high level voltage coupling with the electrocardiograph has to be preferred above in parallel connection to the patient.

An electronic counter for analysis of pulse interval and pulse duration is necessary. These counters are usually incorporated in the pacemaker programmer or in an electrocardiograph, but some small battery operated units are also available. Pulse analysis equipment for visualization of the stimulus artefact is recommended and sometimes integrated in the pacing system analyzer. A passive device which should never be absent from the pacemaker follow-up clinic is a magnet to initiate magnet operation of the pulse generator. Transtelephonic monitoring as part of the follow-up program of cardiac pacemakers is scarcely used in the Netherlands. The relatively short travelling distances and the dense infra structure of pacemaker departments makes transtelephonic monitoring superfluous. To examine the rate response of a rate adaptive pulse generator, an exercise test can be performed using a bicycle ergometer[58], a treadmill[59] or a daily activities protocol.[60]

Arm ergometry[61] as an alternative method of exercise testing, making exercise test equipment superfluous, is unsuitable in testing rate responsive pacemakers. Heavy arm movements are a type of body activity which is disproportional to the general workload. Activity sensing and impedance measuring systems commonly react to this form of exercise with upper rate pacing.

▸ *Data organization.* For obvious logistic and legal reasons, records of patients clinical and pulse generator data must be kept updated, stored safely and easily accessible. After implantation the follow-up record should contain at least the following data:[52]

- ▹ Details of patient: name, identification, gender, address, phone number, day of birth, indication for pacing.
- ▹ Details of pulse generator and lead(s): manufacturer, model, serial number.
- ▹ Details about the implantation: implanting physician, site of implantation, date of implantation, measurements during implant, relevant details.

In Europe a dedicated implant form, containing most of above mentioned administrative data, is sent immediately after implantation to the national pacemaker registry. This 'European Pacemaker Patient Identification Card' is handed out to the patient after implantation and serves as a reference for identification of pulse generator and lead when the patient is admitted to another hospital. It is only possible to add limited follow-up data to this document. In practise it is often not updated during normal follow-up visits and it is not really suitable for continuing documentation. Patients who are travelling to other countries may be given an, updated card together with a handout of the details of the last pacemaker follow-up visit and other data such as diagnosis and medication.

During the follow-up period there has to kept record of:

- ▹ Programmed parameters.
- ▹ Telemetered parameters.
- ▹ Measured parameters.
- ▹ Observations.

The collected data is usually not kept in the patients general out-patient record but in a separate file. In the out-patient record, only important alterations in the programmed parameters or anomalous observations are noted. By its nature, the collected data lends itself well to storage in a computer database. Various computer programs for data management are available, all with their specific advantages and limitations. Despite the ease of storage in computers, data compression is a still necessary. The need to select and compress data will become even more relevant with the increasing diagnostic options presently incorporated in pulse generators. Until the entire follow-up database of the patient is stored for infinity in the pulse generator itself, data storage in every clinic will be a disputed issue. Data organization can carry substantial additional costs if it is not done properly.

Conclusion

During technical follow-up, many abnormalities of pacemaker function can be corrected before becoming clinical relevant. Some minor deviations, eventually leading to malfunction, can be detected by accurate and systematic observation of the pacemaker system. It is not necessary to scrutinize all aspects of the pacemaker system during a routine technical follow-up. It is, however, recommended to create a protocol describing the minimal measurements needed during a routine follow-up visit for each type of pulse generator. The protocol also needs to detail the way in which data is to be administrated and who carries responsibility for organization and decision making. Permanent changes in pulse generator setting may often be a primarily medical decision but some action may be delegated to associated professionals. Delegation of such responsibilities needs special documentation in the technical follow-up protocol. Review of the implanted pacemaker by the technical associate in conjunction with the cardiologist makes optimal pacemaker therapy possible.

A thorough knowledge of the fundamentals of physics, cardiac anatomy and human physiology is needed by the associated professional. Experience in pacemaker trouble shooting and a knowledge of pulse generator specifications and pacemaker technology is obligatory for the responsible cardiologist.

A critical analysis of the quantity and quality of your follow-up program may prove to be cost-effective for the department and should improve the quality of life for pacemaker patients.

Acknowledgement

We thank Telectronics Pacing Systems for their permission to redraw the figures.

Appendix I

The relation between factors determining pacemaker longevity is expressed in the following equation.

$$L = \frac{C.N}{(I_q + I_p).8760.10^{-6}}$$

L	=	Longevity (years)
C	=	Theoretical battery capacity (Ah)
N	=	Cell Usage factor (.9 for 90% of theoretical capacity available)
I_q	=	Quiescent current (uA) (internal circuit drain)
I_p	=	Pacing current (uA)
8760	=	Number of hours in a year

The pacing current can be expressed in:

$$I_p = k.\frac{V_{Pace}.PW.Rate.\%Pace.n}{Z_{lead}.6}$$

I_p	=	Pacing current (uA)
V_{pace}	=	Pacing voltage on lead
PW	=	Pulse width (ms)
Rate	=	Average pacing rate
%Pace	=	Percent of pacing (usually 1.0 for 100% pacing)
n	=	Number of chambers paced (1.0 for SSI, 2 for DDD)
Z_{lead}	=	Lead impedance (Ohm)
k	=	Efficiency constant (1 for 2.5 Volt output, 2.2 for 5.0 Volt output)

References

1. Irnich W, Batz L. Schritttmacher-Infektionen aus der Sicht des Zentralregisters Herzschrittmacher. In: Winter UJ, Zegelman M (eds), Herzschrittmacher- und Defibrillator-Infektionen. Stuttgart, Georg Thieme Verlag, 1994, pp 14-9.
2. Thalen HJ. The Artificial Cardiac Pacemaker. Thesis. Rijksuniversiteit Groningen, 1969, p 331.
3. Bernstein AD, Irwin ME, Parsonnet V, Wilkoff BL, Black WR, Buckingham TA, Maloney JD, Reynolds DD, Saksena S, Singer I, Nickelson DE, Schuring L. Report of the NASPE Policy Conference on Antibradycardia Pacemaker Follow-Up: Effectiveness, Needs, Resources. PACE 1994;17:1714-29.
4. Rodrigo FA, Berg JW van den, Thalen HJ, Koops J. Control of patients with implanted pacemakers. Proceedings of the European Congres of Cardiology, September 1968, Serie C, 70:449-55.
5. Kemp P van der, Schmidt JT, Ruiter R de, Hove JWJ van, Boer TJM de, Schrama T. Pacemakerdata 1993-1994. Oudenhoorn, STIMRO, 1993 (90-71839-03-6).
6. Lampadius MS. Herzschrittmacher-Typenkartei. Kochel am See, FGS-Forschungsgesselschaft Electrostimulation m.b.H., 1994.
7. Sedney MI. The implantable cardiac pacemaker. Thesis. Rijksuniversiteit Leiden, 1986.
8. Anonymous. Reflex Model 8218 physician's manual. Englewood, Colorado, Telectronics Pacing Systems, 1992.
9. Sutton R, Bourgeois IM. The Foundations of Cardiac Pacing Pt. I: An illustrated practical guide to basic pacing. Mount Kisco, New York, Futura Publishing Company, 1991.
10. Levine PA. Holter and pacemaker diagnostics. In: Aubert AE, Ector H, Stroobandt R (eds), Cardiac pacing and Electrophysiology; a bridge to the 21st century. Dordrecht, Kluwer Academic Publishers, 1994, pp 309-24.
11. Cazeau S, Ritter P, Nitzché R, Limousin M, Mugica J. Diagnosis of atrial arrhytmias Using the holter function of a new DDD pacemaker. PACE 1994;17:2106-13.
12. Hayes DL, Vlietstra RE. Pacemaker malfunction. (Review). Annals of Internal Medicine 1993;119:828-35.
13. Levine PA. Differential Diagnosis, evaluation, and management of Pacing System Malfunctioning. In: Ellenbogen KA (ed.), Cardiac Pacing. Boston, Blackwell Scientific Publication, 199, pp 309-82.
14. Hayes DL. Programmability. In: Furman S, Hayes DL, Holmes DR (eds), A Practice of Cardiac Pacing. Mount Kisco, New York, Futura Publishing Compagny, Inc., 1993, pp 635-63.
15. Raitt MH, Stelzer KJ, Laramore GE. Runaway pacemaker during high-energy neutron radiation therapy. Chest 1994;106:955-7.
16. Bourgeois IM. Electromagnetic interference and Cardiac Pacemakers. In: Atlee JL, Gombotz H, Tscheliessnigg KH (eds), Peri-operative management of pacemaker patients. Berlin, Springer Verlag, 1992, pp 70-81 (3-540-53874-7).
17. Knickerbocker G. Guidance article: Cellular telephones and radio transmitters-interference with clinical equipment. Health Devices, Augustus-September 1993;22(8-9):416-8.
18. Siemons GHA. Informatie en advies met betrekking tot mogelijke storing van medische apparatuur door draadloze telefoontoestellen. Staatstoezicht op de Volksgezondheid 1994; GHI/JK/HR 941630:1-2.
19. Marco D, Eisinger G, Hayes DL. Testing of work environments for electromagnetic interference. PACE 1992;15:2016-22.
20. Toivonen L, Valjus J, Hongisto M, Metso R. The influence of elevated 50 Hz electric and magnetic fields on implanted cardiac pacemakers: the role of the lead configuration and programming of the sensitivity. PACE 1991;14:2114-22.

21. Astridge PS, Kaye GC, Whitworth S, Kelly P, Camm AJ, Perrins EJ. The response of implanted dual chamber pacemakers to 50 Hz extraneous electrical interference. PACE 1993;16:1966-74.
22. Rodriguez F, Filimonov A, Henning A, Coughlin C, Greenberg M. Radiation-induced effects in multiprogrammable pacemakers and implantable defibrillators. PACE 1991;14:2143-53.
23. Hemel NM van, Hamerlijnck RPHM, Pronk KJ, Veen EP van der. Upper limit ventricular stimulation in respiratory rate responsive pacing due to electrocautery. PACE 1989;12:1720-3.
24. Gelder LM van, Bracke FALE, El Gamal IH. Upper rate pacing after radiofrequency catheter ablation in a minute ventilation rate adaptive DDD pacemaker. PACE 1994;17:1437-40.
25. Dekker E, Büller J, Schuilenburg RM. Enkele hulpmiddelen bij de diagnostiek van 'pacemaker failure'. Ned T Geneesk 1964;108(45):2160-1.
26. Ruiter JH. Clinical aspects of cadiac pacing for bradyarrhythmias. Thesis. Erasmus University Rotterdam, 1992, p 268.
27. Buys EM, Hemel NM van, Kelder JC, Dessel PFHM van, Bakema H. Unsatisfying results in long-term pacing with a bipolar active fixation atrial lead. PACE 1994;17:2292-6.
28. Goethals MPN, Timmmermans W, Willems R, Andries E, Stroobandt R. Facing the 'faces' of pacing after implantation. In: Andries E, Brugada P, Stroobandt R (eds), How to face 'the faces' of cardiac pacing. Dordrecht, Kluwer Academic Publishers, 1992, pp 139-81.
29. Ko WH, Mugica J, Ripart A (eds), Implantable sensors for closed-loop prosthetic systems. Mount Kisco, New York, Futura Publishing Company, 1985.
30. Zakaria MS, Maue-Dickson W, MacGregor DC. Surgical implantation of dual chamber cardiac pacing systems. TPS Brochure 1988;1:1-10.
31. Stokes K, Staffenson D, Lessar J, Sahni A. A possible new complication of sublcavian stick: conductor fracture. PACE 1987;10:748.
32. Byrd. Safe Introducer Technique for Pacemaker Lead Implantation. PACE 1992;15:262-7.
33. Schuger CD, Mittleman R, Habbal B, Wagshal A, Huang SK. Ventricular lead Transection and Atrial lead damage in a young softbal player shortly after the insertion of a permanent pacemaker. PACE 1992;15:1236-9.
34. Byrd CL, McArthur W, Stokes K, Sivina M, Yahr WZ, Greenberg J. Implant experience with unipolar polyurethane pacing leads. PACE 1983;6:868-82.
35. Furman S, Benedek M. Survival of implantable pacemaker leads. PACE 1990;13:1910-4.
36. Stokes K. Pacing leads for rate adaptive pacing. In: Benditt DG (ed.), Rate adaptive pacing. Oxford, Blackwell Scientific Publications, 1993, pp 31-42.
37. Buckingham TA, Alagona P, Batey R, Belott P, Byrd CL, Gallastegui JL, Hayes DL, Johnson WB, Mead H, Parsonnet V, Reynolds DD, Simonson J, Tonder LM, Wheelan K. The use of impedance measurements to detect pacemaker lead failure during follow-up. Eur JCPE 1994;4:242-6.
38. Berg JW van den, Rodrigo FA, Thalen HJ, Koops J. Photo-analysis of the condition of implanted pacemakers and electrode circuits. Koninkl Nederl Akademie van Wetenschappen 1967, Proceedings Serie C, 70(4):419-47.
39. Amado JB, Trujillo C. Energy requirements during acute endocardial stimulation. A comparative study of different morphology leads. In: Aubert AE, Ector H (eds), Progress in Biomedical Engineering: Pacemaker leads. Amsterdam, Elsevier Science Publishers, 1985.
40. Ellenbogen KA. Cardiac Pacing. Boston, Blackwell Scientific Publication, 1992, p 38.
41. Kay GN. Basic Aspects of Cardiac Pacing. In: Ellenbogen KA, ed. Cardiac Pacing. Blackwell Scientific Publication, Boston, 1992, pp 32-119.
42. Zhdanov AM, Gukov AC, Termosesov SA. Evaluation of the inducability with non-invasive programmed stimulation (NIPS) of atrial arrhythmias in VVI and DDD-R mode. PACE 1993;16:1148.
43. Schneider H. Physical aspects of artificial heart stimulation. Thesis. Rijksuniversiteit Utrecht, 1966, p 111.

44. Sutton R, Guneri S. The impact of steroid eluting leads on long-term pacing in the atrium and ventricle. Eur JCPE 1991;1:10-5.
45. Katritsis D, Jones S, Camm AJ. A rational choice of pacemaker mode. Eur JCPE 1991;1:132-7.
46. Sutton R. Guest Editorial DDDR Pacing. PACE 1990;13:385-7.
47. Furman S. Pacemaker Follow-up. In: Furman S, Hayes DL, Holmes DR (eds), A Practice of Cardiac Pacing. Futura Publishing Company, Mount Kisco, New York, 1993, pp 571-603.
48. Love CJ. Clinical follow-up of rate-adaptive systems. In: Benditt DG (ed.), Rate adaptive pacing. Blackwell Scientific Publications, Oxford, 1993, pp 215-32.
49. Seeger W. Hertzschrittmacher Functionskontrolle. Reinbek, Sachsenwald-Druckerei, 1990.
50. Winter UJ, Zegelman M, Jansen B. Aktuelle Aspekte bei der Prävention, Diagnostik und Therapie von Schrittmacher-Infektionen. In: Winter UJ, Zegelman M (eds), Herzschrittmacher- und Defibrillator-Infektionen. Georg Thieme Verlag, Stuttgart, 1994, pp 1-9.
51. Mechelen R van, Kerckhove Y van der. Atrial capture and dual chamber pacing. PACE 1986;9.
52. Schoenfeld MH. Follow-up of the pacemaker patient. In: Ellenbogen KA (ed.), Cardiac Pacing. Blackwell Scientific Publication, Boston, 1992, pp 419-54.
53. Escher DJW, Furman S. Oscilloscopic and recent other methods of implanted pacemaker follow-up. Ann Cardiol Angéiol 1971;20:503-10.
54. Hayes DL, Furman S. Atrio-ventricular and ventriculo-atrial conduction time in patients undergoing pacemaker implant. PACE 1983;6:38-46.
55. Berkhof MMJ, Snoeck JP, Goethals MPN, Claes MJ. Clinical relevance of histograms in the follow-up of DDDR pacemakers. In: Aubert AE, Ector H, Stroobandt R (eds), Cardiac pacing and Electrophysiology; a bridge to the 21st century. Kluwer Academic Publishers, Dordrecht, 1994, pp 325-31.
56. Lau Chu-P, Leung SK. Clinical usefulness of rate adaptive pacing systems: what should we assess? PACE 1994;17:2233-5.
57. Schuring L. Educational Guidelines, Pacing and Electrophysiology. Futura Publishing Company, Muskegon Michigan, 1994.
58. Lau Chu-P, Mehta D, Toff WD, Stott RJ. Limitations of rate response of an activity sensing rate-responsive pacemaker to different forms of activity. PACE 1988;11:141-50.
59. Lewalter T, MacCarter DJ, Jung W, Schimpf R, Bauer T, Manz M, Funke H, Luderitz B. The 'LITE' protocol for appropriate rate adaptive pacemaker programming. PACE 1994;17:854.
60. Osswald ST, Kiowski W, Leiggener CH, Buser P, Pfisterer M, Burkart F. Adjustment of heart rate response of activity-sensing pacemakers by an exercise protocol mimicking daily activities. Eur JCPE 1993;4:269-77.
61. Froelicher VF. Manual of exercise testing. Mosby-Year Book, St. Louis, Missouri, 1994.

3 PREVENTION OF PACEMAKER COMPLICATIONS

Chapter 8

A Stepwise Approach to Solve Pacemaker Problems*

Berry M. van Gelder and Frank A.L.E. Bracke

Introduction

Normal pacemaker function is characterized by effective stimulation and proper sensing of intrinsic depolarizations of the chamber in which the lead is implanted. Malfunction of the pacing system can only be detected by recording the ECG. Malfunction in single chamber pacing systems is either related to stimulation or sensing of intrinsic depolarizations or both. In dual chamber systems, malfunction in one channel may be related to stimulation or sensing, but also the interaction between the two channels can be a source of malfunction.

Effectiveness of Stimulation

To conclude effective stimulation on the ECG, the interpreter should be able to recognize the pacemaker stimulus and the subsequent depolarization of the adjacent myocardium, caused by this stimulus. If no pacemaker stimulus is visible on the ECG it is defined as no output. For the confirmation of no output there are 2 prerequisites:

1. The programmed pacing rate should be higher than the patient's intrinsic rate, provided that the pacing system has no hysteresis.
2. After fulfilling the first condition magnet application should **not** result in the appearance of pacemaker stimuli. If magnet application results in asynchronous stimulation the phenomenon should be classified as oversensing instead of no output.

* This chapter is part of the coming PhD thesis 'The ECG in the Diagnosis of Pacemaker Function and Malfunction', Berry van Gelder, Eindhoven University of Technology, 1995.

If a pacemaker stimulus is not followed by depolarization it is defined as noncapture. Noncapture should not be caused by refractoriness of the adjacent myocardium, otherwise it should be classified as undersensing instead of noncapture.

No Output

After confirmation of no output by the above mentioned conditions, the causes of no output can be divided into 2 groups:

1. No output due to failure in the electronic circuitry. Failure can be caused by component failure or battery failure; no pulse generation.
2. No output due to discontinuity in the lead system or in the connector block of the pulse generator; no pulse transmission.

Differentiation between no pulse generation and no pulse transmission is relatively easy. If no output is observed and pacemaker programming and telemetry fails, component or battery failure can be concluded. Component failure resulting in no output has been reported after external defibrillation[1], radiofrequency ablation[2], electrocautery[3] and radiation therapy.[4] In case of no output caused by pulse generator malfunction the pulse generator should be replaced. During replacement lead impedance should be checked to exclude an insulation defect, which probably increased battery drain resulting in premature battery failure.

If lead discontinuity (no pulse transmission) is the cause of no output normal communication for programming and telemetry between pulse generator and programmer should be possible. Telemetry of lead impedance will reveal a high impedance often beyond the range of measuring capability of the system. A high lead impedance gives no information about the location of the defect. The lead system integrity can be interrupted at one or more of the following sites:

1. Connection lead - pulse generator
2. Lead connector
3. Lead adapter, if applicable
4. Lead conductor(s)
5. Anodal insulation in unipolar systems
6. Insulation failure

The causes mentioned under 1-4 can best be confirmed by fluoroscopy. In case of intermittent no output provocative maneuvers like pulse generator manipulation might be necessary during fluoroscopy to elucidate the site of interruption.

Anodal insulation caused by subcutaneous air entrapment is rarely encountered in unipolar systems shortly after surgical procedures.[5,6] When air is entrapped between the conduction part of the pulse generator case and the subcutaneous tissue the current pathway is interrupted. This phenomenon is diagnosed by application of some pressure on the overlying skin which results in normal pacing and capture (figure 1).

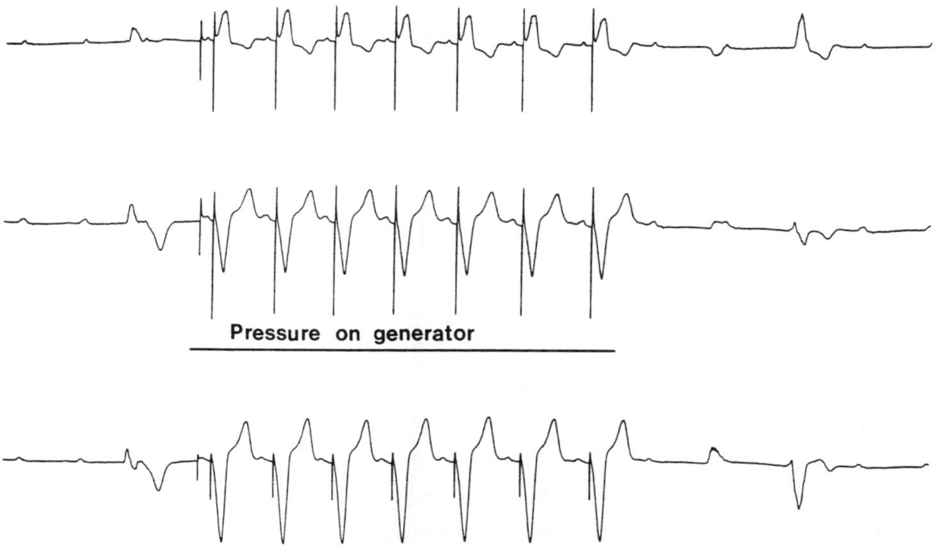

Figure 1. *Three channel ECG (leads I, II, III) of a patient with an implanted unipolar DDD pacemaker. Only during minor pressure on the pulse generator pacing is resumed. After release of pressure no output is recorded. Subcutaneous air insulating the anodal electrode (pulse generator case) was the cause of no output.*

Although high resistance is the main cause of no output, insulation failure forming a short circuit between anodal and cathodal electrode and/or conductor, thus forming a low resistance, may give rise to an ECG showing no output. Although there is transmission of the pacemaker pulse into the lead system the low resistance pathway prevents transmission of the pulse into the myocardium. Because the infinitively short dipole of the short circuit no pacemaker stimulus is recorded.[7]

Noncapture

Causes of noncapture can be divided into the following categories:

1. Position of the stimulation electrode.
2. The cathodal-myocardial interface.
3. The integrity of the lead system.
4. The pulse generator.

Noncapture should not be concluded from a single lead ECG because this sometimes can be confusing (figure 2).

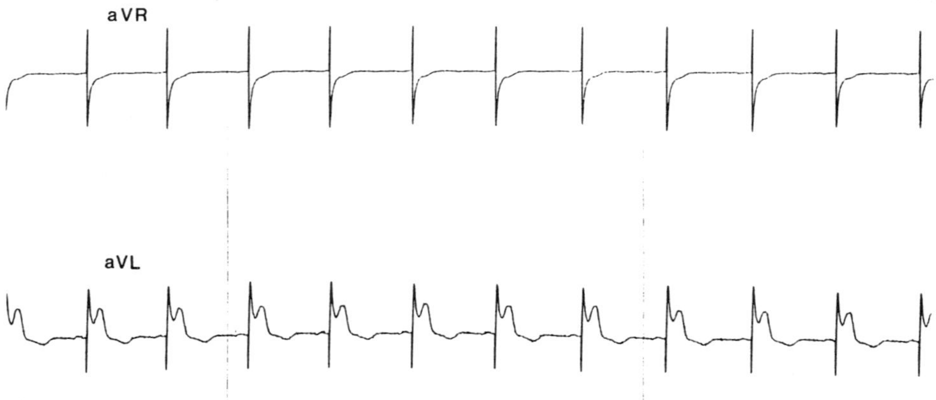

Figure 2. *Two channel ECG, simultaneously recorded, representing pseudo noncapture in the upper tracing (aVR), while the lower tracing (aVL) demonstrates effectual stimulation.*

▸ *Position of the stimulation electrode.* It does not need further explanation that the position of the electrode plays an important role for proper stimulation. Displacement of the lead often results in noncapture. If displacement occurs within the original chamber of implantation, noncapture can be intermittent.

During periods of capture displacement can be concluded from the ECG by a change in morphology of the stimulated complex as compared to previous recordings. Macrodisplacement of the lead resulting in continuous noncapture can be confirmed by fluoroscopy.

Myocardial perforation of the stimulation electrode, which also can be considered as lead displacement, may result in noncapture. Perforation is sometimes hard to identify from X-rays or fluoroscopy but a 'deep' position into the right ventricular apex is suggestive for perforation. Presence of noncapture associated with respiration and direct diaphragmatic stimulation can support the diagnosis.

In bipolar leads used for temporary stimulation, perforation can be illustrated by recording the proximal and distal electrogram and perforation can be confirmed by withdrawal of the lead (figure 3). Care should be taken in withdrawal of a perforated permanent lead associated with pericardial tamponade. In our experience withdrawal of such a lead during thoracotomy revealed excessive bleeding requiring surgical repair of the site of perforation.[8]

Malpositioning of the ventricular lead into the coronary sinus or one of its tributaries may result in noncapture. Placement of the lead into the coronary sinus should be recognized from the ECG during stimulation, which results in a right bundle branch block pattern instead of a left bundle branch block pattern as observed during right ventricular pacing. It usually is associated with higher stimulation thresholds.

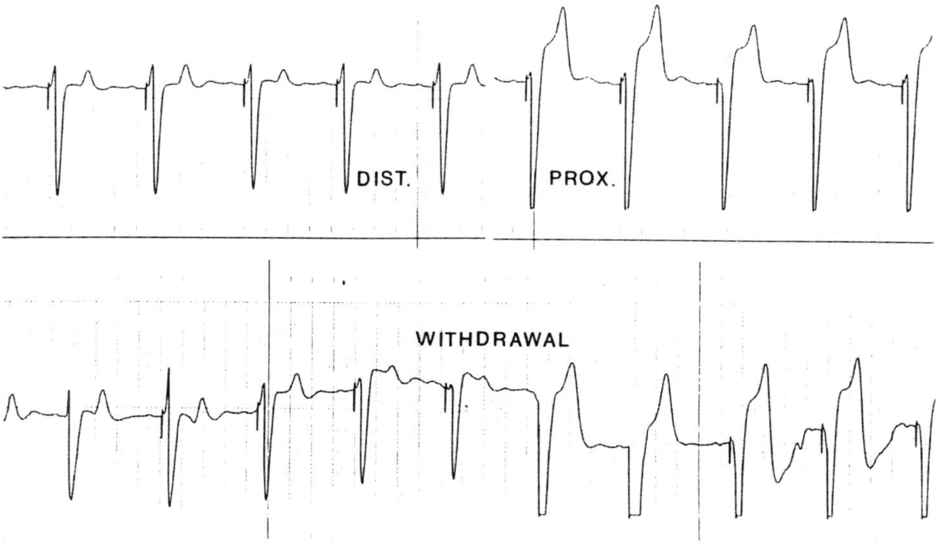

Figure 3. *Intracardiac electrogram recorded from the distal (dist) and proximal (prox) electrode of a bipolar lead for temporary pacing. The electrograms show a higher amplitude of the QRS complex from the proximal electrode than from the distal electrode. An injury pattern is observed at the proximal electrode, indicating that this electrode is in contact with the myocardium. These observations are suspect for lead perforation, which is confirmed by the distal electrogram during withdrawal of the lead.*

▸ *The cathodal-myocardial interface.* The electrode-myocardial interface is influenced by local processes that occur around the interface but also by the general state of excitability of the myocardium. Both may lead to noncapture or intermittent noncapture.

The local process is determined by the local tissue reaction after lead implantation and includes necrosis, cellular infiltration, and fibrosis. The layer formed by this process consists of conductive but non excitable cells, which extend the distance between the stimulation electrode and the excitable myocardium. Excessive rise in stimulation threshold above the maximum output level of the pulse generator without displacement of the stimulation electrode is named exit block. Electrodes employing active (screw-in) fixation are more prone to rise in stimulation threshold as a result of progressive reaction around the electrode.[9]

Local ischemia and DC countershock can give rise to a (temporarily) increase in stimulation threshold and intermittent noncapture.[10,11,12]

The general state of excitability of the myocardium is affected by the physiological state, the sympathetic and parasympathetic tone. A rise in stimulation threshold can be observed during electrolyte disturbance (hyperkalemia) and application of antiarrhythmic agents.[13]

▸ *Integrity of the lead system.* Any increase in lead impedance reduces the stimulation current through the myocardium according to Ohm's law. Only in case of complete interruption with infinitely high impedance no output is observed. Noncapture will occur if the decrease in stimulation current, due to an increase in impedance, falls below the stimulation threshold. If noncapture is intermittent, periods of noncapture are often associated with attenuation of the pacemaker stimulus on the ECG (figure 4). The attenuation of the pacemaker stimulus generally indicates decrease in stimulation current by an increase in lead impedance. Fluoroscopy should be used to determine the site of discontinuity.

Insulation defects, except from those creating a complete short circuit, rarely cause noncapture. Because the pacemaker pulse is a voltage pulse, failure to capture will only occur if the current through the insulation defect exceeds the maximum capacity of the pulse generator, thus reducing the current through the myocardium. The parallel impedance through the insulation break should be extremely low and before this level is reached sensing abnormalities will be observed.

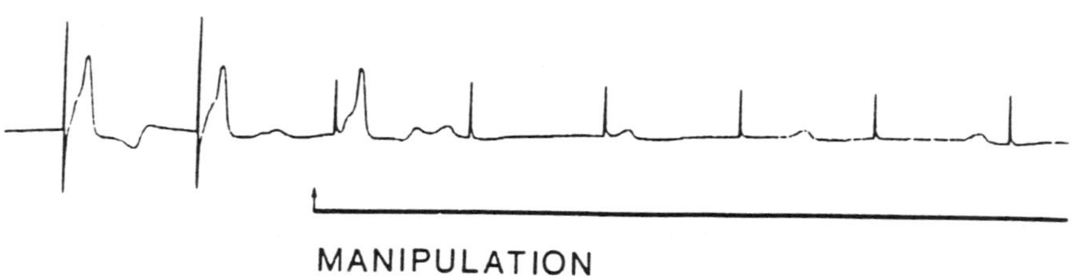

Figure 4. *ECG lead I during manipulation of the pulse generator showing attenuation of the pacemaker stimulus with loss of capture. This indicates a high lead resistance caused by a conductor break, which was provoked by manipulation.*

▸ *Pulse generator.* Noncapture due to pulse generator malfunction can be encountered in case of battery exhaustion. Battery exhaustion is easily recognized by measuring battery voltage by telemetry, or a change in pacing parameters (e.g. mode, rate, pulse width) indicating battery status. Loss of capture can be encountered in a normally functioning pulse generator in which one of the output parameters (pulse width and/or voltage or current) has been inappropriately programmed.

Sensing Abnormalities

Timing intervals on the ECG play an essential role in the evaluation of pacemaker sensing. The escape interval, which is defined as the time between a paced or sensed cardiac event and the subsequent pacing stimulus in the same chamber, is the most important parameter in pacemaker sensing. For inhibited systems a general rule is that prolongation of the escape interval is called oversensing. A coupling interval between an intrinsic cardiac event and the following pacemaker stimulus shorther than the escape interval is defined as undersensing.

Oversensing

If prolongation of the escape interval is caused by oversensing, regular pacing with a fixed stimulus interval will be observed after application of a magnet or by programming the pacemaker system to the asynchronous mode (figure 5).

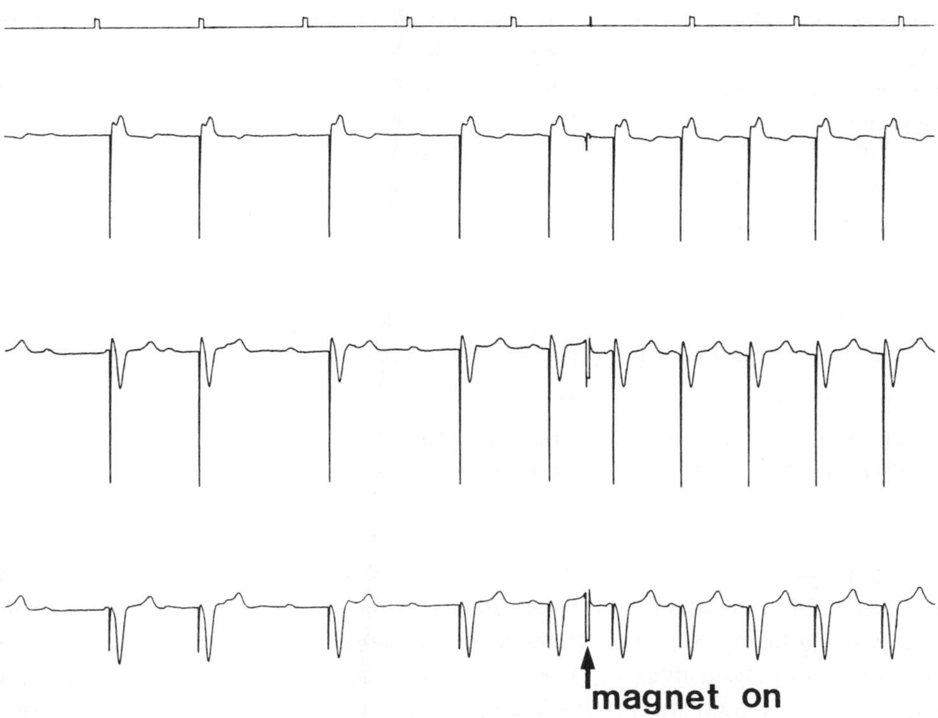

Figure 5. *Three channel ECG (leads I, II, III) of a patient with an implanted VVI pacemaker showing prolongation of the escape interval (shortest pacing interval). Regular pacing is restored after magnet application, indicating oversensing.*

Basically all causes of oversensing have in common that a voltage across the anodal and cathodal electrode of a pacemaker is built up and reaches or exceeds a certain level. This level is determined by the sensitivity of the pulse generator. Sources of interference, responsible for oversensing, can be divided into two groups:

1. Interference from exogenous signals.
2. Interference from endogenous signals.

▸ *Interference from exogenous signals.* Exogenous signals are defined as signals whose origin is located outside the human body. Exogenous signals can be coupled to the pacing system directly due to a direct contact between the interference source and the patient or indirectly by a magnetic or electromagnetic field.[14] Examples of directly coupled interference sources, frequently encountered in the hospital environment, are electrocauterization or coagulation equipment and, nerve or muscle stimulators. Application of current in medical practice should always be monitored reliably and throughout the whole procedure.[15]

The effect of magnetic or electromagnetic interference sources on pacing systems is difficult to predict. The influence is determined by the intensity of the interference source itself, the distance to the pacemaker patient, implant configuration, electrode configuration, shielding and sensitivity of the pulse generator.[16] Because of the variety of electromagnetic interference sources and situations in which they are encountered, it is not possible to generalize about the electromagnetic immunity of even a particular pacemaker. Pacemaker patients with a high electromagnetic interference work environment present a unique situation and should ideally be evaluated individually.[17]

▸ *Interference from endogenous signals.* Endogenous signals are defined as signals whose origin is located within the human body. The sources for interference from endogenous signals can be divied into 3 groups:

1. Signals from intracardiac origin.
2. Physiological signals from extracardiac origin.
3. Signals generated by the pacing system.

Oversensing by intracardiac signals. T wave oversensing, sensing of the last portion of the T wave by the ventricular electrode, can be encountered in VVI pacemakers and is usually seen after paced beats rather than spontaneous beats. T wave oversensing is characterized by prolongation of the escape interval with a more or less constant interval. T wave oversensing, which is relatively benign, can be prevented by reducing pacemaker sensitivity or if this fails by prolongation of the refractory period.

Similar to T wave sensing, far-field R wave sensing can be encountered in AAI pacemakers (figure 6). It is rarely seen in bipolar systems and it also can be prevented by reducing sensitivity or prolongation of the refractory period.

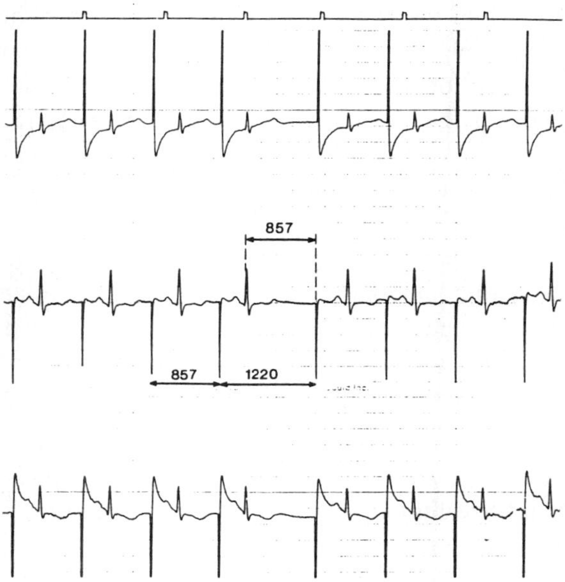

Figure 6. *Three channel ECG (leads I, II, III) of a patient with an implanted AAI pacemaker. The escape interval is programmed at 857 ms. Prolongation of the escape interval (1220 ms) is observed; the time of oversensing corresponds with the preceding R wave (far-field R wave sensing).*

P wave oversensing is rarely encountered in VVI pacemakers. It can be encountered in bipolar systems in which the proximal electrode is located in the vicinity of the tricuspid valve, thus enabling P wave sensing (figure 7). Such a position of the lead combined with a high sensitivity setting of the pulse generator is necessary to evoke P wave oversensing.[18,19]

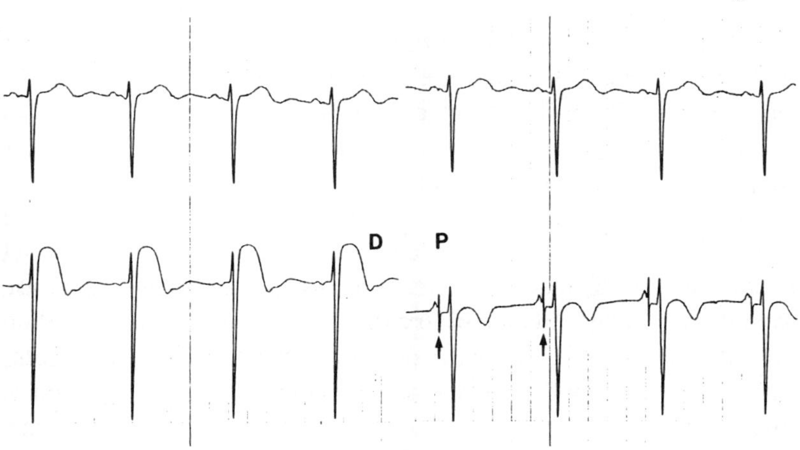

Figure 7. *Unipolar electrograms from a bipolar lead for permanent ventricular pacing; electrode separation 25 mm. The electrode was implanted in the right ventricular inflow tract. The distal electrogram (D) shows a normal pattern; in the proximal electrogram (P) a sharp deflection (arrows) of the atrial depolarization was recorded in the last part of the P wave.*

▸ *Oversensing from extracardiac physiological signals (myopotentials).* All skeletal muscles generate electrical potentials during contraction. When the muscle is in direct contact with or in the direct vicinity of one of the electrodes of the pacing system, these potentials can be detected by the sensing amplifier.[20] Myopotential oversensing is frequently encountered in unipolar systems. In unipolar systems the myopotentials are detected by the case of the pulse generator (the anodal electrode), that is in contact with one of the skeletal muscles, e.g. the pectoral muscle. The reported incidence of musculoskeletal inhibition of unipolar pacemakers is up to 69% during normal daily activity, objectivated by Holter recording.[21] However, only in 12% of these patients inhibition was associated with symptoms. On rare occasions oversensing from myopotentials can occur at the cathodal electrode of ventricular pacemakers, either unipolar or bipolar. The ventricular electrode, traditionally implanted in the right ventricular apex, is in the direct vicinity of the diaphragm, which also generates myopotentials during inspiration. Circumstances enabling sensing of myopotentials generated by the diaphragm are:

1. Perforation of the pacing electrode.[22]
2. Thin wall of the right ventricular myocardium.
3. High sensitivity of the pulse generator.[23]

Myopotential oversensing can be prevented by reducing sensitivity[24], provided that sensing of intrinsic activity is maintained. If this fails symptomatic inhibition can be prevented by programming the system to the triggered mode (AAT,VVT).

▸ *Oversensing from signals generated within the pacing system.* Oversensing from signals generated within the pacing system are in the majority of cases caused by abrupt changes in lead impedance. The changes in lead impedance can be due to interruption in the conductor or connector of the lead. Partial fracture can occur in multifilar leads, where one of the conductor strands is broken and the intermittent contact between the broken strands is responsible for the impedance variation. Changes in system impedance can also occur in an electrically intact electrode that touches a second (inactive) electrode.[25] Also insulation defects are a source for impedance changes that can create oversensing.[26] An insulation defect between the anodal and the cathodal conductor of a bipolar lead enables intermittent contact between both conductors resulting in spurious signals responsible for pacemaker inhibition (figure 8).

Because these signals are in general not visible in the standard ECG, telemetry of the intracardiac electrogram is a valuable diagnostic tool to detect signals responsible for oversensing.

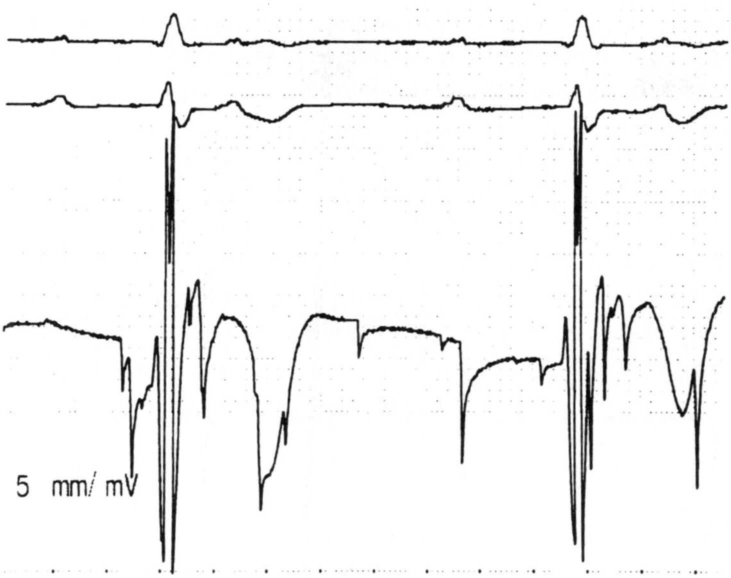

Figure 8. *Intracardiac electrogram recorded from the distal electrode of a bipolar ventricular lead. Spurious signals are generated by intermittent contact between anodal and cathodal conductor due to an insulation defect, causing oversensing in the pacing system.*

Undersensing

Shortening of the coupling interval between intrinsic activity and subsequent pacemaker stimuli, electrocardiographically known as undersensing can be divided into 3 categories, related to the cause of undersensing:

1. The intrinsic intracardiac electrogram is of sufficient amplitude to be sensed by the pacemaker but occurs in the refractory period of the pacing system.
2. The intrinsic intracardiac electrogram is not of sufficient amplitude and/or slew rate to be sensed by the pacemaker at the programmed sensitivity level.
3. The intrinsic intracardiac electrogram is of sufficient amplitude and/or slew rate to be sensed by the pacemaker but the signal is attenuated by electrical dysfunction of the lead or pulse generator.

▸ *Effect of the refractory period.* Every paced or sensed event initiates a refractory period. The refractory period is divided in an absolute refractory period (blanking period) followed by a relative refractory period also called noise sampling period. A sense event occurring in the absolute refractory period is completely ignored by the pacing system. A sensed event during the relative refractory period, however, does not affect the escape interval but prolongs the refractory period with a certain interval. This prolongation is type and manufacturer related. This mechanism may induce electrocardiographic undersensing caused by oversensing as illustrated in figure 9.

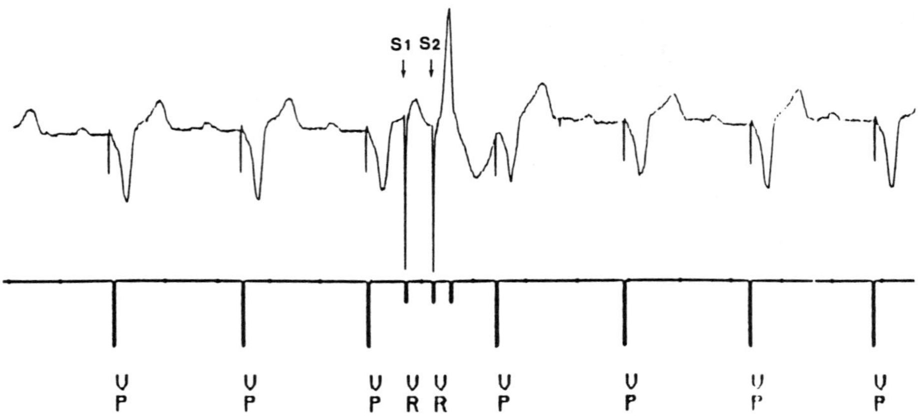

Figure 9. *One channel ECG (lead II) of a patient with an implanted VVI pacemaker demonstrating the effect of the relative refractory period. Two programmed chest wall stimuli (S1, S2) with a coupling interval of 300 and 220 ms respectively are applied to the patient. The total refractory period is 325 ms. The marker channel illustrates sensing in the relative refractory period (VR); VP = ventricular pacing. See text for further explanation.*

Two programmed chest wall stimuli with a coupling interval of 300 and 220 ms respectively were applied to the patient. The total refractory period of the pulse generator was 325 ms. The first chest wall stimulus (in the relative refractory period) initiated an additional refractory period. In the relative part of this refractory period, the second chest wall stimulus was sensed. The latter again initiated a refractory period in which the ventricular premature contraction took place. The ventricular premature contraction was also sensed in the relative refractory period and the escape interval was not affected by any of the three sensed events. This example demonstrates that undesired sense events, which are often invisible on the surface ECG, can cause an electrocardiographic pattern of undersensing.[27-29] If undersensing is evident on the ECG, oversensing should be excluded first as the possible cause.

▸ *Inadequate intracardiac electrogram.* If a signal cannot be sensed by a pulse generator at its maximum sensitivity, without oversensing of other cardiac related signals, it should be considered to be an inadequate signal. Although the electrogram amplitude expressed in mV and the sensitivity of the pulse generator are used as a standard for proper sensing, the use of only these two criteria has limitations. It is not only the amplitude but also the spectral content of the signal, as well as the characteristics of the input amplifier, that determine sensing function.[30] An indication for the frequency spectrum of the intracardiac signal can be obtained from the slew rate or voltage amplitude versus time (dv/dt).

An inadequate electrogram can be caused by displacement of the electrode, myocardial fibrosis formation around the electrode, myocardial infarction and changes in intraventricular conduction (figure 10).

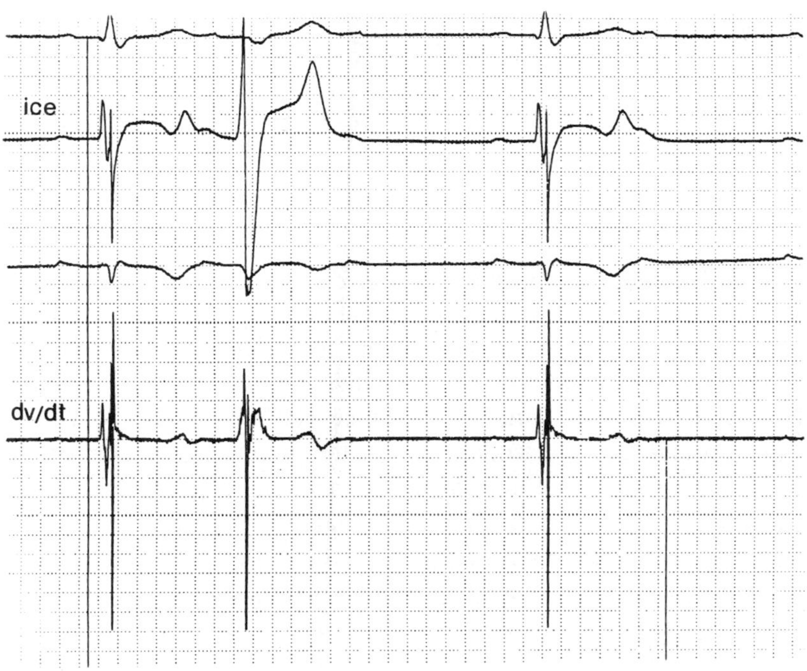

Figure 10. *Four channel recording showing the unipolar intracardiac electrogram (ICE) and the slew rate of this electrogram (dv/dt). It illustrates that the slew rate of the ventricular premature beat is much lower than the slew rate of the sinus beats, inspite of a higher amplitude of the ventricular premature beat. Remaining tracines show ECG lead I (top) and lead III.*

In those cases where an inadequate signal is considered to be the cause of undersensing, this should be confirmed by recording the intracardiac electrogram.[31] If this option is not available in the implanted pacing system, the diagnosis should be made by elimination of the other causes (refractoriness of the pacing system, dysfunction of the lead or pulse generator).

▸ *Attenuation of the intracardiac electrogram by the pacing system.* The intrinsic electrogram can be of sufficient amplitude and slew rate but can be attenuated by dysfunction of the lead system or pulse generator. To illustrate this mechanism a simplified electrical diagram of the pacing system is represented in figure 11.

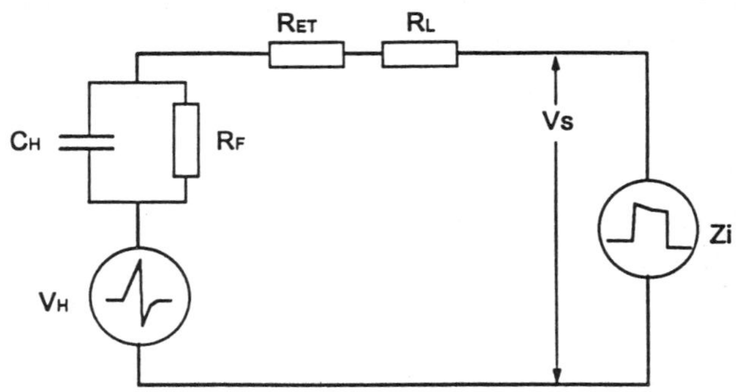

Figure 11. *Diagram of the simplified equivalent circuit model, in which the heart is the signal source (Vh); the Helmholtz capacitance (CH), the Faraday resistance (RF) and the electrode-tissue resistance (Ret) are the components of the electrode-tissue interface, Rl is the conductor resistance, Zi is the input impedance of the pulse generator, Vs is the signal sensed by the pulse generator.*

The myocardial depolarization may be regarded as a voltage source (Vh). This voltage source is connected to the pulse generator by the lead impedance (Zl). The latter is formed by the conductor of the lead (Rlead), the resistance of the electrode tissue interface (Ret) and a capacitive component (Helmholz capacitance, CH) parallel with the Faraday resistance (RF) both due to concentration polarization around the electrode.[32] Zi is the input impedance of the pulse generator and Vs is the amplitude of the intracardiac electrogram sensed by the pulse generator. It will be clear from this diagram that if Zi >> Zl, that the difference between Vh and Vs is neglectible, which is the ideal situation.

An increase in Zl (e.g. partial lead fracture) will decrease the signal sensed by the pulse generator. If for instance lead impedance is increased to the value of Zi (Zl = Zi) the signal sensed by the pulse generator is half the amplitude of the intracardiac electrogram. Because Zi is in the order of 20 KΩ or higher the stimulation current is dramatically reduced (0.25 mA at 5 V pacemaker output), so noncapture will become manifest before undersensing will be observed.

A decrease in lead impedance caused by an insulation defect between anodal and cathodal conductor or electrode is demonstrated in figure 12. The insulation defect forms a low resistance pathway (Rid) between anodal and cathodal conductor or electrode. Rid is parallel with Zi. The total resistance (Zt) is equal to Zi.Rid/Zi+Rid. If Zt is equal to Zl, the signal sensed by the pulse generator is half the amplitude of the intracardiac signal Vh.[33] Because pulse generators are constant voltage sources, stimulation threshold will hardly be affected by insulation defects. This implies that an insulation defect mainly affects pacemaker sensing while stimulation is maintained.

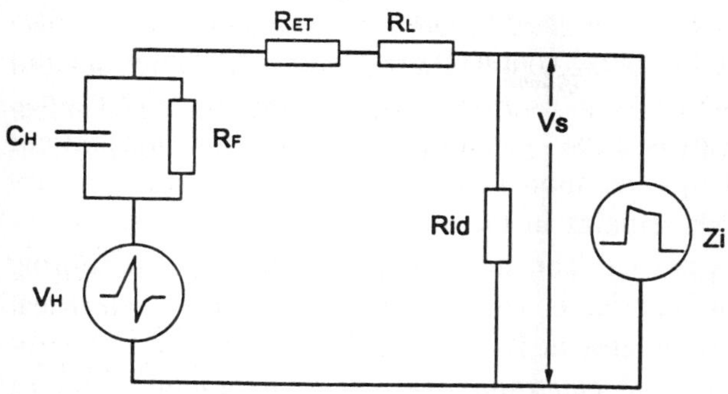

Figure 12. *Same diagram as figure 11 with an additional resistor (Rid) across the input impedance (Zi) of the pulse generator. This resistor simulates an insulation defect of the lead. The effect of the insulation defect on the sensed signal (Vs) is explained in the text.*

The influence of an insulation defect on the amplitude and morphology of the sensed signal is demonstrated in figure 13 by placing an external resistor between anodal and cathodal conductors, thus imitating an insulation defect. The signal is measured with an electrocardiograph with a high input impedance, so the signal loaded with 20 KΩ (which is in the order of pulse generators input impedance), is comparable with the signal sensed by the pulse generator. Loading the signal with 5 and 1 KΩ respectively shows attenuation and differentiation of the signal.

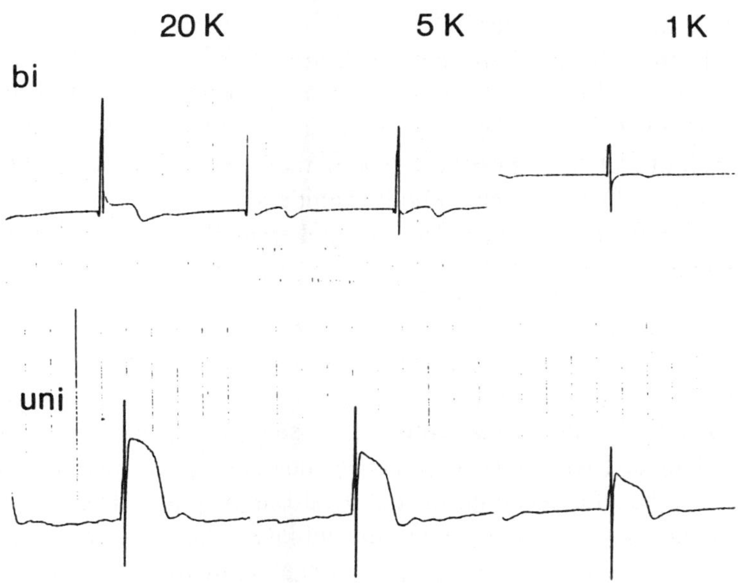

Figure 13. *Recording of a unipolar and bipolar electrogram from the same bipolar lead. The signal is loaded with 20, 5, 1 KΩ respectively, the latter two simulating an insulation defect. Note the attenuation and differentiation (change in morphology) of the sensed signal. Differentiation is more pronounced in the bipolar configuration.*

▸ *Undersensing due to pulse generator malfunction.* An adequate intracardiac signal, in terms of amplitude and spectral characteristics, and a normally functioning lead can be ignored by a defective pulse generator resulting in undersensing. Undersensing by a malfunctioning pulse generator is rarely an intermittent phenomenon. It can be caused by a component failure in the electrical circuitry or a defective reed switch, which remains in the closed position.[34] In both cases this will result in asynchronous pacing. The best tool to diagnose undersensing caused by pulse generator malfunction is chest wall stimulation. If electrical stimuli applied by an external stimulator at its maximum output to skin electrodes close to the anodal and cathodal electrode, are unable to inhibit a pacing system, pulse generator malfunction can be concluded. Before this test electrical integrity of the lead system should be confirmed.

Pacemaker Malfunction in Dual Chamber Systems

In dual chamber systems atrial and ventricular pacing and sensing should be separately assessed, in a similar way as in a single chamber system, to be certain that normal function of both channels exists. However, it will be possible that stimulation or failure to capture or sense in one channel affects the function of the other channel. Because of this interaction between both channels timing intervals can be complex and determination of normal pacing and sensing from the surface ECG can be difficult.[35] On some occasions the explanation of the ECG can be difficult or impossible without the recording of a marker channel, indicating sense and pace events in both chambers.

The following paragraphs describe pacemaker malfunction specifically related to dual chamber systems.

Cross Talk

Cross talk is defined as inappropriate sensing of the atrial stimulus in the ventricular channel (figure 14). In practice, however, it is not the atrial output pulse itself but the afterpotential of the atrial output pulse. This is explained by the fact that all modern pulse generators initiate a ventricular blanking period during atrial stimulation, which period is longer than the duration of the atrial pulse. The ventricular blanking period is a temporary disabling of the ventricular sensing amplifier following delivery of an atrial output pulse. Because crosstalk can still be encountered in pacemakers with ventricular blanking periods, the atrial output pulse itself can be excluded as the cause of crosstalk.

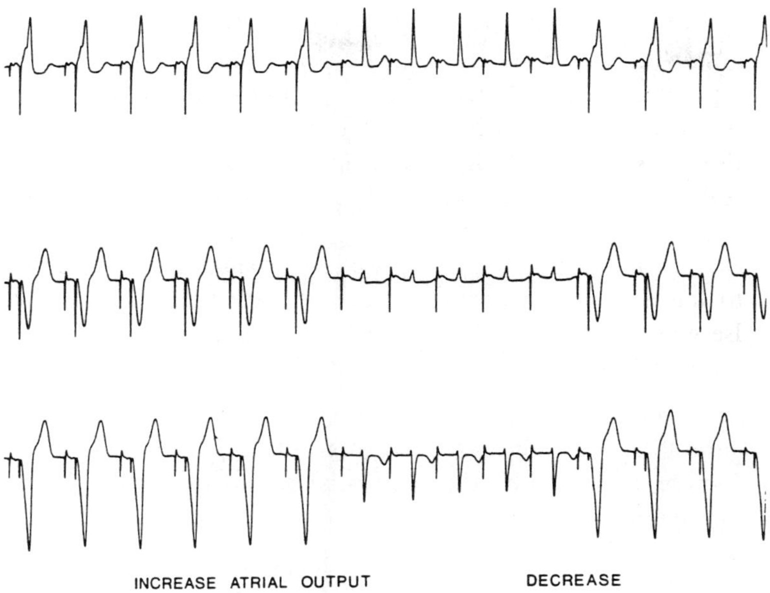

Figure 14. *Three channel ECG (leads I, II, III) of a patient with an external DVI pacemaker. During atrial output increase cross talk with inhibition of the ventricular stimulus is observed. After decreasing atrial output, normal pacemaker function is restored.*

The following factors can have effect on cross talk:

1. Atrial output (pulse width, amplitude).
2. Ventricular sensitivity.
3. Duration of the ventricular blanking period.
4. Electrode configuration (unipolar/bipolar).
5. Location and distance of the atrial and ventricular electrode.
6. The stimulation rate.[36]
7. Pulse generator circuitry.[37]
8. Lead impedance.

Because of the numerous factors that can affect cross talk, cross talk cannot completely ruled out by the ventricular blanking period. Therefore a second protection mechanism to prevent inhibition of the ventricular channel is incorporated in the majority of today's pulse generators. This mechanism is called ventricular safety pacing.

Ventricular Safety Pacing

This feature is designed to augment the ventricular blanking function to ensure that cross talk inhibition will not occur. If for some reason the ventricular blanking period is too short, the cross talk sensing window, which begins at the end of the ventricular blanking period, serves as a backup. Any signals sensed in the ventricular channel during this interval are interpreted as cross talk, and cause the pulse generator to deliver a ventricular output at the end of this interval (ventricular safety pacing). The duration of this interval is determined by the specifications of the pulse generator. In practice this interval is between 100 - 110 ms.

If the AV interval after an atrial paced event is programmed longer than the safety pacing interval, cross talk will be signalled on the ECG in the form of recurrent 'early' ventricular pacing, or AV sequential pacing with a shortened AV interval (figure 15). This indicates that cross talk is present and that the atrial output (amplitude, pulse width), the ventricular sensitivity or the blanking period may need adjustment.[38,39]

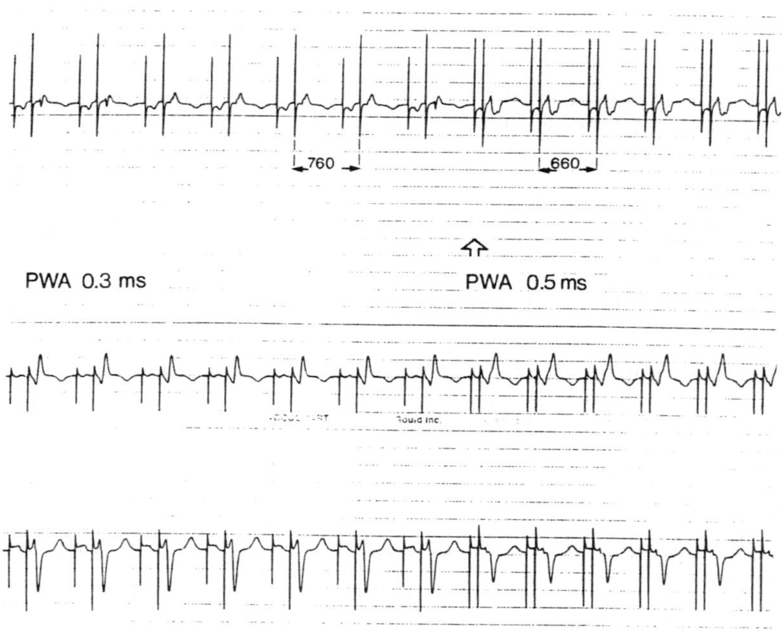

Figure 15. *Three channel ECG (leads I, II, III) of a patient with an implanted DDD pacemaker. After programming the atrial pulse width from 0.3 to 0.5 ms, cross talk is signalled on the ECG in the form of recurrent 'early' ventricular pacing, or AV sequential pacing with a shortened AV delay (ventricular safety pacing). Shortening of the AV interval results in shortening of the A-A interval (from 760 to 660 ms) in this atrial based timing system.*

Electrocardiographic Consequences of Ventricular Safety Pacing and Ventricular Blanking

Ventricular events occurring during the ventricular blanking period will be ignored by the ventricular channel and the ventricular stimulus will be emitted at the end of the programmed AV interval, provided no other ventricular sensed events occur in the remaining part of the AV interval. Figure 16 (pannel A) shows an ECG of a patient with a DDD pacemaker, stimulating at a lower rate of 100 ppm and an AV interval of 125 ms. A ventricular premature beat occurs more or less simultaneously with the atrial stimulus. The following AV interval is equal to the programmed interval of 125 ms, indicating that the moment of ventricular sensing occurs during the blanking period and the AV interval is not affected. However, the ECG can be easily misinterpreted as ventricular undersensing. In the same patient an identical ventricular premature beat with a longer coupling interval to the preceding ventricular paced beat illustrated proper ventricular sensing. In this recording (figure 16, pannel B) the ventricular sense event occurs during the ventricular safety pacing interval, which results in shortening of the AV interval, thus confirming ventricular safety pacing. In figure 16 (pannel C) the same ventricular premature beat occurs with a longer coupling interval than in the middle tracing. The atrial stimulus is now just preceeding the ventricular premature beat. Ventricular sensing occurs outside the ventricular safety pacing period and the ventricular output pulse is inhibited. All three ECG's illustrate the relationship between the moment of the ventricular sense event during the different parts of the AV interval and the reaction of the ventricular channel. To summarize, a ventricular sense event during the blanking period will not affect the programmed AV pace interval. A ventricular sense event during the ventricular safety pacing interval will evoke a ventricular stimulus with a shortened AV interval. A ventricular sense event during the AV interval outside the blanking and safety pacing interval will inhibit the ventricular ouput pulse.

Ventricular safety pacing can be sometimes misleading in the ECG interpretation, especially when ventricular safety pacing is caused by ventricular premature beats originating from the left ventricle. The detection time for these premature beats, by the right ventricular electrode, is relatively late. This implies that the atrial stimulus still can be emitted late in the QRS complex. Emission of the atrial impuls initiates a blanking period followed by the ventricular safety pacing period. The ventricular stimulus can be emitted in the first portion of the intrinsic T wave.

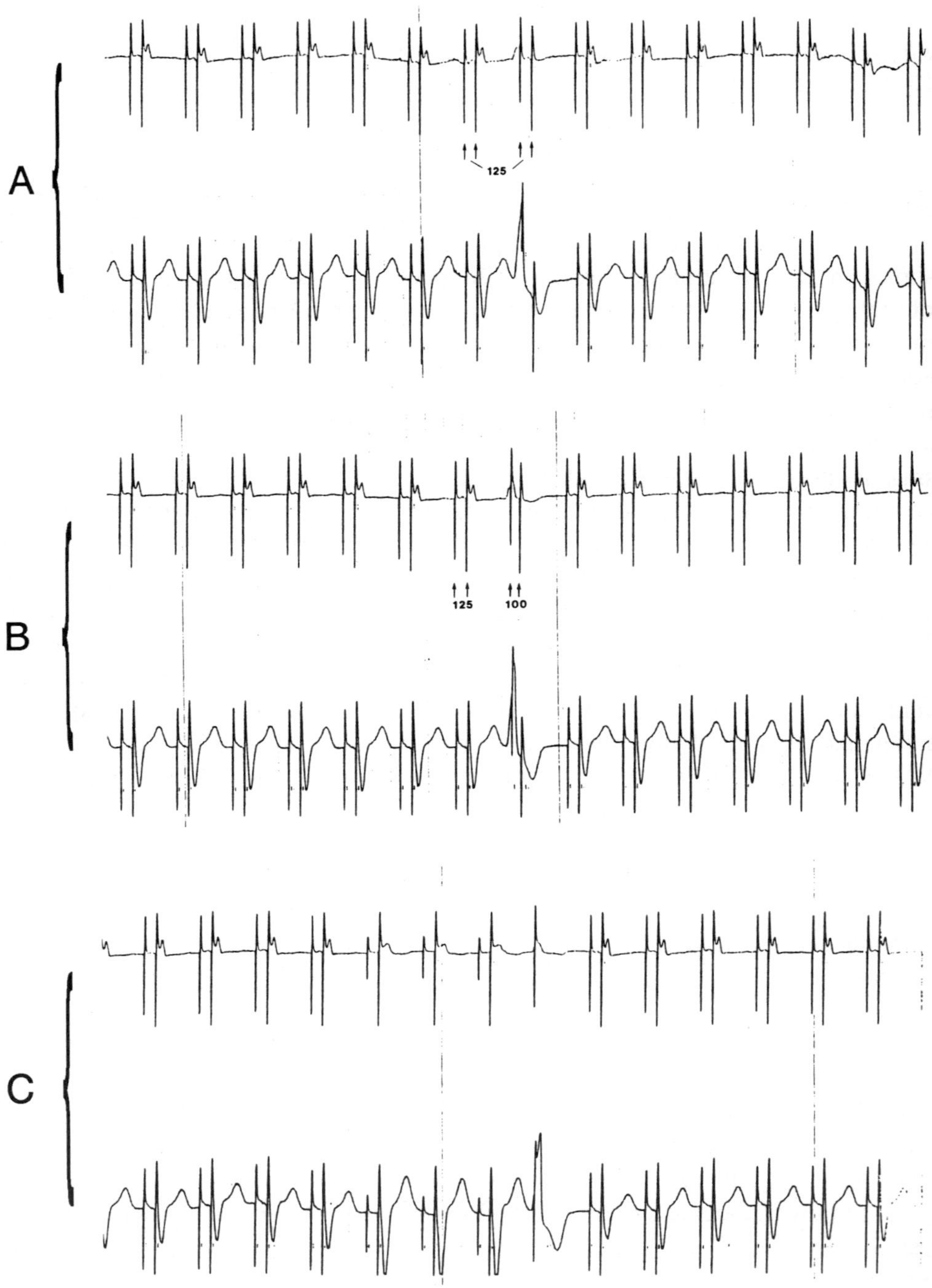

Figure 16. *Two channel ECG (leads I, II) of a patient with an implanted DDD pacemaker. In panel panel A the ventricular premature beat occurs during the ventricular blanking period, not affecting the AV interval (125 ms). In pannel B the coupling interval between the ventricular premature beat and the preceding QRS complex is slightly longer. The ventricular premature beat now occurs in the ventricular*

safety pacing interval resulting in shortening of the AV interval (100 ms). In panel C the coupling interval again is slightly longer, the ventricular premature beat occurs after the ventricular safety pacing interval and ventricular stimulation is inhibited. This example illustrates the different effects of ventricular events during the AV interval.

Effect of Ventricular (Over)sensing on Atrial Sensing in Dual-Chamber Systems During the VA Interval

From the timing system in dual chamber systems, it is understood that a ventricular sense or pace event temporarily disables the atrial channel by initiation of the postventricular atrial refractory period (PVARP). However, it is not only the real pace and sense events that initiate PVARP but every false signal, detected by the ventricular channel. This means that every possible cause of ventricular oversensing initiates a PVARP and in the majority of cases it is not only initation of PVARP, but this PVARP will be extended as well, due to the fact that the event causing ventricular oversensing will be interpreted by the pacemaker as a PVC. Because an important proportion of the signals responsible for false ventricular inhibition (and thus initiation of PVARP) are invisible on the normal ECG, PVARP can be initated without awareness of the interpreter. The result of ventricular oversensing is often that an intrinsic P wave following ventricular oversensing is ignored by the pacemaker due to the initiation of the (extended) PVARP.[40] The patient will present with electrocardiographical atrial undersensing, while the cause of atrial undersensing is ventricular oversensing (figure 17).

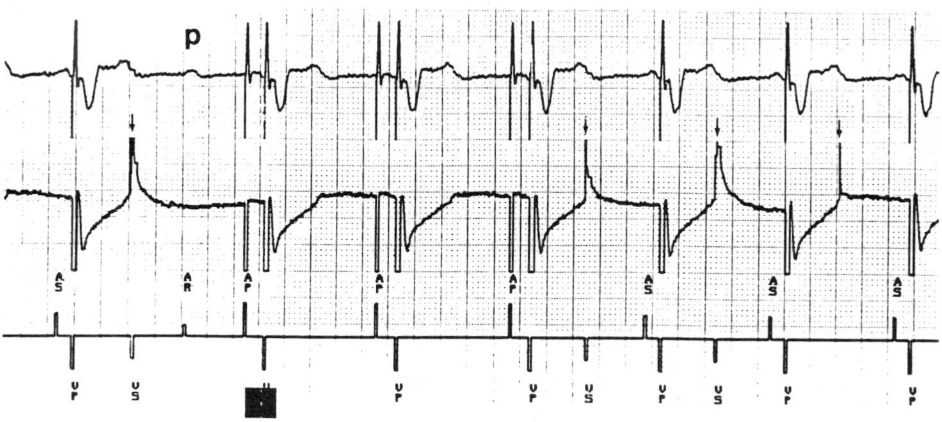

Figure 17. *Three channel recording of the ECG lead II (upper tracing), intracardiac ventricular electrogram (middle tracing), and marker channel (lower tracing) from a patient with an implanted bipolar DDD pacemaker. The ECG shows an intrinsic P wave (P) not followed by ventricular stimulation, suggestive for atrial undersensing. The marker channel, however, indicates that this P wave occurs during the atrial refractory period (AR). This atrial refractory period is initiated by oversensing in the ventricular channel (VS). The intracardiac electrogram shows signals (arrows) caused by an intermittent contact in the ventricular lead, responsible for oversensing. AP = atrial pacing; AR = atrial sense event during the atrial refractory period; AS = atrial sensing; VP = ventricular pacing.*

When atrial undersensing is present in the ECG of a patient with a dual chamber pacemaker, ventricular oversensing should be excluded as the cause, by recording of the marker channel and/or the intracardiac electrogram, if these options are available in the pacing system. If none of the options are available in the pacing system and atrial undersensing is observed one can consider programming the pacing system to the VVI mode. If in the VVI mode prolongation of the escape interval is recorded, ventricular oversensing is the most likely explanation of atrial undersensing.

Analysis of Pacemaker Malfunction

For the analysis of pacemaker function or malfunction a systematical stepwise approach can be used. To analyze a pacemaker problem, the problem first should be identified. After identification a strategy for the problem solution should be described. For the description of the identification and the stepwise strategy a flow diagram or flow chart can be used.

In the design of a flow chart for the diagnosis of pacemaker malfunction or apparent malfunction it appears that there are a large number of possibilities that have to be confirmed or excluded before the final diagnosis can be made. If a flow chart is designed as a decision tree, it rapidly grows to a size unsuitable for book publishing and not practical for the ECG interpreter.

In the draft of the flow chart we will use a schematic presentation of the pacemaker ECG illustrating malfunction, followed by the steps used for the analysis. In these steps smaller, but surveyable decision trees can be used. It has to be easy for the interpreter to find the schematic ECG, corresponding with the actual ECG. This approach links up best with the practical situation.

For the analysis the following assumptions are made:

1) The interpreter knows the specifications of the pulse generator and the programmed pacing mode.
2) Lead impedance can be measured by pacemaker telemetry or pulse waveform analysis.
3) Depolarization following stimulation can be established on the ECG.

In the flow chart the motivation for the queries will be ommitted or only indicated by key words. For the sake of compactnesss, the same will be done for the answers and the final diagnosis. If two or more conditions are mentioned they all have to be fulfilled, unless otherwise stated.

The flow chart is divided into the following electrocardiographic manifestations of pacemaker malfunction:

Single-Chamber Systems

1.1 Continuous no output
1.2 Intermittent no output
1.3 Continuous noncapture
1.4 Intermittent noncapture
2.1 Oversensing; fixed prolongation escape interval
2.2 Oversensing; varying prolongation escape interval
3 Undersensing

Dual-Chamber Systems

4 Atrial oversensing
5 Atrial undersensing
6.1 Ventricular oversensing; ventricular safety pacing
6.2 Ventricular oversensing during AV interval
6.3 Ventricular oversensing during VA interval
7.1 Ventricular undersensing during AV interval (premature beat, shortening AV interval)
7.2 Ventricular undersensing during AV interval (premature beat, normal AV interval)
7.3 Ventricular undersensing during AV interval (conducted beat)
7.4 Ventricular undersensing during VA interval terminated by atrial pacing
7.5 Ventricular undersensing during VA interval terminated by atrial sensing

1.1 Continuous no Output (Single-Chamber System)

ECG : No pacemaker stimuli visible.

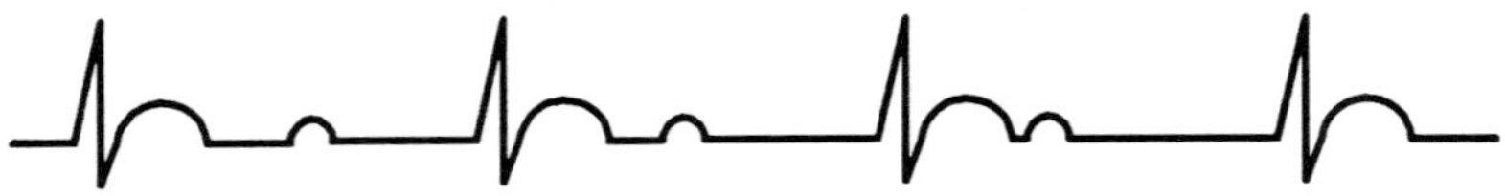

Conditions:
1) RR interval > escape or hysteresis interval.
2) No pacemaker stimuli after magnet application (12 lead ECG and supplementary modified chest leads). If magnet application results in pacemaker stimuli proceed to oversensing.

Communication by telemetry:
Not possible → pulse generator failure.
Check lead impedance during replacement to exclude lead malfunction (low impedance) as the cause of generator failure (battery depletion).

Still possible → measure lead impedance.

High Lead Impedance (>2000 Ω)

- Conductor break.
- Improper lead connection.
- Air entrapment, unipolar system.

If manipulation results in pacemaker stimuli on the ECG, the galvanic discontinuity is located between pulse generator and venous entry.
Use fluoroscopy to determine the site of discontinuity.
Program a bipolar system in the unipolar configuration, if available. If no effect, discontinuity is located in the *cathodal* conductor or its connection. If pacemaker stimuli are observed, discontinuity is located in the *anodal* conductor or its connection.
Recurrence of pacemaker stimuli after application of slight pressure on the generator indicates air entrapment. This problem is only observed in unipolar systems shortly after surgical procedures.

Low Lead Impedance (<100 Ω)

- Short circuit, insulation defect.

In unipolar systems located between pulse generator and cathodal conductor.
In bipolar systems located between anodal and cathodal conductor. If programmable in unipolar configuration, stimulation can be restored; increased stimulation threshold, increased current drain → accelerated battery depletion!

1.2 Intermittent no Output (Single-Chamber System)

ECG: Intermittent pacemaker stimuli.

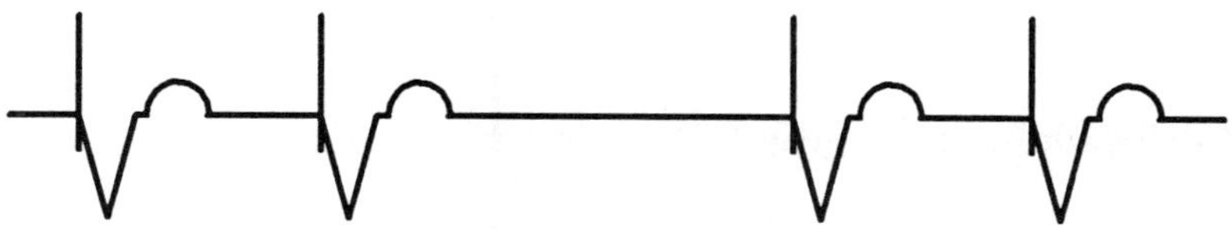

Conditions
1) Prolonged interval is an exact multiple of the escape interval.
2) Not affected by magnet application.
If condition 1 or 2 is not fulfilled, proceed to oversensing.

Measure lead impedance
Repetitive measurements might be necessary to determine lead impedance during no output.

High Lead Impedance (>2000 Ω)

- Conductor break.
- Improper lead connection.

If manipulation results in aggravation of the problem or restoration of continuous pacing, the galvanic discontinuity is located between pulse generator and venous entry.
Use fluoroscopy to determine the site of discontinuity.
Program a bipolar system in the unipolar configuration, if available. If no effect, discontinuity is located in the *cathodal* conductor or its connection. If continuous pacing is observed, discontinuity is located in the *anodal* conductor or its connection.

Restoration of regular stimulation after application of slight pressure on the pulse generator indicates air entrapment. This problem is only observed in unipolar systems shortly after surgical procedures.

Low Lead Impedance (< 100 Ω)

▸ Short circuit, insulation defect.

In unipolar systems located between pulse generator and cathodal conductor.
In bipolar systems located between anodal and cathodal conductor. If programmable in unipolar configuration stimulation can be restored; increased stimulation threshold, increased current drain → accelerated battery depletion!

1.3 Continuous Noncapture (Single-Chamber System)

ECG: Pacemaker stimuli not followed by depolarization

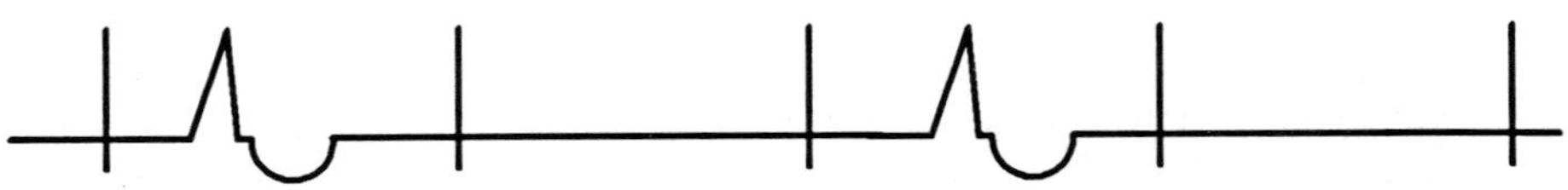

Conditions
1) Myocardium is not refractory at the time of pulse delivery.
2) Proper output setting, not inadvertently programmed below stimulation threshold.
3) Battery depletion excluded.

Additional observations
1) Sensing from another chamber than the original implantation site → macrodislocation.
2) Sudden onset of diaphragmatic stimulation → lead displacement or perforation.

If none of these two observations are present:

Measure lead impedance

Lead Impedance Within Normal Limits

- Admistration of threshold elevating drugs?
- Electrolyte imbalance?
- Myocardial infarction?
- Immediately after cardioversion or defibrillation?
- Cardioplegia during open heart surgery?

If none of above mentioned causes applicable:
Fluoroscopy for lead displacement or perforation. Usually shortly after implantation.

If none of above mentioned causes applicable → exit block.

High Lead Impedance

- Conductor break (fluid bridge between both ends).
- Improper lead connection.

If manipulation results in (intermittent) capture the defect is located between pulse generator and venous entry. Use fluoroscopy to determine the site of the defect.
Program a bipolar system in the unipolar mode, if available. If no effect, the defect is located in the *cathodal* conductor or its connection. If capture is restored, defect is located in the *anodal* conductor or its connection.

Low Lead Impedance

- Insulation defect.

In unipolar systems located between pulse generator and cathodal conductor. In bipolar systyems located between anodal and cathodal conductor. If programmable in unipolar configuration capture can be restored; increased stimulation threshold, increased current drain → accelerated battery depletion!

NOTE:
Intrinsic events following a noncaptured stimulus, within the refractory period, will show apparent undersensing.

1.4 Intermittent Noncapture (Single-Chamber System)

ECG: Pacemaker stimuli intermittently followed by depolarization

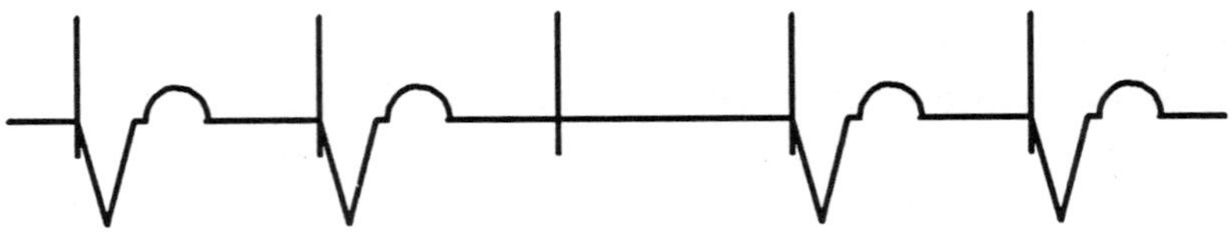

Conditions

1) Myocardium is not refractory at the time of pulse delivery.
2) Proper output setting, not inadvertently at the level of the stimulation threshold.
3) Battery depletion excluded.

Additional observations

1) Changes in the morphology of the stimulated depolarization in comparison with previous recordings → lead displacement or perforation.
2) Attenuation of the pacemaker stimulus during noncapture → intermittent galvanic discontinuity (high lead impedance) or insulation defect (low lead impedance).

If none of these two observations are present:

Measure lead impedance

Repetetive measurements might be necessary to determine lead impedance during noncapture.

Lead Impedance Within Normal Limits

- Administration of threshold elevating drugs?
- Electrolyte imbalance?
- Myocardial infarction?
- Observed immediately after DC shock?

If none of above mentioned causes applicable:
Fluoroscopy for lead displacement. Usually shortly after implantation.
If none of above mentioned causes applicable → fibrous tissue formation around stimulation electrode.

High Lead Impedance

- Conductor break with intermittent contact and fluid bridge between both ends.
- Improper lead connection.

If manipulation results in aggravation of the problem or restoration of continous capture, the defect is located between pulse generator and venous entry.
Program a bipolar system in the unipolar configuration, if available. If no effect, the defect is located in the *cathodal* conductor or its connection. If continuous capture is restored, defect is located in the *anodal* conductor or its connection.

Low Lead Impedance

- insulation defect

In unipolar systems located between pulse generator and cathodal conductor.
In bipolar system located between anodal and cathodal conductor. If programmable in unipolar configuration stimulation can be restored; increased stimulation threshold, increased current drain → accelerated battery depletion!

NOTE:
Intrinsic events following a noncaptured stimulus within the refractory period will show apparent undersensing.

2.1 Oversensing (Single-Chamber System)

ECG: More or less fixed prolongation of the escape interval.

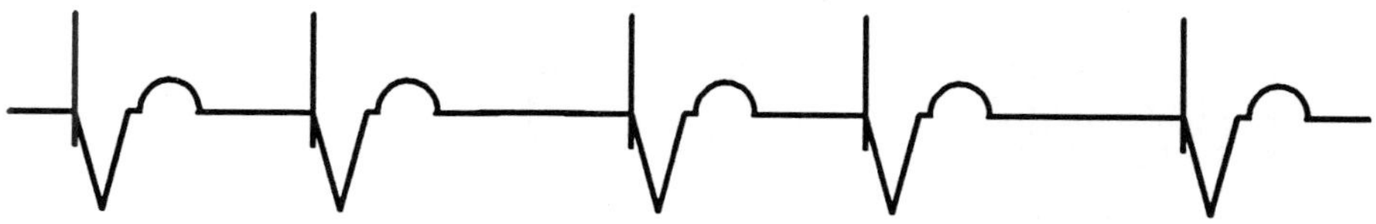

Conditions:
1) Prolonged interval is not a multiple of the escape interval.
2) Prolonged interval after intrinsic depolarization > hysteresis interval.

3) Magnet application results in regular asynchronous pacing at a preset interval. If there is no effect, then irregular pulse formation is concluded (pulse generator failure). Unlikely in currently available pulse generators.
4) Electroc Magnetic Interference (EMI) from the patient's environment is excluded as the cause of oversensing.
5) Disable hysteresis.

Additional observation

More or less fixed prolongation of the escape interval, but shorter than twice the escape interval → prolongation of escape interval is related to stimulation or cardiac response to stimulation.

Intracardiac Electrogram (IEGM)

The IEGM will elucidate the nature of signals responsible for oversensing.

- T wave sensing (VVI pacemaker).
- R wave sensing (AAI pacemaker).
- Afterpotential sensing.
- Spurious signals, caused by abrupt changes in lead impedance, provoked by atrial or ventricular contraction (lead malfunction). A second (abandoned) lead touching the functioning lead may evoke these signals. Fluoroscopy.

No IEGM available → Measure lead impedance

Lead Impedance Within Normal Limits

- T wave sensing (VVI pacemaker)
- R wave sensing (AAI pacemaker)
- Afterpotential sensing

Afterpotential sensing can be confirmed by normalizing the escape interval after reducing pacemaker output or by shortening the prolonged escape interval by reducing the refractory period.

Oversensing can be corrected by reducing sensitivity or extending the refractory period.

High or Low Lead Impedance

Impedance changes are caused by either a conductor defect (high lead impedance) or insulation defect (low lead impedance) but provoked by atrial or ventricular contraction. The latter implies that the defect is located within the heart, which only can be corrected by implantation of a new lead. Differentiation between insulation and conductor defect has no practical value.

2.2 Oversensing (Single-Chamber System)

ECG: Varying prolongation of the escape interval

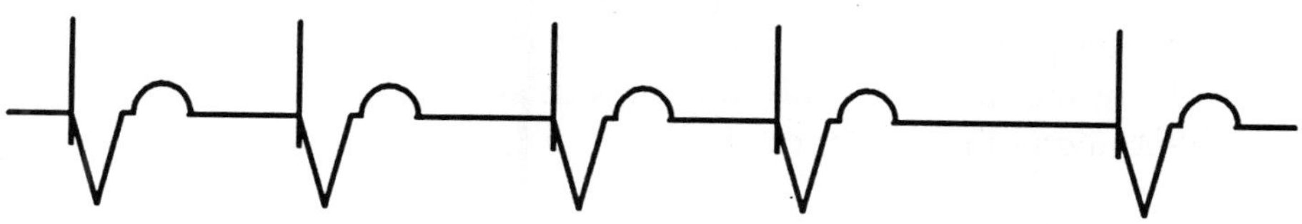

Conditions

1) Prolonged interval after intrinsic depolarization > hysteresis interval
2) Magnet application results in regular asynchronous pacing at a preset interval. If no effect, irregular pulse formation (pulse generator failure). Unlikely in currently available pulse generators.

Intracardiac Electrogram (IEGM)

The IEGM will elucidate the nature of signals responsible for oversensing.

- P wave sensing (VVI pacemaker).
- Spurious signals, caused by abrupt changes in lead impedance (lead malfunction) or by intermittent contact of the functioning lead with an abandoned lead. Fluoroscopy.

Marker channel

If sense markers coincide with P waves (VVI pacemaker) → P wave oversensing.

Sense markers randomly distributed over cardiac cycle → spurious signals, lead malfunction. Intermittent contact abandoned lead.

Triggered mode
If neither IEGM nor marker channel is available program to triggered mode. P-synchronous pacing → P wave sensing. Pacing with a varying interval → purious signals.

Measure lead impedance

High Lead Impedance

- intermittent contact in conductor
- unstable lead connection

If manipulation results in aggravation of oversensing, the defect is located between pulse generator and venous entry. If a bipolar system is programmed in the unipolar configuration with abolition of oversensing, the defect is located in the anodal conductor.

Low Lead Impedance

- insulation defect

In bipolar systems located between anodal and cathodal conductor (chapter V, figure 5.23). Insulation defect in the outer insulation will be indicated by 'unipolarization' of the pacemaker stimulus. In unipolar systems, chest wall stimulation can be used to confirm and to localize the insulation defect.

NOTE:
If an event caused by oversensing preceeds an intrinsic event with a coupling interval shorter than the refractory period, the ECG may show undersensing.

3. Undersensing (Single-Chamber System)

ECG: Interval between an intrinsic event and subsequent paced event is shorter than the escape interval.

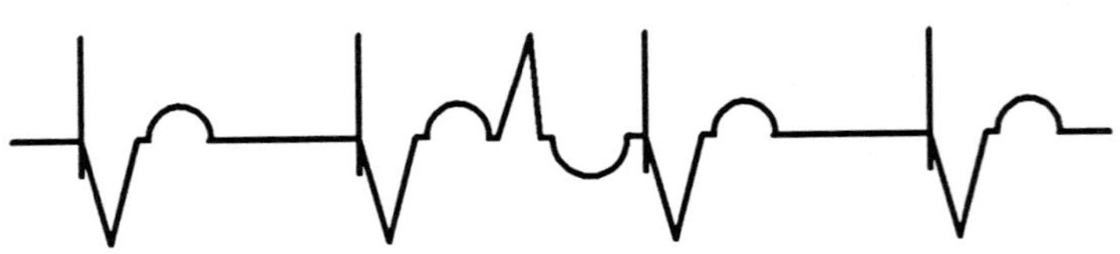

Conditions:

1) The unsensed intrinsic depolarization occurs outside the refractory period initiated by a paced event.
2) Pacemaker is not in the asynchronous mode by magnet application or inadvertently programmed in the asynchronous mode.

Exclude oversensing

- marker channel
- triggered mode, if no marker channel available

If oversensing is present proceed to oversensing 2.2.

Measure lead impedance

Lead Impedance Within Normal Limits

- Pacemaker not inhibited by chest wall stimuli → pulse generator failure
- Morphology of the stimulated depolarization is changed compared with previous recordings → electrode displacement
- Morphology of the stimulated depolarization is not changed compared with previous recordings → fibrous tissue formation; increased stimulation threshold.

  Exclude changes in medication, electrolyte disturbances and myocardial infarction as the cause of undersensing.

High Lead Impedance

- Conductor failure with intact insulation. Always associated with an increase in stimulation threshold. For unipolar systems use fluoroscopy to determine the site of the conductor failure.

  Program a bipolar system in the unipolar configuration, if available. If lead impedance returns to normal the defect is located in the anodal conductor, if not it is located in the cathodal conductor.

Low lead impedance

- Insulation defect.

In unipolar systems, chest wall stimulation can be used to confirm and localize the insulation defect.

In bipolar systems the insulation defect is located between *anodal* and *cathodal* conductor.

4. Atrial Oversensing (Dual-Chamber System)

ECG: Ventricular paced event not preceded by a P wave.

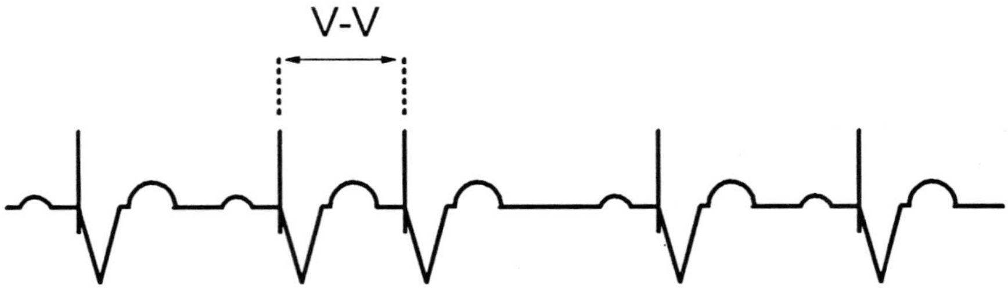

Conditions

1) No atrial depolarization is preceding Vpace. Use precordial leads or the intracardiac electrogram, if available, to exclude atrial premature contraction.
2) The V-V interval is shorter than the lower rate interval. If the V-V interval is equal to the lower rate interval and condition 1 is fulfilled → atrial no output.
   Proceed to 1.2 for the atrial channel.

Sensing of far-field ventricular activity?

1) Confirm the presence of far-field ventricular activity detected at the atrial electrode by recording of the intracardiac electrogram and/or the marker channel.
2) If none of these two options are available, program PVARP to an interval longer than the total duration of ventricular depolarization. If oversensing disappears, far-field sensing of ventricular depolarization can be concluded.

Sensing of far-field ventricular activity excluded → proceed to oversensing 2.2 for the atrial channel.

5. Atrial Undersensing (Dual-Chamber System)

ECG: P wave not followed by inhibition of the atrial stimulus and ventricular stimulation at the preset AV interval.

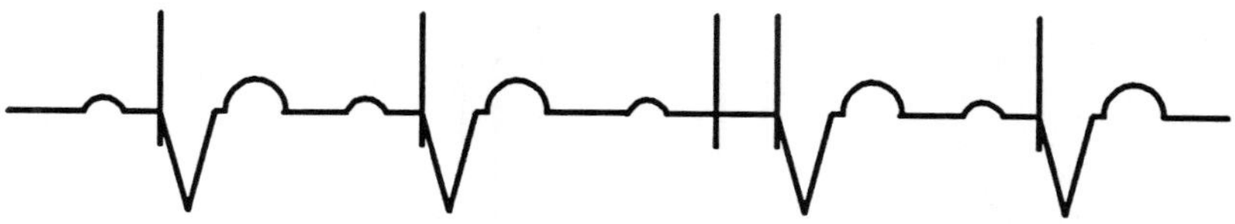

Conditions

1) P waves occur outside PVARP or extended PVARP.
2) Pacemaker is not in the asynchronous mode by magnet application, back-up mode pacing or inadvertently programmed in the asynchronous mode.

Exclude ventricular oversensing

Ventricular oversensing initiates or prolongs PVARP, which may result in an ECG showing atrial undersensing. (See figure 17)

Ventricular oversensing excluded by

1) Marker channel recording.
2) If not available, program to the VVI mode. Normal escape interval excludes ventricular oversensing.

If ventricular oversensing is present proceed to 2.1 or 2.2 for the ventricular channel.

If ventricular oversensing is excluded proceed to 3 for the atrial channel.

NOTE:

1) The ECG may show atrial noncapture due to atrial stimulation during the refractoriness of the atrial myocardium.
2) Atrial undersensing may be overlooked if the RR interval is shorter than the programmed VA interval! If the RR interval is shorter than the VA interval, the lower rate times will be reset (by R wave sensing) before emission of the atrial stimulus, thus potentially masking atrial undersensing.

6.1 Ventricular Oversensing; Ventricular Safety Pacing

ECG: Shortening of the Apace-Vpace interval. (See figure 15)

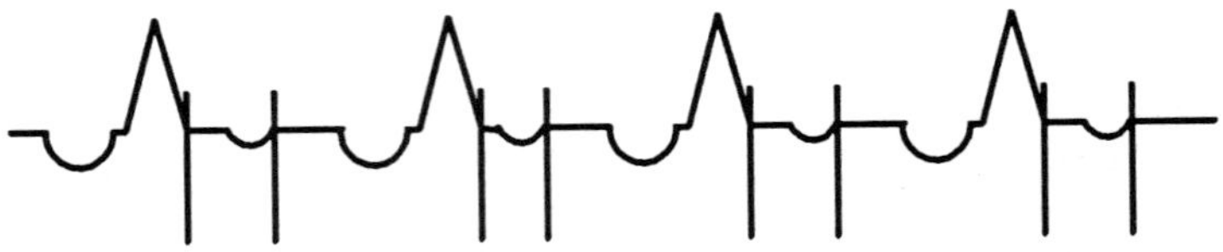

Conditions
1) Ventricular safety pacing present for cross talk protection.
2) Atrial stimulation not followed by intrinsic ventricular activity.
3) The programmed AV interval is longer than 110 ms.

Program the pacing system in the VVI mode
If the escape interval remains constant and is equal to the preset lower rate interval, oversensing is caused by atrial stimulation and cross talk can be concluded. The ventricular safety pace mechanism is activated by cross talk resulting in shortening of the Apace-Vpace interval. Ventricular safety pacing is characterized by an AV interval between 100 and 110 ms.

If the escape interval shows prolongation or is longer than the programmed lower rate interval oversensing in the ventricular channel is concluded. Proceed to 2.1 or 2.2 for the ventricular channel.

Prevention of cross talk
1) Reduce atrial output (pulse amplitude or pulse width).
2) Reduce ventricular sensitivity.
3) Program bipolar electrode configuration, if available.*
4) Extend the ventricular blanking period.

* NOTE:
In some pulse generators (Intermedics, Inc.) cross talk can be aggravated when programming the atrial lead configuration from unipolar to bipolar.

6.2 Ventricular Oversensing During AV Interval Outside Ventricular Safety Pace Interval

ECG: Atrial stimulus not followed by a ventricular stimulus at the preset AV interval.

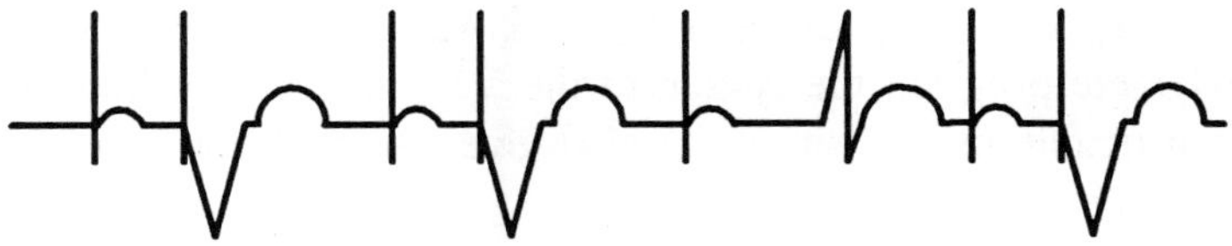

Conditions

1) Ventricular safety pacing present for cross talk protection
2) Interval between atrial stimulus and intrinsic ventricular activity (if present) is longer than the programmed AV interval

Ventricular safety pacing absent or not activated

Exclude cross talk, see 6.1.

Proceed to oversensing 2.1 or 2.2 for the ventricular channel.

NOTE:
Ventricular oversensing during the AV interval initiates a ventricular refractory period. Intrinsic events occurring during this refractory period may give rise to an ECG pattern of ventricular undersensing.

6.3 Ventricular Oversensing During VA Interval

ECG: Prolongation of the VA interval

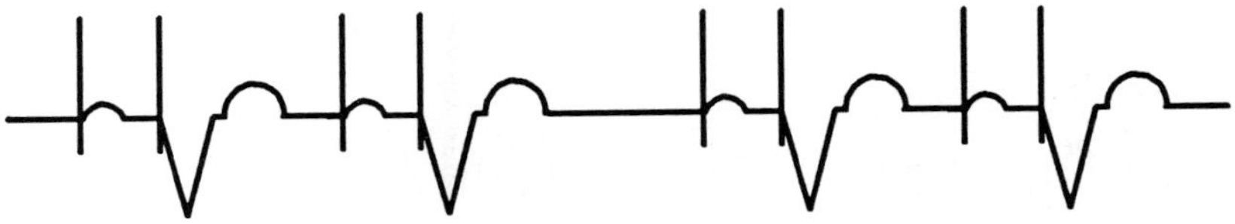

If the prolongation of the VA interval is a more or less fixed interval, proceed to 2.1 for the ventricular channel.

If the prolongation of the VA interval is a varying interval, proceed to 2.2 for the ventricular channel.

NOTE:
1) Ventricular oversensing can be masked if the interval between two consecutive atrial sensed, ventricular paced events is shorter than the VA interval. If this condition exists, record the marker channel and if not available program the system to the VVI mode to exclude oversensing.
2) Ventricular oversensing may also give rise to a pattern of atrial undersensing!

7.1 Ventricular Undersensing During the AV Interval Initiated by Atrial Stimulation

ECG: Intrinsic ventricular depolarization during the AV interval followed by a ventricular stimulus with shortening of the AV interval.

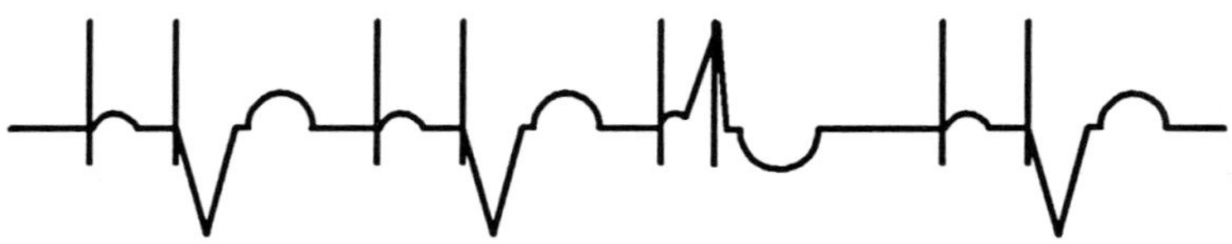

Conditions
1) Intrinsic ventricular depolarization is a premature ventricular contraction.
2) Intrinsic ventricular depolarization is preceded by an atrial stimulus.
3) AV interval is shortened to 100-110 ms.

Conclusion
Premature ventricular contraction occurs during the ventricular safety pacing interval resulting in shortening of the AV interval and an ECG pattern of ventricular undersensing. Normal pacemaker function.

7.2 Ventricular Undersensing During the AV Interval Initiated by Atrial Stimulation

ECG: Intrinsic ventricular depolarization during the AV interval followed by a ventricular stimulus at the preset AV interval. (See figure 16, pannel A)

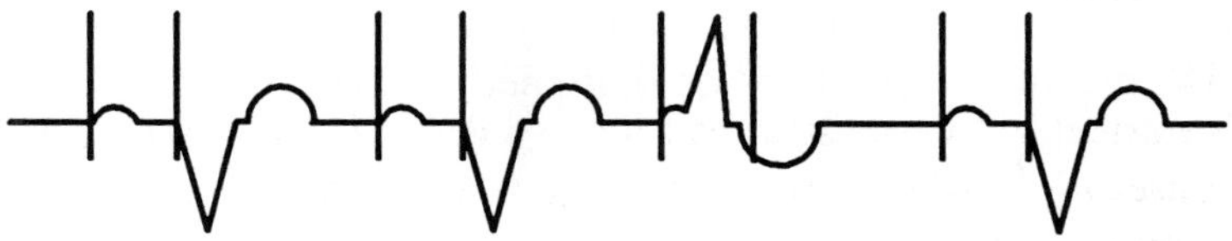

Conditions

1) Intrinsic ventricular depolarization is a ventricular premature contraction.
2) Intrinsic ventricular depolarization is preceded by an atrial stimulus.
3) AV interval is unchanged.

Exclude real ventricular undersensing

Exclude real ventricular undersensing by programming the system to the VVI or VVT mode to verify proper sensing of ventricular premature contractions.

If real ventricular undersensing is present, proceed to 3 for the ventricular channel.

Conclusion

Premature ventricular contraction occurs during the ventricular blanking period resulting in an ECG pattern of ventricular undersensing. Although this is normal pacemaker function, programming a long AV interval should be avoided under these conditions (chapter VI, 6.7).

7.3 Ventricular Undersensing During the AV Interval Initiated by Atrial Stimulation

ECG: Intrinsic conducted beat preceded by atrial stimulation and followed by a ventricular stimulus with a shortened or unchanged AV interval.

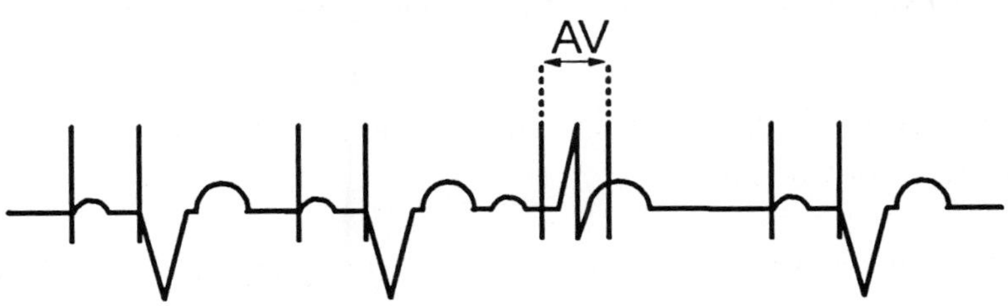

Conditions

1) Intrinsic ventricular depolarization is a conducted beat.
2) Intrinsic ventricular depolarization is preceded by an atrial stimulus.
3) AV interval is unchanged or shortened to 100-110 ms.

Conclusion

Ventricular depolarization is not sensed because it occurs during the ventricular blanking period initiated by the atrial stimulus (AV interval unchanged).

Ventricular stimulus is evoked by the ventricular depolarization occurring in the ventricular safety pacing interval (AV interval shortened).

In both cases the primary cause of the ventricular stimulus following intrinsic depolarization is failure to sense the intrinsic P wave.

Proceed to undersensing 3 for the atrial channel.

7.4 Ventricular Undersensing During the VA Interval

ECG: Interval between intrinsic ventricular event and subsequent paced atrial event shorter than the programmed AV interval.

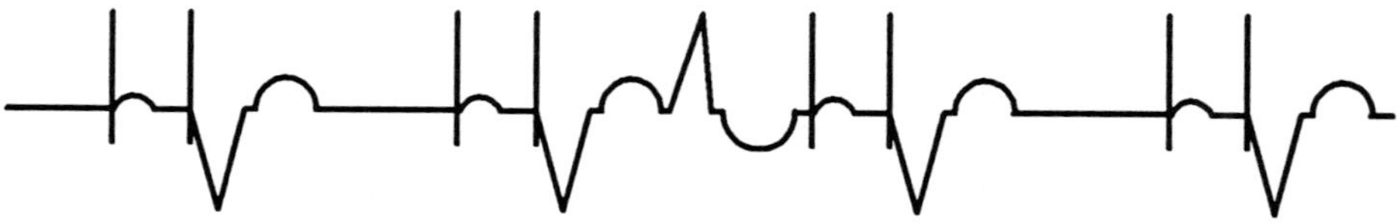

Conditions

1) Intrinsic ventricular depolarization occurs outside the ventricular refractory period initiated by the preceding ventricular paced event.
2) Pacemaker is not in the asynchronous mode by magnet application, back-up mode pacing or inadvertently programmed in the asynchronous mode.

Proceed to undersensing 3 for the ventricular channel.

7.5 Ventricular Undersensing During the VA Interval

ECG: Intrinsic ventricular depolarization followed by atrial sensing ventricular pacing.

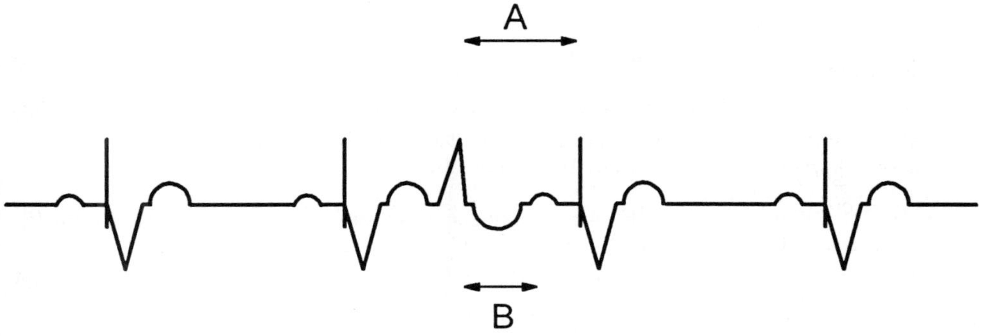

Condition
Intrinsic ventricular activity occurs outside the ventricular refractory period initiated by the preceding ventricular paced event.

Ventricular undersensing is present, if

1) The coupling interval (A) between the intrinsic ventricular depolarization and subsequent ventricular pace event is shorther than the upper rate interval.

or

2) The coupling interval (B) between the intrinsic ventricular depolarization and the subsequent atrial depolarization is shorter than the (extended) PVARP.

If one of both conditions is fulfilled proceed to 3 for the ventricular channel.
If none of the two conditions is fulfilled → normal pacemaker function.
In case of doubt, program the system to the VVT mode, which confirms presence or absence of ventricular sensing.

References

1. Gould L, Patel S, Gomes GI, Chokshi AB. Pacemaker failure following external defibrillation. PACE 1981;4:575-77.
2. Vaniero G, Maloney J, Rashidi R, Mccowan R, Castle L, Morant V, Wilkoff B, Simons T. The effects of percutaneous cathter ablation on preexisting permanent pacemakers. PACE 1990;13:1637-45.
3. Gould L, Chandrakandt P, Betzu R. Pacemaker failure following electrocautery. Clin Prog Pacing Electrophysiol 1986;4:53-5.
4. Adamec R, Haefliger JM, Kllisch JP, Niederer J, Jaquet P. Damaging effect of therapeutic radiation on programmable pacemakers. PACE 1982;5:146-50.
5. Lasala AF, Fieldman A, Diana DJ, Humphrey CB. Gas pocket causing pacemaker malfunction. PACE 1979;2:183-5.
6. Kreis DJ, LiCalzi L, Shaw RK. Air entrapment as a cause of transient cardiac pacemaker malfunction. PACE 1979;2:641-44.
7. Gelder BM van, Bracke FALE, El Gamal MIH. Adapter failure as a cause of pacemaker malfunction. PACE 1993;16:1961-5.
8. Bracke F, Gelder B van. Treatment of perforation and cardiac tamponade in the chronic phase after implantation of a tined ventricular lead. Neth J Cardiol 1993;6:128 (abstract).
9. Gelder LM van, El Gamal MIH, Tielen CHJ. Long term follow up of myocardial screw-in electrodes. PACE 1989;12:1201 (abstract).
10. Snow N. Acute myocardial ischemia during pacemaker implantation: Implication for threshold determination and potential complications. PACE 1983;6:35-7.
11. Aylward P, Blood R, Tonkin A. Complications of defibrillation with permanent pacemaker in situ. PACE 1979;2:462-4.
12. Palac RT, Hwang MH, Klondnycky ML, Loeb Hs. Delayed pulse generator malfunction after D.C. countershock. PACE 1981;4:163-7.
13. Dohrmann ML, Goldschlager N. Metabolic and pharmacological effects on myocardial stimulation threshold in patients with cardiac pacemakers. In SS Barold (Ed.). Modern Cardiac Pacing. Mount Kisco, New York, USA. Futura Publishing Company, 1985, p 162-166.
14. Irnich W. Interference in pacemakers. PACE 1984;7:1021-47.
15. Levine PA, Balady GJ, Lazar HL, Belott PH, Roberts AJ. Electrocautery and pacemakers: Management of the paced subject to electrocautery. Ann Thoracic Surg 1986;41:313-7.
16. Toivonen L, Valjus J, Hongisto M, Metso R. The influence of elevated 50 Hz electric and magnetic fields on implanted cardiac pacemakers: The role of the lead configuration and programming of the sensitivity. PACE 1991;14:2114-22.
17. Marco D, Eisinger G, Hayes DL. Testing of work environments for electromagnetic interference. PACE 1992;15:2016-22.
18. Gelder LM van, El Gamal MIH, Tielen CHJ. P wave sensing in VVI pacemakers: Useful or a problem ? PACE 1988;11:1413-8.
19. Gelder BM van, Bracke FALE, El Gamal MIH. P wave oversensing in a unipolar VVI pacemaker. PACE 1995;18;370-3.
20. Wirtzfeld A, Lampadius M, Ruprecht EO. Unterdruckung von Demand-Schrittmachern durch Muskelpotentiale. Dtsch Med Wochenschr 1972;97:61-6.
21. Breivik K, Ohm OJ. Myopotential inhibition of unipolar QRS-inhibited (VVI) pacemakers, assessed by ambulatory Holter monitoring of the electrocardiogram. PACE 1980;3:470-8.
22. El Gamal M, Gelder B van. Suppression of an external demand pacemaker by diaphragmatic myopotentials: A sign of electrode perforation? PACE 1979;2:191-5.
23. Gelder LM van, El Gamal MIH, Bracke FALE. Are bipolar systems prone to oversensing at high sensitivity setting? PACE 1991;14:1991 (abstract).

24. Berger R, Jacobs W. Myopotential inhibition of demand pacemakers: Etiology, diagnostic, and therapeutic considerations. PACE 1979;2:596-602.
25. Waxman HL, Lazarra R, El-Sherif N. Apparent malfunction of demand pacemakers due to spurious potentials generated by contact between two endocardial electrodes. PACE 1978;1: 531-4.
26. Gelder LM van, El Gamal MIH. False inhibition of an atrial demand pacemaker caused by an insulation defect in a polyurethane lead. PACE 1983;6:834-9.
27. Warnowicz MA, Goldschlager N. Apparent failure to sense (undersensing) caused by oversensing: Diagnostic use of a noninvasively obtained intracardiac electrogram. PACE 1983;6:1341-3.
28. Falkoff M, Ong LS, Heinle RA, Barold SS. The noise sampling period: A new cause of apparent sensing malfunction of demand pacemakers. PACE 1978;1:250-53.
29. Gelder LM van, El Gamal MIH. Undersensing in VVI pacemakers detected by Holter monitoring. PACE 1988;11:1507-11.
30. Barold SS, Ong LS, Heinle RA. Demand pacemakers: Normal and abnormal mechanisms of sensing. In: Samet P and El-Sherif N (Eds), Cardiac Pacing. Grune & Stratton, New York, 1980, p 559.
31. Sarmiento. Clinical utility of telemetered intracardiac electrograms in diagnosing a design dependent lead malfunction. PACE 1990;13:188-95.
32. Bornzin G, Stokes K. The electrode-biointerface: sensing. In: Barold SS (Ed.): Modern Cardiac Pacing, Futura Publishing Company, Mount Kisco, New York, 1985, p 79.
33. Beek GJ van, Dulk K den, Lindemans FW, Wellens HJJ. Detection of insulation failure by gradual reduction in noninvasively measured electrogram amplitudes. PACE 1986;9:772-5.
34. Driller J, Barold SS, Parsonnet V. Normal and abnormal function of the pacemaker magnetic reed switch. J Electrocardiol 1976;9:283-8.
35. Gelder BM van, Mechelen R van, Dulk K den, El Gamal MIH. Apparent P wave undersensing in a DDD pacemaker post exercise. PACE 1992;15:1651-6.
36. Byrd CL, Schwartz SJ, Gonzales M, Ciraldo RJ, Yahr WZ, Sivina M, Greenberg JJ. Rate responsive pacemakers and cross talk. PACE 1988;11:798 (abstract).
37. Combs WJ, Reynolds SJ, Shrama AD, Bennett TD. Cross talk in bipolar pacemakers. PACE 1989;12: 1613-21.
38. Barold SS, Ong LS, Falkoff MD, Heinle RA. Cross talk or selfinhibition in dual chamber pacemakers. In: Barold SS (Ed.), Modern cardiac pacing. Futura Publishing Company, Mount Kisco, New York, 1985, p 618.
39. Levine PA, Mace RC. Assessment and management of cross talk. In: Pacing Therapy: A guide to cardiac pacing for optimum hemodynamic benefit. Futura Publishing Company, Mount Kisco, New York, 1983, pp 239-251.
40. Mechelen R van, 't Hart C, Boer H de. Failure to sense P waves during DDD pacing. PACE 1986;9:498-502.

3 PREVENTION OF PACEMAKER COMPLICATIONS

Chapter 9

Cardiac Arrhythmias and the Interaction with Pacemakers

Luc Jordaens

Introduction

Pacemakers were initially designed to treat bradyarrhythmias. Later, the medical community realized the importance of pacemaker therapy in relation to 'sudden death'. This was probably due to the fact that pacing in patients with heart block and sinus node disease prevented ventricular tachyarrhythmias in some of the patients. Therefore, modern pacemakers can be important as well as effective instruments in the treatment of tachyarrhythmias. However, as is well known from antiarrhythmic drugs, pacemakers can be arrhythmogenic, and they can cause arrhythmias in certain conditions. This was already recognized in the fixed rate (VOO) pacemaker and was an important stimulus to develop the ventricular demand pacemaker, which responds to the electrical activity of the heart, and avoids asynchronous pacing.[1]

Table 1. **Pacemakers and (Tachy-)Arrhythmias**

- Prevention of arrhythmias
- Termination of arrhythmias
- Provocation or aggravation of arrhythmias
  - by interaction with the substrate
  - by the pacing system
- Coping with arrhythmias
- Interference with arrhythmia treatment
- Interpretation of arrhythmias

In this chapter we will try to describe how pacemakers can cause arrhythmias, and how arrhythmias and anti-arrhythmic therapy interfere with normal pacemaker function (Table 1). Preventive pacing and antitachycardia pacing (ATP) are beyond the scope of this study. ATP is a potentially important feature of cardiac stimulation. The advances in ablative interventions have limited the application of this technology to acute and complex situations.[2] Some indications for ATP still exist. Therefore ATP should possibly be incorporated in permanent pacemakers. Nevertheless,

ATP can also cause arrhythmias. It seems that e.g. atrial flutter is not infrequent in patients after DDD implantation.[3] We and others observed in the past that atrial fibrillation occurred in at least one third of the patients with conventional indications for ATP.[2]

However, these mechanisms of proarrhythmia caused by pacing, such as acceleration, degeneration, etcetera, will not be discussed further in this study. We now have implantable cardioverter-defibrillators (ICD's) with ATP facilities for the treatment of potentially lethal ventricular arrhythmias. We have experienced that these devices, which are implanted as pacemakers transvenously, have some proarrhythmic features which are also common to pacemakers. We will discuss these complications which are clearly due to the pacing dysfunction of such devices.

It can be anticipated that some parts of the discussion will be redundant, as the interaction of a pacemaker with an arrhythmia is sometimes very complicated, and several explications at different levels can be necessary to explain a single problem. The mechanism of these arrhythmias can be related to an interaction of substrate and both hardware and software of the pacemaker (figure 1). Furthermore, arrhythmias can occur at both the atrial and the ventricular level, or result from the integration of information from both levels in the pacemaker. Whether the underlying technical error is a pacing or sensing malfunction, or a consequence of both, the basic electrophysiological mechanisms often remain the same, and correction at the level of the latter (i.e. correction of electrolyte disturbances, ischaemia, antiarrhythmic treatment or reposition of an electrode) is sometimes more important than reprogramming the pacemaker. However, a clear understanding of the pacemaker function and programming remains a prerequisite in the inevitable trouble-shooting.

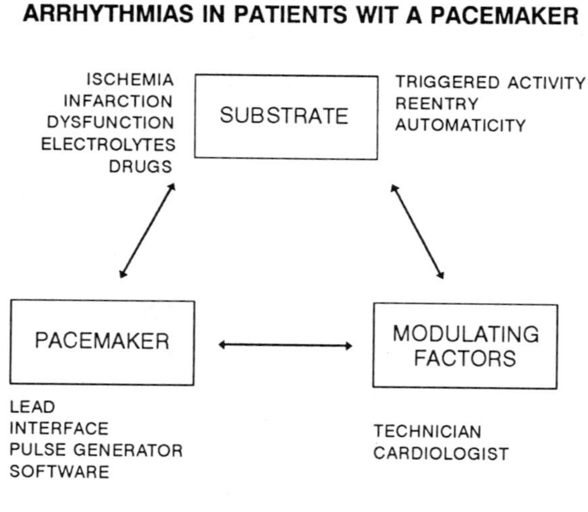

Figure 1. *Substrate, triggering and modulating factors in the pathogenesis of arrhythmias after implantation of a pacemaker. We propose to identify as many of the underlying factors before correction of the problem.*

Arrhythmias Due to Interaction of the Substrate and the Pacemaker System

Pacemaker implantation itself, normal or abnormal pacemaker function and erroneous programming can provoke arrhythmias. Figure 1 illustrates how arrhythmias occur by an interaction of several factors. As for all arrhythmias, triggering and modulating factors can be identified. An overview of interaction related problems is given in table 2.

Mechanically Induced Arrhythmias

It is very uncommon to provoke life threatening events during pacemaker implantation. In contrast, atrial fibrillation occurred several times in our experience, just by introducing a J-shaped atrial lead. Most cardiologists have also experienced this event while using temporary catheters during routine electrophysiology studies.[4] On the other hand, it is common to observe asymptomatic ventricular arrhythmias in the first few days after a pacemaker implantation. It is believed that the positioning of the catheter and its movement over the tricuspid valve plays an important role in the genesis of such arrhythmias. Furthermore, it can be assumed that triggered activity arising in valvular cells contributes to these arrhythmias.[5]

Table 2. **Arrhythmias Due to Interaction of Substrate and Pacemaker System**

- Caused by mechanical factors or interaction at the interface electrode-myocardium
- Caused by pacing or pacing failure
  - failure to pace (noncapture by various reasons)
  - slow pacing
  - hysteresis
  - fast pacing
  - inappropriate rate response
  - competitive pacing
  - asynchronous pacing
- Caused by disturbances in sensing
  - undersensing
  - oversensing
- Caused by AV mismatch
  - absence of AV synchrony due to stimulation or inhibition at one level causes arrhythmias at the other level
- Caused by AV harmony
  - presence of AV synchrony with
    - ·· pacing as the cause of other arrhythmias
    - ·· sensing as the cause of inhibition or asystole

The right ventricular apex is the conventional site for electrode placement, and it is suspected that other sites, e.g. the right ventricular outflow tract, are more arrhythmogenic (figure 2). Arrhythmias of this genesis usually do not lead to serious events, but could eventually explain the high incidence of ventricular tachyarrhythmias in patients with a substrate for sudden death early after implan-

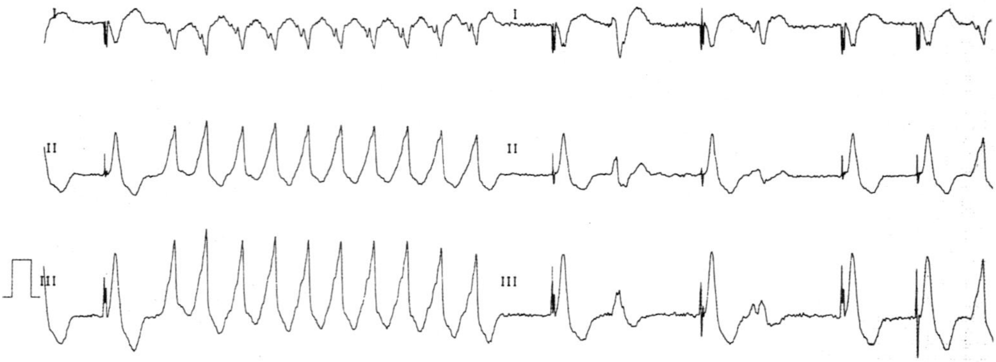

Figure 2. *Short ventricular tachycardia, with left bundle branch block morphology and inferior axis, initiated by pacing in the right ventricular outflow tract in a patient with complex congenital heart disease. The paced complex has the same morphology as the subsequent ventricular complexes, indicating that the origin of the arrhythmias is located near the electrode tip.*

tation of a transvenous ICD.[6] An exacerbation of asymptomatic spontaneous arrhythmias in patients receiving a pacemaker can trigger a subsequent reentrant tachycardia when a substrate is present. Therefore, extended hospitalization is advocated by patients with organic heart disease after implantation of a device.

Arrhythmias and the Interface of Electrode and Myocardium

The interaction between the electrode tip and the myocardium is not completely understood, but the Minute trauma during implantation can certainly cause microreentrant phenomena that initiate arrhythmias. Apart from biological effects, electrical phenomena can play a role at the interface. It is thought that cathodal pacing is less arrhythmogenic than anodal pacing, the anodal pacing with the pacing electrode positive, relative to the indifferent electrode. Anodal pacing is possible with shorter coupling intervals than cathodal pacing, and this might explain some arrhythmias.[7] The clinical importance of anodal pacing and what can happen in some conditions is not known.[8] It is unlikely that high output stimulation alone, with a correctly positioned catheter provokes more arrhythmias than stimulation at twice the diastolic threshold.[9]

Arrhythmias Caused by Pacing or Pacing Failure

Regular pacing can protect against arrhythmias caused by abnormal automaticity, reentry or triggered automaticity. Torsades de pointes is a typical example. From a clinical point of view, regular pacing protects against accelerated ventricular arrhythmias during exercise.[10] Rate responsive pacing could therefore play a role in prevention of exercise related death in patients with a pacemaker. The importance of reliable and relatively fast pacing immediately after His bundle ablation was demonstrated recently by several groups.[11,12] Whether the possibility of torsades de pointes persists during long-term follow-up is not known.

▸ *Pacing failure.* All mechanisms interfering with the maintenance of regularity can trigger arrhythmias under certain conditions. Pauses, hysteresis, slow pacing, failure to pace for various reasons such as metabolic disturbances and anti-arrhythmic drugs can be sufficient to initiate a reentrant tachycardia or to reveal a spontaneous cardiac pacemaker activity that was otherwise suppressed by the pacemaker.

▸ *Fast pacing.* Fast pacing might induce arrhythmias e.g. by enhancing triggered activity in the presence of digitalis toxicity.[13]

▸ *Competitive or asynchronous pacing.* Asynchronous pacing occurs when normal sensing is disturbed, and reentrant arrhythmias may be triggered by stimulation in the vulnerable period. Similarly, arrhythmias can arise when during the electrophysiology study or the pacemaker implantation, the pacemaker and the ICD compete (figures 3 and 4).

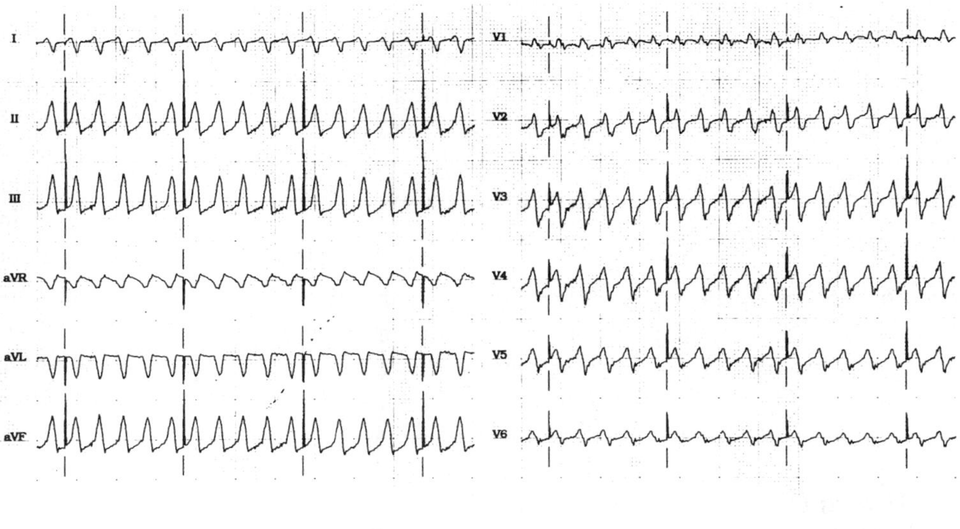

Figure 3. *Undersensing of ventricular tachycardia by a VVI pacemaker in a patient with dilated cardiomyopathy.*

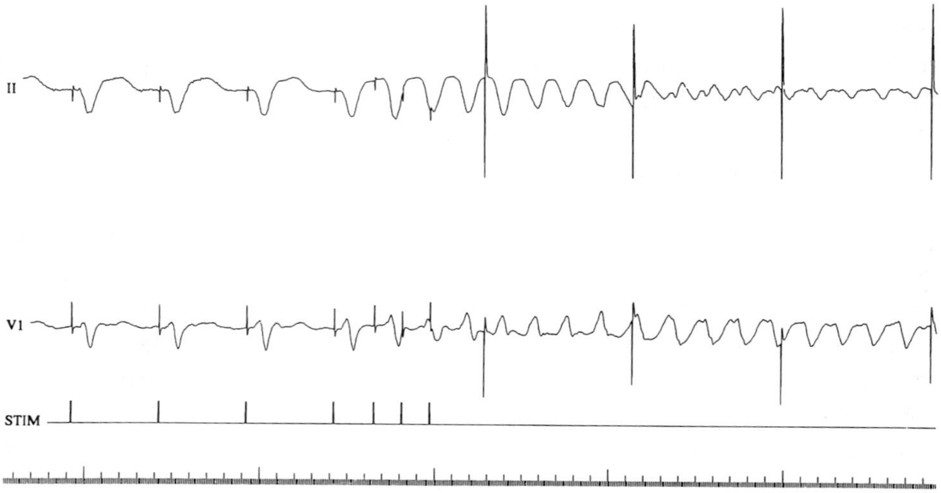

Figure 4. *Programmed electrical stimulation. After premature stimuli (S1S4) tachycardia is induced. This is not sensed by the unipolar VVI pacemaker, accelerating the arrhythmia with its second spike, hereby degenerating the tachycardia to fibrillation (same patient as in figure 3). The stimulus channel (STIM) shows when stimuli were given by the external pacemaker.*

Arrhythmias Caused by Sensing or Sensing Failure

Both bipolar and unipolar pacing systems are prone to sensing problems. However, it is generally accepted that bipolar configurations are more reliable in this respect, and will less often cause sensing problems. On the other hand, bipolar leads are more vulnerable and their long-term reliability is not so clearly demonstrated.[14] Sensing problems can be avoided by carefully measuring intracardiac electrograms at the time of implantation and by selecting other sites for the lead when the initial site is not reliable. However, changes in the substrate may occur due to infarction or metabolic changes.

▸ *Absence of sensing and undersensing.* Asynchronous or competitive pacing can happen during magnet application or when the programmed sensitivity is too low. Pacing may occur in the relative refractory period or in the supernormal phase of the action potential. This may cause atrial and ventricular tachyarrhythmias that could initiate ventricular flutter and fibrillation.

▸ *Oversensing.* Pauses may be harmful, as they can trigger escape rhythms, which may be atrial or ventricular tachyarrhythmias as well as slow escape rhythms. It is not unlikely that such a mechanism is present in some cases of sudden cardiac death after pacemaker implantation, especially when a dilated cardiomyopathy is the underlying disease.[15] Pauses may occur by inhibition of pacing by external or internal sources of interference. Myopotentials, external magnetic fields, diathermy, and medical technology in general are well known causes of pacemaker inhibition.

Arrhythmias Caused by Atrioventricular Mismatch

Information and events from both atrial and ventricular levels can be conflicting, and pacing may become arrhythmogenic because a pacemaker cannot respect the normal atrial and ventricular sequencing while receiving, technically speaking, the correct information. This technical interaction can be undesirable from the electrical or hemodynamical point of view, and such a situation can therefore be considered as 'atrioventricular mismatch'.

An inappropriate pacing mode, such as VVI for the sick sinus syndrome, is an example. In this condition, retrograde conduction with abnormal atrial activation primarily caused by ventricular stimulation, can cause atrial arrhythmias. This is probably the reason for an increased incidence of atrial fibrillation in sick sinus syndrome patients treated with VVI.[16]

The association of antegrade conduction delay and the presence of retrograde conduction with reentrant junctional arrhythmias is another example. This may cause pacemaker bigeminy with important hemodynamic repercussions. The programming of long refractory periods or the presence of a long blanking period in two-chamber pacemakers promotes AV mismatching and can be associated with an increased incidence of arrhythmias, not recognized at the level where they should be sensed. We observed how a long PVARP was associated with high ventricular rates during atrial flutter.[17] As only every second flutter wave was sensed, this arrhythmia is also to be considered as AV mismatch. Specialized algorithms to recognize ventricular premature beats with subsequent programming of synchronous atrial stimulation can also provoke similar arrhythmias when AV synchrony is not respected.[18]

Arrhythmias Caused by Attempted Atrioventricular Harmony

In contrast to the former, synchronization between both levels can be successful, but can also cause arrhythmias. Some cases of pacemaker mediated tachycardia are an example of AV harmony. Tracking of supraventricular arrhythmias can cause fast pacing at the ventricular level in normal VDD, DDD or DDDR pacemakers.[19] This also occurs when noise is sensed at the atrial level. Both mechanisms may result in a 'pseudo endless loop tachycardia'.[20] In patients with a substrate for arrhythmias, fast ventricular pacing because of such sensed events can induce serious rhythm disturbances (figure 5). Cross talk is the result of sensing by the ventricular channel with subsequent inhibition of atrial spikes.[21] In the presence of conduction disease, this can result in inappropriate bradycardia, due to ventricular pacing inhibition, with asystole.

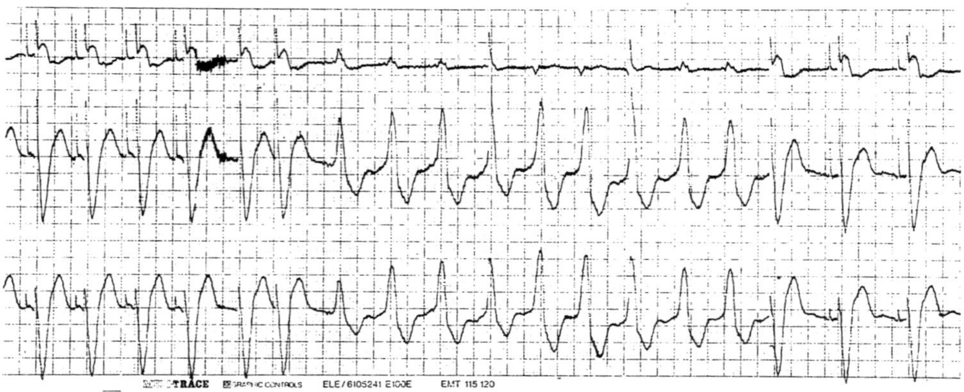

Figure 5. *Short ventricular tachycardia after reprogramming (noise) of a DDD pacemaker, in a patient with sinus node disease, treated with amiodaron for sustained ventricular tachycardia. The tachycardia terminates with atrial synchronous ventricular pacing, followed by dual-chamber pacing.*

Arrhythmias Due to Problems Related to the Pacemaker Alone

It is possible that normal function or dysfunction of a pacemaker in the presence of a normal substrate, can initiate arrhythmias (Table 3). In these instances, the response of the myocardium is always modulated by its own properties such as refractory periods, susceptibility for ventricular arrhythmias and ischemia.

Table 3. **Arrhythmias Caused by Pacemaker Function**

- *Dysfunction*
  - runaway
    - .. intrinsic (component failure)
    - .. extrinsic cause
- *Normal function*
  - electronic circus movement tachycardia
    - .. orthodromic
    - .. antidromic
  - sensor mediated tachycardia
    - .. interference by noise
    - .. positive feedback (activity, QT, temperature)

Runaway Pacemakers

Today it has become very uncommon to observe a runaway pacemaker. Runaway may occur with fixed rate pacing but it is also a possibility with modern pacemakers. The rate is usually regular, and often the output is insufficient to capture the myocardium (figure 6). Electrocautery and external equipment can cause runaway, but component failure due to leakage of body fluids in the pacemaker was the most frequent cause of this arrhythmia.[22]

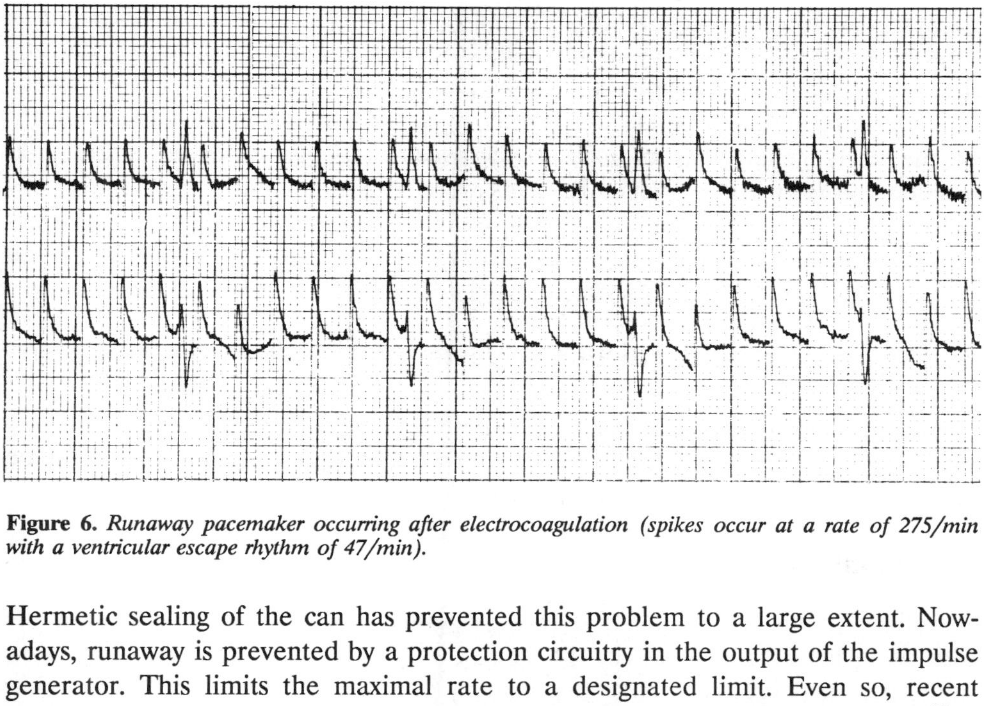

Figure 6. *Runaway pacemaker occurring after electrocoagulation (spikes occur at a rate of 275/min with a ventricular escape rhythm of 47/min).*

Hermetic sealing of the can has prevented this problem to a large extent. Nowadays, runaway is prevented by a protection circuitry in the output of the impulse generator. This limits the maximal rate to a designated limit. Even so, recent incidents of runaway pacemakers have been reported with a high fatality rate.[23]

Pacemaker Mediated Tachycardia

Pacemaker mediated tachycardia (PMT), endless loop tachycardia, and electronic or artificial circus movement tachycardia were a major obstacle in the early years of VDD and DDD pacing.[20] PMT is basically initiated when retrogradely conducted P waves are sensed and when normal ventricular pacing follows after the programmed AV interval. The pacing rate is usually at the programmed upper rate. However, other sensed events such as myopotentials, flutter waves, noise and external signals can also be responsible for fast ventricular pacing. These arrhythmias are often also called PMT but are in fact examples of interaction of pacemaker and environment. Modern dual-chamber pacemakers can usually prevent and, when required, terminate conventional PMT.[24] This electronic arrhythmia was no matter of concern in surveys of our population.[3,25]

Sensor Mediated Pacemaker Tachycardia

Correct interpretation of sensor information by inappropriate signals can also trigger symptomatic rate increase.[26] This has been described for various sensors such as activity sensing while patients drive a car. Some tachycardias cause a positive feedback on the sensor input (QT shortening) and maintain in this way the tachycardia. An occasional interaction between arrhythmias and sensor function is termination of the arrhythmia by sensor activation with fast pacing.[27] In the early generations of QT driven pacemakers we observed a potential problem, as ventricular premature beats were sometimes not sensed when they fell in the QT sensing window. This was eliminated in later generations. Information to the ventricular sensor from the atrial rate identified by a third sensor, can be used to terminate PMT ('sensor cross-checking').

The Influence of Antiarrhythmic Treatment on Pacemaker Behaviour

Pacemaker behaviour is influenced by both pharmacologic and nonpharmacologic therapy. While the effects of antiarrhythmic drugs are reversible, some physical effects of electrical therapies may cause permanent pacemaker damage.

Drugs and Sensing

Antiarrhythmic drugs, and to a lesser extent ß-blocking agents, may alter the rate of tachycardia, and affect the quality of electrograms.[28] Some drugs slow intra-atrial and intraventricular conduction. This may affect the upstroke (slew rate) of the atrial or ventricular electrogram, and therefore cause undersensing. Changes in atrioventricular conduction or in the repolarization may be important with respect to sensing whereas interactions with refractory period and blanking window are not impossible. T wave sensing is not uncommon, certainly not in defibrillators which often automatically adjust sensitivity to high levels, and can also be influenced by antiarrhythmic drugs.

Drugs and Pacing

Class Ic drugs (encainide, flecainide, propafenone) increase the threshold for stimulation. This can render efforts to terminate tachycardia by useless pacing,

→ **Figure 7.** *Ventricular fibrillation in a patient with an implanted (unipolar) VVI pacemaker, during implantation of an ICD. Undersensing of ventricular fibrillation by the unipolar pacemaker. After the shock, exit block occurs during four seconds. After a bipolar paced complex with ventricular capture (given by the ICD), one more spike of the unipolar pacemaker is not followed by ventricular activation, but thereafter normal pacing resumes. Same patient as in figure 3. The pacemaker was removed after the ICD implantation.*

and has important consequences for patients who need bradycardia support.[28,29]

Drugs and Antitachycardia Pacing

Drugs may adversely affect the efficacy of ATP because they may decrease the excitable gap in the reentry circuit.[30] Furthermore, besides the described loss of capture, drugs can render ATP ineffective by altering the cycle length of the tachycardia, bringing the rate below the selected criterium for ATP intervention.[30]

Cardioversion and Defibrillation

Defibrillation can cause changes at the interface of electrode and the myocardium, but also damage to circuitry and software of devices.[31] This may result in acute elevation of the pacing thresholds, sensing problems, runaway and end-of-life behaviour. Less serious are reprogrammings to another pacing mode or interference with sensor systems. These can be permanently damaged as well. Unipolar systems are more vulnerable than bipolar systems. It is advisable to have a temporary pacemaker in standby when a cardioversion is performed on a patient with a pacemaker. It is also desirable to program maximal output and sensitivity, and the device should be checked after the shocks. The same problems can occur when shocks from ICD's are given in patients with a pacemaker (figure 7).[28]

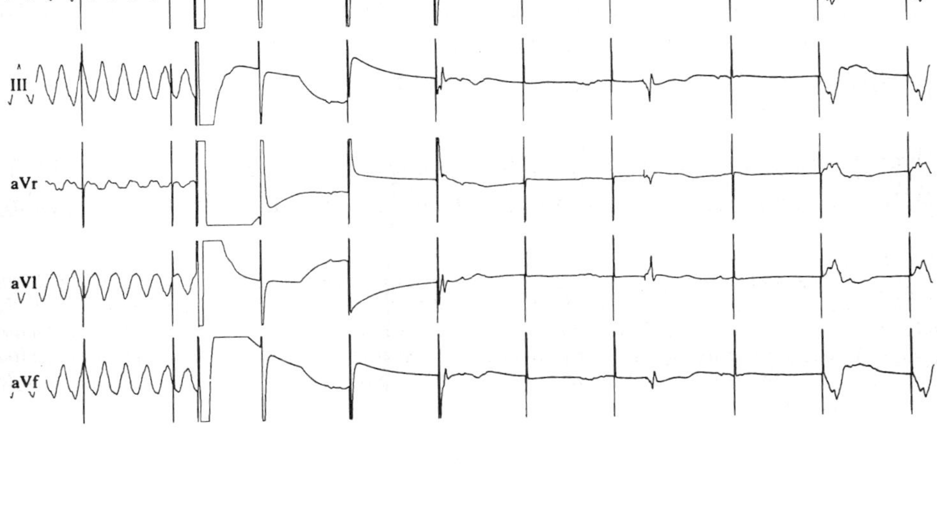

Radiofrequency Ablation

Electrocautery and radiofrequency ablation are similar energy sources.[33] Injury to the myocardium-electrode interface has been described as well as damage to microprocessors and circuitry. 'Deprogramming' to another pacing mode is a minor defect compared to the former disturbances. Animal data show that recently developed pacemakers are prone to interaction with radiofrequency energy.[34] If possible, it seems wise to avoid radiofrequency ablation when a patient already has a pacing system (figure 8). Reports that pacemakers are unharmed after ablation procedures should be considered as anecdotal.

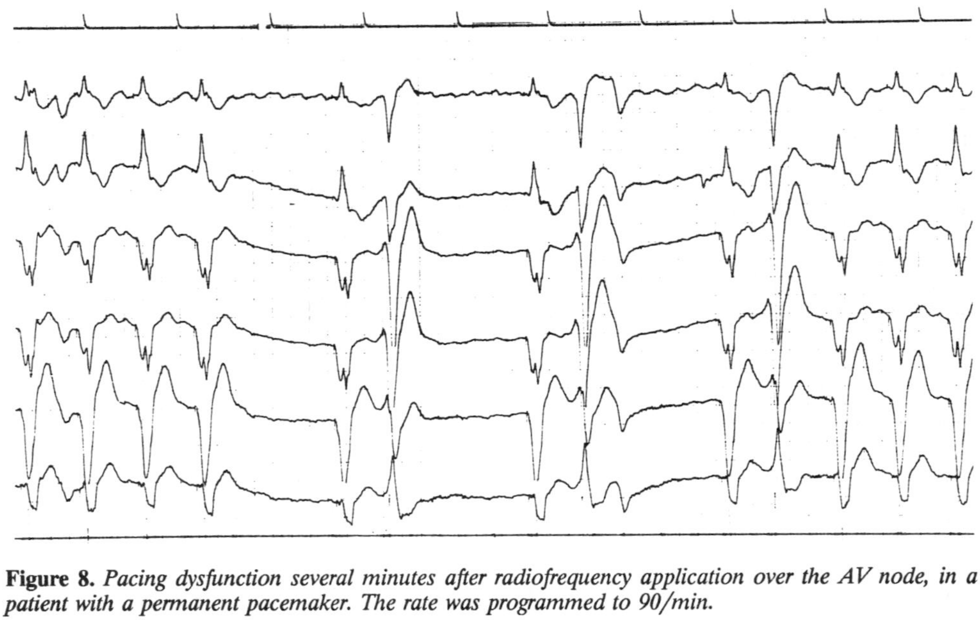

Figure 8. *Pacing dysfunction several minutes after radiofrequency application over the AV node, in a patient with a permanent pacemaker. The rate was programmed to 90/min.*

Algorithms to Modify the Impact of Spontaneous Arrhythmias

Algorithms can be conceived to minimize the deleterious effects on cardiac output of regular and irregular high rates in the atrium. In most cases these high rates are caused by atrial fibrillation[3], which cannot be treated by ATP, in contrast to atrial flutter. This can cause important problems for the selection of the optimal device: should priority be given to ATP when atrial flutter has been documented, or should 'mode switching' be preferred, as it is thought that atrial flutter usually progresses atrial fibrillation.[35] The possibilities of ablation of atrial flutter or preventive pacing are not always effective or available, reason why the described dilemma with the present available devices remains crucial.

Mode Switching

Some DDD pacemakers revert to VVI pacing when atrial arrhythmias are recognized, or gradually lower the pacing rate (fallback).[36,37] The actual approach to maintain AV synchrony during sinus rhythm, and to achieve a maximal hemodynamic stability during supraventricular tachyarrhythmias is automatic adaptation of the stimulation mode to the changing status of the atria. This provides regular stimulation in the ventricle, also during atrial arrhythmias, and in the better scenario adapted to the hemodynamic needs of the patient.[38] The algorithm for this 'mode switching' should have sufficient sensitivity and specificity to cope with all situations such as emotion and exercise.[17] Several systems showed shortcomings, for example conversion to VVIR after atrial extrasystoles. Furthermore, fast resynchronization is necessary after return to sinus rhythm, and delay in resynchronization has been reported to provoke new arrhythmias by retrograde conduction. In our observation, atrial fibrillation was always detected, but in some cases atrial flutter was causing problems because every second f wave coincided with the post ventricular atrial refractory period of the pacemaker.[17]

'Preventive' Pacing

While prevention of arrhythmias by pacing seemed to be an important topic in the early eighties, much less attention was given to this subject at the end of the decade. Nevertheless, some algorithms that can modulate the heart rate in such a way that atrial fibrillation occurs less frequently in some patients than in patients without the algorithm, are now available. Recognition of isolated extrasystoles is necessary for proper functioning.[39] Therefore, this algorithm is responding to an arrhythmia and should not be considered strictly 'preventive'.

Interpretation of Cardiac Arrhythmias with Telemetered Electrograms

Pacing becomes very complex today. The interpretation of arrhythmias interacting with pacemaker functions can be simplified by several tools, implemented in simple or more sophisticated pacemaker systems.[40] Events can be clarified by telemetered data, namely numeric, with counters; graphic, in its most elementary form with marker channels; or in a sophisticated form, displaying a tracing that resembles an electrogram and is called an electrogram, even when it is reconstructed from numeric data. All these tools can be used to show on-line diagnostic information or can store information concerning a particular event. These functions become important to understand whether mode switching was properly used in a pacemaker (figure 9), and in particular whether antitachycardia func-

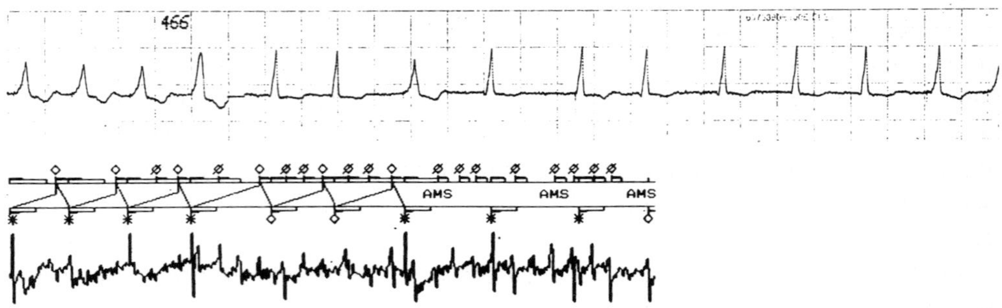

Figure 9. *Arrhythmia strip from a DDD pacemaker with print out of programmer (Meta 1254, Telectronics). Atrial fibrillation, with fusion beats in the ventricle. The upper channel of the printout with the ladder diagram indicates that mode switching (AMS) to VVI(R) occurred after an initial episod when P-waves were tracked. The lower strip with the on-line electrogram of the atrial lead clearly shows atrial fibrillation.*

tions were appropriately activated (ATP, shocks in ICD's). Storage of long segments consumes an enormous amount of energy. Therefore, some companies preferred to show snapshots of a few seconds, rather than complete rhythm strips from the seconds before and after the shock. These electrograms became important features to understand more of the mechanisms and triggers involved in the pathogenesis of ventricular arrhythmias (figure 10).[41] Reprogramming to avoid shocks during atrial fibrillation and because of T wave or noise sensing

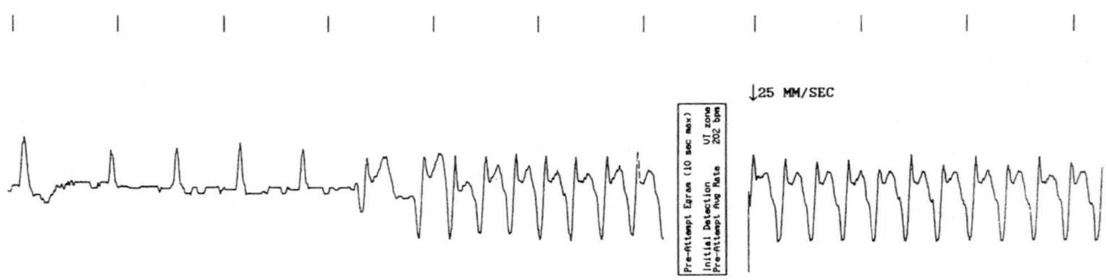

Figure 10. *Electrogram at initial detection of a monomorphic ventricular tachycardia. The arrhythmia is initiated by a late coupled ventricular premature beat (Ventak 1720).*

becomes easier.[42,43] Information on short arrhythmias can become useful to tailor antiarrhythmic drug therapy, and the effect of drug therapy can be assessed with stored data.

Conclusion

The problems caused by interaction of pacemakers and arrhythmias are numerous. Sudden death remains one of the most important mechanisms of death in patients with a pacemaker. Data in literature on proarrhythmia by pacemakers are scarce. Most information is anecdotal and not the result of a systematic study. Furthermore, when interactions are encountered, fast and correct troubleshooting is mandatory, and several simultaneous corrections of the environment and the substrate are performed.

In the post-CAST era, antiarrhythmic drugs became less and less important, but when these drugs are prescribed, they can cause sensing and pacing problems. The new antiarrhythmia technologies such as radiofrequency ablation, intracardiac cardioversion and defibrillation, will not be without drawbacks in this field. However, it can be anticipated that the advent of automatic reprogramming of output and sensitivity can already prevent excessive problems. The availability of stored data with high quality electrograms of events, which were not completely understood by the pacemaker, can be a help for the cardiologist in further problem solving. At least they show that the cardiologist is not completely redundant in the management of patients with a pacemaker.

References

1. Singer E, Gooch AS, Morse D. Exercise-induced arrhythmias in patients with pacemakers. J Am Med Ass 1974;244:1515-18.
2. Vertongen P, Van Wassenhove E, Jordaens L. Antitachycardia pacing for supraventricular tachycardia: limited long-term efficacy due to atrial fibrillation. Eur JCPE 1992;2:90-5.
3. Detollenaere M, Van Wassenhove E, Jordaens L. Atrial arrhythmias in dual-chamber pacing and their influence on long-term mortality. PACE 1992;15:1846-50.
4. Josephson ME. Electrophysiologic investigation: technical aspects. In: Josephson ME (ed.), Clinical cardiac electrophysiology. Philadelphia, Lea & Febiger, 1993, pp 5-21.
5. Rozanski G, Jalife J. Automatic activity in atrioventricular valve leaflets of rabbit heart. Am J Physiol 1986;250:H397-406.
6. Jordaens L. Specific use of antitachyarrhythmia device alternatives; the European perspective. Cardiol in the elderly 1994;2:560-6.
7. Orias O, Brooks C, Suckling EE, Gilbert JL, Siebens AA. The excitability of the mammalian ventricle throughout the cardiac cycle. Am J Physiol 1950;163:272-9.

8. Sutton R, Bourgeois I. What is a pacemaker? In: Sutton R, Bourgeois I (eds), The foundations of cardiac pacing: an illustrated practical guide to basic pacing. Futura Publishing Inc., Mount Kisco, 1991, pp 45-122.
9. Weissburg PL, Broughton A, Harper RW, Young A, Pitt A. Induction of ventricular arrhythmias by programmed electrical stimulation: A prospective study on the effects of stimulation current on arrhythmiua induction. Br Heart J 1987;58:489-94.
10. Jordaens L, Vandekerckhove Y, Van Wassenhove E, Clement DL. Does rate-responsive pacing suppress exercise-related ventricular arrythmias? Stimucoeur 1986;14:93-8.
11. Peters RH, Wever EF, Hauer RN, Wittkampf FH, Robles de Medina EO. Bradycardia-dependent QT-prolongation and ventricular fibrillation following catheter ablation of the atrioventricular junction with radiofequency energy. PACE 1994;17:108-12.
12. Jordaens L, Rubbens L, Vertongen P. Sudden death and long-term survival after His bundle ablation. Eur JCPE 1993;3:232-7.
13. Rosen MR, Reder RF. Does triggered activity have a role in the genesis of cardiac arrhythmias? Ann Int Med 981;94:794-801.
14. Breivik K, Ohm OJ, Engedal H. Long-term comparison of unipolar pacing and sensing, using a new multiprogrammable pacemaker system. PACE 1983;6:592-600.
15. Luu M, Stevenson WG, Stevenson LW, Baron K, Walden J. Diverse mechanisms of unexpected cardiac arrest in advanced heart failure. Circulation 1989;80:1675-80.
16. Rosenqvist M, Brandt J, Schüller H. Long-term pacing in sinus node disease: effects of stimulation mode on cardiovascular morbidity and mortality. Am Heart J 1988;116:16-22.
17. Provenier F, Jordaens L, Verstraeten T, Clement DL. The "Automatic Mode Switch Function" in successive generations of minute ventilation sensing dual chamber rate responsive pacemakers. PACE 1994;17:1913-19.
18. Heijer P den, Crijns HJ, Binsbergen EJ van, Ebels T, DeJongste MJ, Lie KI. Orthodromic pacemaker circus movement tachycardia. PACE 1987;10:955-7.
19. McCabe JB. Pacemaker-mediated tachycardia: Tracking of atrial fibrillation during DDD pacing. Ann Emerg Med 1986;15:83-5.
20. Barold SS. Repetitive reentrant and non-reentrant ventriculo-atrial synchrony in dual chamber pacing. Clin Cardiol 1991;14:754-63.
21. Brandt J, Fahraeus T, Schüller H. Far-field QRS complex sensing via the atrial pacemaker lead. II. Prevalence, clinical significance and possibility of intraoperative prediction in DDD pacing. PACE 1988;11:1540-4.
22. Gelder LM van, El Gamal MIH. Externally induced irreversible runaway pacemaker. PACE 1981;4:578-81.
23. Mickley H, Andersen C, Nieelsen LH. Runaway pacemaker: a still existing complication and therapeutic guidelines. Clin Cardiol 1989;12:412-4.
24. Dulk K den, Lindemans F, Wellens HJ. Management of pacemaker circus movement tachycardia. PACE 1984;7:346-55.
25. Jordaens L, Robbens E, Van Wassenhove E, Clement DL. Incidence of arrhythmias after atrial or dual-chamber pacemaker implantation. Eur Heart J 1989;10:102-7.
26. Lau CP. Sensors and pacemaker mediated tachycardias. PACE 1991;14:495-8.
27. Dulk K den, Brugada P, Wellens HJJ. Tachycardia termination with a rate-respoinsive pacemaker. Am J Cardiol 1987;59:1424-26.
28. Singer I, Guarnieri T, Kupersmith J. Implanted automatic defibrillators: effects of drugs and pacemakers. PACE 1988;11:2250-62.
29. Bianconi L, Boccadamo R, Toscano S, Serdoz R, Carpino A, Iesi AP, Altamura G. Effects of oral propafenone therapy on chronic myocardial pacing threshold. PACE 1992;15:148-54.
30. Fisher JD, Kim SG, Waspe LE, Matos JA. Mechanisms for the success and failure of pacing for termiation of ventricular tachycardia: clinical and hypothetical considerations. PACE 1983;1094-1105.

31. Naccarelli GV, Zipes DP, Rahilly GT, Heger JJ, Prystowsky EN. Influence of tachycardia cycle length and anti-arrhythmic drugs on pacing termination and acceleration of ventricular tachycardia. Am Heart J 1983;105:1-5.
32. Levine PA, Barold SS, Fletcher RD, Talbot P. Adverse acute and chronic effects of electrical defibrillation and cardioversion on implanted unipolar cardiac pacing systems. J Am Coll 1983;1:1413-22.
33. Caseau S, Theret D, Lascault G, Gougne G, Ritter P, Ripart A. Environnement et stimulation cardiaque définitive. Arch Mal Coeur 1992;85:77-81.
34. Chin MC, Rosenqvist M, Michael AL, Griffin JC, Langberg JJ. The effect of radiofrequency catheter ablation on permanent pacemakers: an experimental study. PACE 1990;13:23-9.
35. Dulk K den, Wylick AR van, Kersemakers J, Wellens HJJ. Do all pacemakers need both antibradycardia and antitachycardia features? Am J Cardiol 1985;55:593-4.
36. Mahaux V, Verboven Y, Waleffe A, Kulbertus H. Clinical interest of a sensor driven algorithm limiting ventricular pacing rate during supraventricular tachycardia in dual-chamber pacing. PACE 1992;15:1862-6.
37. Mayumi H, Uchida T, Shinozaki K, Matsui K. Use of a dual-chamber pacemaker with a novel fallback algorithm as an effective treatment for sick sinus syndrome associated with transient supraventricular tachyarrhythmia. PACE 1993;16:992-1000.
38. Lau CP, Tai YT, Fong PC, Li JPS, Chung FLW. Atrial arrhythmia management with sensor controlled atrial refractory period and automatic mode switching in patients with minute ventilation sensing dual chamber rate adaptive pacemakers. PACE 1992;15:1504-14.
39. Murgatroyd FD, Nitzsché R, Slade KB, Limousin M, Rosset N, Camm AJ, Ritter P, fot the Chourus Multicentre Study Group. A new pacing algorithm for overdrive suppression of atrial fibrillation. PACE 1994;17:1966-73.
40. Sarmiento JJ. Clinical utility of telemetered intracardiac electrograms in diagnosting a design dependent lead malfunction. PACE 1990;13:188-95.
41. Roelke M, Garan H, McGovern BA, Ruskin JN. Analysis of the initiation of spontaneous monomorphic ventricular tachycardia by stored intracardiac electrograms. J Am Coll Cardiol 1994;23:117-22.
42. Birgersdotter-Green U, Rosenqvist M, Lindemans FW, Rydèn L, Radegran K. Holter documented sudden death in a patient with an implanted defibrillator. PACE 1992;15:1008-114.
43. Jordaens L, Van Belleghem Y, Herregods L. Removal of endocardial defibrillation leads. PACE, in press.

4 MISCELLANEOUS ASPECTS

Chapter 10

Cardiac Stimulation as Nonpharmacological Treatment of Heart Failure

Patricia F.A. Bakker

Introduction

Heart failure constitutes a growing problem. The number of patients presenting with pump failure continues to increase due to progressive aging of the population and prevention of premature death by improved medical and nonpharmacological treatment, particularly of coronary artery disease, hypertension, valvular heart disease, and malignant ventricular tachyarrhythmias.

The clinical syndrome of heart failure is characterized by serious morbidity and impaired quality of life due to depressed myocardial function. Mortality rates are high in most series of patients with an advanced stage of heart failure.[1-4] Current treatment options for heart failure are summarized in Table 1. The mainstay of treatment is drug therapy. Despite the progress in pharmacological agents, a substantial number of patients still have moderate to severe drug-refractory symptoms. In a selected group of patients, myocardial function can be improved and symptoms reduced by percutaneous transluminal angioplasty, coronary artery bypass grafting, valve repair or replacement, left ventricular aneurysmectomy, or a combination of these treatment modalities. An even smaller subset of patients is eligible for heart transplantation. Recently two experimental therapies have made their entry into clinical practice: dynamic cardiomyoplasty and the application of assist devices. The latter have been generally used as bridge to transplant, but more recently also for permanent assist. The use of skeletal muscle ventricles for circulatory assistance, is still

Table 1. **Current Treatment Options in Heart Failure**

- Medication
- Percutaneous transluminal angioplasty
- Coronary artery bypass grafting
- Heart valve repair or replacement
- Cardiac transplantation
- Dynamic cardiomyoplasty
- Cardiac assist devices

confined to the experimental laboratory, but also shows promise for the future.

In view of the limited availability of donor hearts and the growing patient population with heart failure, there is a strong need for alternative therapeutic approaches.

Recent progress in cardiac pacing has focused on improvement of cardiac performance, also in patients with heart failure irrespective of its etiology. Pacing modalities devised to treat pump failure are summarized in Table 2.

Table 2. **Pacing Modalities to Treat Pump Failure**

- Rapid atrial pacing
- Dual-chamber pacing with short atrioventricular delay
- Septal short atrioventricular delay pacing
- Atrial synchronous biventricular pacing

The following paragraphs of this chapter will outline the background, results, specific indications, and future prospects of pacing as nonpharmacological treatment for heart failure.

Heart Failure and Cardiac Pacing: General Aspects

In patients with heart failure, various electrocardiographic abnormalities can be observed. Sinus bradycardia or sinus tachycardia can be present at rest. Prolongation of the PR interval and QRS complex are frequent findings. Several patients with resting sinus bradycardia show chronotropic incompetence during exercise, due to sinus node dysfunction or secondary to drug therapy.

The inability to appropriately increase heart rate with exercise limits exercise capacity due to insufficient increase in cardiac output to meet increased tissue demands for oxygen supply and removal of metabolites. In patients with dilated cardiomyopathy, an increase in cardiac output almost exclusively results from a rise in heart rate, since preload reserve is nearly exhausted.

Prolongation of the PR interval affects the timing of atrial systole in relation to ventricular systole. This can alter the contribution of atrial contraction to ventricular filling. In addition, early closure of the atrioventricular valves as well as atrioventricular valve regurgitation have been described.[5,6] In severe congestive heart failure, the diastolic filling period can be so short that stroke volume is limited. Presystolic atrioventricular valve regurgitation contributes to shortening of the effective diastolic filling period, and by itself reduces forward stroke volume. The presystolic component of mitral and tricuspid regurgitation is especially prominent in patients with prolonged atrioventricular conduction times.[7]

QRS duration is positively correlated with the duration of mitral regurgitation.[8] A prolonged QRS complex reduces peak dP/dt and prolongs overall duration of the pressure pulse, the time to peak rate of rise in pressure, and relaxation time. A coordinated pattern of contraction and relaxation is a prerequisite for optimal cardiac function. Depolarization and repolarization, contraction and relaxation are tightly coupled. An altered sequence of electrical activation results in changes in contraction and relaxation.

There is a growing understanding of mechanisms that play a role in heart failure and we are seeking for interventions that aim at preserving or restoring myocardial function. Artificial cardiac stimulation can be used to increase heart rate, to alter the temporal relation between atrial and ventricular contraction and to alter ventricular activation sequence.

Both in pacing for hypertrophic cardiomyopathy and in pacing for dilated cardiomyopathy basically the same concepts are used, but applied in a different manner. In hypertrophic cardiomyopathy, pacing is used to produce an abnormal activation pattern and to reduce the force of contraction of the myocardium while maintaining atrioventricular synchrony. Pacing for dilated cardiomyopathy is applied to optimize atrioventricular delay and restore ventricular activation sequence in order to improve contraction synchrony between the left and right ventricle.

Pacing in Hypertrophic Cardiomyopathy

Background

Hypertrophic cardiomyopathy is characterized by pronounced hypertrophy of the myocardium with a variable distribution pattern with regard to the extent and the site of hypertrophy. Disproportionate involvement of the interventricular septum is common. Systolic ventricular function is typically preserved, while diastolic function is depressed due to impaired relaxation and increased chamber stiffness.[9] Dynamic subaortic obstruction to left ventricular outflow is present in approximately 25% of patients.[10] The mechanism of dynamic left ventricular outflow obstruction is a systolic anterior motion of the anterior mitral leaflet, which is caused by a Venturi effect in the narrowed outflow tract and by anatomical anterior displacement of the subvalvular apparatus of the mitral valve.[11,12]

Hypertrophic cardiomyopathy has a significant morbidity and mortality. Clinical manifestations vary considerably, ranging from an asymptomatic status to severe dyspnea, heart failure, angina pectoris, palpitations, and syncope. The most common causes of mortality are arrhythmic sudden death and congestive heart failure.[13]

Medical treatment with beta-adrenergic blockers, calcium channel blockers, or disopyramide has been the therapy of choice for many years both in obstructive and nonobstructive hypertrophic cardiomyopathy. These medications aim at reducing oxygen demand, decreasing myocardial contractility, and correcting abnormal calcium kinetics to improve left ventricular relaxation and filling. Patients with subaortic obstruction who do not sufficiently respond to medication or develop side effects, can be surgically treated by transaortic septal myectomy to relieve left ventricular outflow tract obstruction. Mitral valve replacement is performed in the presence of serious structural mitral valve disease. Surgical skills, that are closely related to sufficient experience with septal myectomy, greatly determine success in reducing outflow tract gradient and preventing morbidity and mortality.[14]

Although medical and surgical treatment are successful in relieving symptoms in the majority of patients, a substantial number of patients remain symptomatic or develop side effects to medications. Particularly for these subgroups of patients, alternative therapies are needed.

Dual-chamber pacing with an atrioventricular delay that is sufficiently short to result in pre-excitation of the right ventricular apex ensures an altered ventricular activation sequence that causes the interventricular septum to move paradoxically during systole. Thereby, left ventricular outflow tract dimensions may increase, and blood flow velocity and the Venturi effect decrease. Systolic anterior motion of the anterior mitral leaflet is diminished concomitantly, which is associated with a decrease in mitral regurgitation and further relief of outflow tract obstruction. Another mechanism that may contribute to the reduction in subaortic gradient is the electrically induced impairment of contraction velocity and depressed force of contraction.[15] It has been postulated that dual-chamber pacing may as well exert a beneficial effect on diastolic ventricular function in hypertrophic cardiomyopathy.

Results of Dual-Chamber Pacing in Symptomatic Obstructive Hypertrophic Cardiomyopathy

Several studies show that dual-chamber pacing with a shortened atrioventricular delay improves exercise tolerance and clinical symptoms in patients with obstructive hypertrophic cardiomyopathy during short-term follow-up. Jeanrenaud *et al*, and Fananapazir *et al* reported an average acute reduction in peak pressure gradient of approximately 40 mmHg at the optimum atrioventricular interval.[16,17] During short-term follow-up (1.5 to 3 months), the gradient in patients from the study by Fananapazir *et al* was further reduced, concurrently with significant increase in cardiac output and systemic arterial pressures. In the series of Jeanrenaud, a further reduction of the gradient was observed at mid-term (mean: 11

months), and long-term follow-up (mean: 44 months). At mid-term follow-up, the pressure gradient during sinus rhythm was not reduced as compared to pre-implant baseline values, in contrast to the reduction in gradient of 36 mmHg at the end of follow-up. This was associated with a decrease in left ventricular ejection fraction in 4 of 7 patients. Also, there may be a component of ventricular remodelling, as suggested by enlargement of the ventricular cavity and decreased ejection fraction in some of these patients during long-term follow-up.

Results of Dual-Chamber Pacing in Symptomatic Nonobstructive Hypertrophic Cardiomyopathy

In 12 patients with hypertrophic cardiomyopathy without resting left ventricular outflow gradient, and a provocable gradient of <30 mmHg who were symptomatic despite drug treatment, a dual-chamber pacemaker was implanted and cardiac medications were stopped.[18] Approximately 4 months after initiation of dual-chamber pacing, significant improvement by at least one New York Heart Association (NYHA) functional class and increase in mean exercise duration from 6.8 to 8.5 minutes ($p=0.007$) was noted. However, hemodynamic parameters did not improve. These findings were believed to possibly reflect the beneficial effects of discontinuation of medications on functional capacity, rather than an effect of pacing. There was one death 3 months post-implantation, and one patient was lost to follow-up. During long-term (>1 year) follow-up, worsening of symptoms necessitated reinstitution of drug therapy in 6 out of 10 patients, and additionally, discontinuation of pacing in one patient.

In another combined series of 11 patients similar results were obtained.[19] A significant improvement in mean exercise duration from 7.69 to 10.05 minutes ($p=0.021$) was found at short-term (8 days) follow-up. Exercise tests were performed off drugs.

Indications and Prospects

It has been proposed that dual-chamber pacing should be tried before surgery in patients with obstructive hypertrophic cardiomyopathy who have drug-refractory symptoms.[17] Current results of transaortic septal myectomy compare favorably with those of previous reports: septal myectomy can now be performed with a very low mortality (<1.2%).[14,20,21] Mortality rates are higher in the aged and in those undergoing coronary artery bypass grafting or valve surgery.[22] After myectomy, there is a greater decrease in pressure gradient (87%) than has been achieved by dual-chamber pacing (56%), and the mean residual gradient is less with surgery (9 vs 38 mmHg). Mitral regurgitation, when severe, is usually significantly improved after myectomy alone.[20,23] The relatively high residual gradient with pacing may be an important marker for complications during follow-up, since a residual gradient >15 mmHg is an independent predictor of mortality after transaortic septal myectomy.[20] Moreover, a reduced annual mortality rate has been reported after septal myectomy as compared to medical treatment.[14] Before definitive conclusions can be drawn with regard to the preferred treatment modality in the individual patient with obstructive hypertrophic cardiomyopathy, further studies are needed to elucidate the precise mechanisms of the various therapeutic approaches, and to prospectively compare their impact on functional capacity, survival and potential arrhythmogenic effects.

It is concluded that implantation of a dual-chamber pacemaker in patients with nonobstructive hypertrophic cardiomyopathy and drug-refractory symptoms can as yet not be routinely recommended.

Rapid Atrial Pacing in Dilated Cardiomyopathy

Background

In patients with dilated cardiomyopathy and advanced congestive heart failure, the Frank-Starling curve is shifted to the right and is often relatively flat. Little decrease in stroke volume occurs with considerable decrease in end-diastolic volume. The latter is associated with decreased wall stress and improved myocardial perfusion.

The effect of rapid atrial pacing is explained by a decrease in diastolic filling period, thereby reducing end-diastolic volume and wall stress, and improving myocardial perfusion. The increased heart rate with rapid atrial pacing is expected to more than compensate for the reduction in stroke volume, and to result in increased cardiac output. A decrease in left ventricular size with rapid atrial pacing in patients with dilated cardiomyopathy, may also result in a decrease in secondary mitral and tricuspid regurgitation.

Results of Rapid Atrial Pacing

Several authors reported a decrease in left ventricular size and end-diastolic pressure as well as an increase in contractility with rapid atrial pacing in patients with coronary artery disease. However, Feldman and colleagues[27] demonstrated little or no improvement in systolic and diastolic ventricular function during atrial pacing tachycardia in 7 patients with idiopathic dilated cardiomyopathy and congestive heart failure (LVEF: 0.19 ± 0.11). A minimal increase in left ventricular peak filling rate and absence of a leftward shift of the end-systolic pressure-volume relationship, and minimal to absent downward shift of the diastolic pressure-volume relationship were found. Their results suggest a depression of both inotropic and lusitropic reserve. These findings are in agreement with two other studies in patients with dilated cardiomyopathy. Grossman and coworkers[28] observed depression of negative dP/dt and no increase in velocity of circumferential fiber lengthening or shortening during rapid atrial pacing. Erbel *et al*[29] observed no change in left ventricular end-systolic or end-diastolic volumes, whereas left ventricular ejection fraction was significantly reduced.

Indications and Prospects

There are no conclusive data supporting the hypothesis formulated by Iskandrian[30] that rapid atrial pacing is beneficial in patients with dilated cardiomyopathy. Moreover, rapid atrial pacing can only be applied in patients without sinus tachycardia at rest and severe coronary artery disease, since even a modest increase in heart rate may increase myocardial oxygen demand to such an extent as to cause myocardial ischemia. It is conceivable, though, that some patients with poor left ventricular function, sinus bradycardia at rest and compromised ability to increase heart rate during exercise could benefit from a rate-modulating atrial pacing system.

Dual-Chamber Pacing with Short Atrioventricular Delay

Background

Prolonged duration of ventricular depolarization in the dilated heart may create an unfavorable relationship between atrial and ventricular systole, due to the delay in onset of left ventricular contraction. Pacing with a relatively short atrioventricular interval (100 ms) may be beneficial by pre-exciting the ventricular apex to overcome the delay in apical activation caused by left ventricular dilatation. Thus atrioventricular synchrony is improved.[31] Since appropriate timing of atrial contraction is an important factor for left ventricular filling, especially during late diastole, dual-chamber pacing may improve ventricular filling in dilated cardiomyopathy. Also a reduction in regurgitation of the mitral and tricuspid valve is expected. Functional systolic and presystolic atrioventricular valve regurgitation may shorten the diastolic filling period to the extent that stroke volume is limited. Regurgitation can be diminished or abolished by improved atrioventricular synchrony.

From a theoretical point of view, potential adverse effects of right ventricular pacing in the VDD mode may be a limitation to its expected benefits. Cardiac pacing from the right ventricular apex is known to result in asynchronous ventricular contraction and relaxation sequences. Particularly onset of left ventricular contraction is delayed and interventricular septal motion is abnormal. Karpawich demonstrated a nearly normal pattern of ventricular emptying during septal pacing at or close to the His bundle in dogs with complete atrioventricular block.[32] By contrast, delayed ventricular emptying during apical pacing was found. Therefore, dual-chamber pacing with a short atrioventricular interval may be hemodynamically more beneficial when a stimulation site at the interventricular septum close to the His bundle is used, rather than at the right ventricular apex.

Results of Dual-Chamber Pacing with Short Atrioventricular Delay

Hochleitner *et al* studied 16 patients with end-stage idiopathic dilated cardiomyopathy.[31] A dual-chamber pacemaker was implanted with the ventricular lead positioned in the right ventricular apex. A short atrioventricular delay of 100 ms was programmed. During short-term follow-up (2 to 14 days), NYHA functional class improved from 3.6±0.4 to 2.1±0.5, cardiothoracic ratio decreased form 0.60±0.06 to 0.56±0.05. Tricuspid regurgitation diminished, mitral regurgitation reduced from grade 2.0±0.4 to 0.9±0.4, and left ventricular ejection fraction increased from 16±8.4 to 25.6±8.6%. Systolic and diastolic blood pressures also increased significantly. Clinical improvement persisted in 12 patients during a one-year observation period. Four patients died, 3 suddenly and 1 due to stroke. The long-term efficacy of this pacing therapy was evaluated by Hochleitner *et al*[33] in 17 patients with end-stage idiopathic dilated cardiomyopathy in a longitudinal study with up to 5 years of follow-up. The median survival time was 22 months, and 3 patients were alive after 5 years. The significant clinical and hemodynamic improvement observed in their previous study[31] persisted in most patients during follow-up or until death. Ten patients died during follow-up, and 4 underwent a cardiac transplantation. Death occurred suddenly in 9 patients, and the cause of death was a thromboembolic event in 4 of them, and unknown in the remaining 5 patients. One patient died from adenocarcinoma.

Brecker and colleagues[34] evaluated the acute effects of dual-chamber pacing at various short atrioventricular delays in 12 patients, using a temporary or a permanent pacing system. The etiology of heart failure was idiopathic dilated cardiomyopathy in 9 patients and ischemic heart disease in the other 3. The shortest programmable atrioventricular delay (6 to 31 ms) yielded optimal results. Mitral and tricuspid regurgitation became significantly shorter in duration and both left and right ventricular filling times became significantly longer, and concomitantly cardiac output increased. Presystolic mitral regurgitation was largely eliminated. A striking improvement in exercise duration was noted.

Auricchio *et al*[35] reported beneficial effects of atrial synchronous pacing with an atrioventricular delay of 100 ms on hemodynamics and clinical condition in 2 patients with end-stage congestive heart failure due to ischemic heart disease. Other studies on the effects of dual-chamber pacing at short atrioventricular delay in patients with congestive heart failure due to ischemic heart disease or nonischemic heart disease did not show a benefit.[36,37]

In the single clinical report on septal short atrioventricular delay pacing, acute hemodynamic data were obtained in 15 patients.[38] Left ventricular function was impaired due to ischemic heart disease (n=10) or nonischemic dilated cardiomyopathy (n=5). Mean left ventricular ejection fraction measured 0.32. During VDD pacing, delays of 50, 100, and 150 ms were tested. Two ventricular stimulation sites were compared: the right ventricular apex and the interventricular septum close to the His bundle. Cardiac output increased from 4.1 to 4.45 l/min (n.s.) during stimulation at the right ventricular apex, whereas septal stimulation resulted in an increase in cardiac output from 4.1 to 4.6 l/min ($p=0.037$). Both apical and septal pacing were associated with a significant increase in mean arterial blood pressure. The best results with both stimulation sites were obtained at atrioventricular delays of 50 and 100 ms.

Indications and Prospects

From the literature, inconclusive data are obtained with regard to the benefits and indications of dual-chamber pacing with a short atrioventricular delay. Nonetheless, promising results have been reported in several studies, showing significant improvement in hemodynamics and clinical condition both in patients with nonischemic and ischemic dilated cardiomyopathy, and severe congestive heart failure. Differing results may be explained by patient selection, and lacking knowledge of mechanisms of heart failure that play a role in the individual patient. Echocardiography is probably a valuable tool to assess some of these mechanisms and to select the optimal atrioventricular delay.

Biventricular Pacing

Background

Normal cardiac performance requires atrioventricular synchrony as well as synchronous ventricular contraction.[39] Several studies have shown that a normal contraction pattern is a prerequisite for preservation of both systolic and diastolic ventricular function. Atrioventricular and interventricular asynchrony may contribute to hemodynamic impairment in heart failure. Restoration of synchronous contraction of the right and left ventricle together with optimization of the atrioventricular delay may result in hemodynamic and clinical improvement in patients with heart failure due to dilated cardiomyopathy. Based upon these concepts a new pacing modality was recently introduced: atrial synchronous biventricular stimulation.[40] A dual-chamber pacemaker is implanted with an endocardial right ventricular and an epicardial left ventricular electrode for simultaneous stimulation of both ventricles. In addition, atrioventricular synchronization is optimized.

Results of Biventricular Pacing

Beneficial effects of biventricular pacing with short atrioventricular interval (100 ms) have been reported in 5 patients with end-stage congestive heart failure due to dilated cardiomyopathy.[40,41] All patients had a prolonged PR interval and a left-sided conduction delay. Preoperative left ventricular ejection fraction measured 0.05-0.23. Acutely, significant hemodynamic improvement was found. After 3 months follow-up, 4 patients had improved at least 1 NYHA functional class, the dose of furosemide was reduced in 3 of them by 340-625 mg, and left ventricular ejection fraction (mean±SD) increased by 0.8±0.2. Echocardiographic

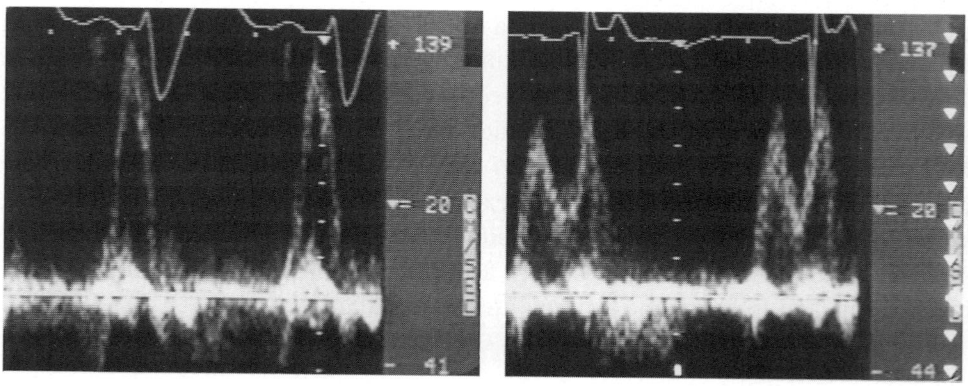

Figure 1. *Pulsed Doppler recordings of transmitral velocity pattern in a patient with end-stage dilated cardiomyopathy, at base line (left hand panel), and at 6 weeks after institution of permanent biventricular pacing (right hand panel). An increase in diastolic filling period from 150 ms (left panel) to 260 ms (right panel) is noted as well as a change in mitral flow velocity curve from a single filling wave to a separate E and A wave. Although Doppler measurements of ventricular filling are to some extent affected by changes in heart rate, the decrease in heart rate from 105 bpm (left panel) to 87 bpm does not sufficiently explain the significant increase in diastolic filling period.*

studies revealed an increase in diastolic filling period (figure 1) of 90±56 ms and 12±3 ml. The degree of mitral regurgitation decreased from severe to moderate in 2 patients. In 1 patient in whom capture of the left ventricle was lost during the third postoperative month, all variables relapsed to base line values. The effects of atrial synchronous biventricular pacing on functional capacity has been prospectively assessed in 6 patients with dilated cardiomyopathy.[42] Three months after pacemaker implantation, median NYHA functional class had significantly improved from 4 to 2.5. Peak bicycle exercise capacity significantly improved: mean peak oxygen uptake increased by 4.4 ml/min/kg, and anaerobic threshold by 3.8 ml/min/kg.

Indications and Prospects

The aforementioned data are preliminary, but the results are encouraging. The hemodynamic, echocardiographic and clinical observations suggest that this subset of patients has benefitted from biventricular pacing at short atrioventricular delay. Continuing collection and analysis of data will further reveal whether this pacing modality is also beneficial in the long term. In addition, specific indications need to be defined.

Acknowledgement

The contribution of H.W.J. Meijburg, MD, regarding the echocardiographic studies is gratefully acknowledged.

References

1. Saxon LA, Stevenson WG, Middelkauff HR, Fonarow G, Woo M, Moser D, Stevenson LW. Predicting death from progressive heart failure secondary to ischemia or idiopathic dilated cardiomyopathy. Am J Cardiol 1993;72:62-5.
2. Stevenson LW, Tillish JH, Hamilton M, Luu M, Chelimsky-Fallick C, Moriguchi J, Kobashigawa J, Walden J. Importance of hemodynamic response to therapy in predicting survival with ejection fraction <20% secondary to ischemic or nonischemic dilated cardiomyopathy. Am J Cardiol 1990;66:1348-54.
3. The consensus trial study group. Effects of enalapril on mortality in severe congestive heart failure. New Eng J Med 1987;316:1429-35.
4. Schocken DD, Arrieta MI, Leaverton PE, Ross EA. Prevalence and mortality rate of congestive heart failure in the United States. J Am Coll Cardiol 1992;20:301-6.
5. Mehta D, Gilmour S, Ward DE, Camm AJ. Optimal atrioventricular delay at rest and during exercise in patients with dual-chamber pacemakers: a non-invasive assessment by continuous wave Doppler. Br Heart J 1989;61:161-6.

6. Iwase M, Sotobata I, Yokota M, Takagi S, Jing HX, Kawai N, Hayashi H, Murase M. Evaluation by pulsed Doppler echocardiography of the atrial contribution to left ventricular filling in patients with DDD pacemakers. Am J Cardiol 1986;58:104-9.
7. Panidis IP, Ross J, Munley B, Nestico P, Mintz GS. Diastolic mitral regurgitation in patients with atrioventricular conduction abnormalities: a common finding by pulsed Doppler echocardiography and its association with complete heart block. Am J Cardiol 1986;57:692-4.
8. Xiao HB, Brecker SJD, Gibson DG. Effects of abnormal activation on the time course of the left ventricular pressure pulse in dilated cardiomyopathy. Br Heart J 1992;68:403-7.
9. Wigle ED. Impaired left ventricular relaxation in hypertrophic cardiomyopathy: Relation to the extent of hypertrophy. J Am Coll Cardiol 1990;15:814-5.
10. Pierce GE, Morrow AG, Braunwald E. Idiopathic subaortic stenosis: III. Intraoperative studies of the mechanism of obstruction and its hemodynamic consequences. Circulation 1964;30(suppl IV):IV-152-IV-213.
11. Wigle ED, Sasson Z, Henderson MA, Ruddy TD, Fulop J, Rakowski H, Williams WG. Hypertrophic cardiomyopathy. The importance of the site and the extent of hypertrophy: A review. Prog Cardiovasc Dis 1985;28:1-83.
12. Cape EG, Simons D, Jimoh A, Weyman AE, Yoganathan AP, Levine RA. Chordal geometry determines the shape and the extent of systolic anterior mitral motion: In vitro studies. J Am Coll Cardiol 1989;13:1438-48.
13. Shah PM, Adelman AG, Wigle ED, Gobel FL, Burchell FB, Hardarson L, Curiel R, Calzada CS de la, Oakley CM, Goodwin JF, Yu PN. The natural (and unnatural) history of hypertrophic obstructive cardiomyopathy: a multicenter study. Circ Res 1974;35(suppl II):II-179-II-195.
14. Ten Berg JM, Suttorp MJ, Knaepen PJ, Ernst JMPG, Vermeulen FEE, Jaarsma W. Hypertrophic obstructive cardiomyopathy. Initial results and long-term follow-up after Morrow septal myectomy. Circulation 1994;90:1781-5.
15. Duck HJ, Hutshenreiter W, Pankau H, Trenchmann R. Vorhofsynchrone Ventrikelstimulation mit verkurzter AV Verzögerungszeit als Therapieprinzip der hypertrophischen obstructiven Kardiomyopathie. Z Gesamte Inn Med 1984;39:437-47.
16 Jeanrenaud X, Goy J-J, Kappenberger L. Effects of dual-chamber pacing in hypertrophic obstructive cardiomyopathy. Lancet 1992;339:1318-23.
17. Fananapazir L, Cannom RO III, Tripodi D, Panza JA. Impact of dual-chamber pacing in patients with obstructive hypertrophic cardiomyopathy with symptoms refractory to verapamil and beta-adrenergic blocker therapy. Circulation 1992;85:2149-61.
18. Cannon RO III, Tripodi D, Dilsizian V, Panza JA, Fananapazir L. Results of permanent dual-chamber pacing in symptomatic nonobstructive hypertrophic cardiomyopathy. Am J Cardiol 1994;73:571-6.
19. McDonald K, McWilliams E, O'Keeffe, Maurer B. Functional assessment of patients treated with permanent dual-chamber pacing as primary treatment for hypertrophic cardiomyopathy. Eur Heart J 1988;9:893-8.
20. Mohr R, Schaff HV, Danielson GK, Puga FJ, Tajik AJ. The outcome of surgical treatment of hypertrophic obstructive cardiomyopathy: experience over 15 years. J Thorac Cardiovasc Surg 1980;97:666-74.
21. Cohn LH, Trehan H, Collins JJ Jr. Long-term follow-up of patients undergoing myotomy/myectomy for obstructive hypertrophic cardiomyopathy. Am J Cardiol 1992;70:657-60.
22. Cooper MM, Tucker E, McIntosh CL, Cannon RO III, Clark RE. Effect of left ventricular septal myectomy on concomitant mitral regurgitation. Ann Thor Surg 1989;48:251-6.
23. McIntosh CL, Maron BJ. Current operative treatment of obstructive hypertrophic cardiomyopathy. Circulation 1988;78:487-95.
24. Iskandrian AS, Hakki AH, Bemis CE, Kane SA, Boston B, Amenta A. Left ventricular end-

diastolic pressure-volume relation: a combined radionuclide and hemodynamic study. Am J Cardiol 1983;51:1057-61.
25. Iskandrian AS, Bemis CE, Hakki AH, Heo J, Kimbiris D, Mintz GS. Ventricular systolic and diastolic impairment during pacing-induced myocardial ischemia in coronary artery disease: simultaneous hemodynamic, electrocardiographic and radionuclide angiographic evaluation. Am Heart J 1986;112:382-91.
26. Aroesty JM, McKay RG, Heller GV, Royal HD, Als AV, Grossman W. Simultaneous assessment of left ventricular systolic and diastolic dysfunction during pacing-induced ischemia. Circulation 1985;71:889-900.
27. Feldman MD, Alderman JD, Aroesty JM, Royal HD, Ferguson JJ, Owen RM, Grossman W, McKay RG. Depression of systolic and diastolic myocardial reserve during atrial pacing tachycardia in patients with dialted cardiomyopathy. J Clin Invest 1988;82:1661-9.
28. Grossman W, McLaurin LP, Rolett EL. Alteration in left ventricular relaxation and diastolic compliance in congestive cardiomyopathy. Cardiovasc Res 1979;13:514-22.
29. Erbel R, Schweizer P, Krebs W, Langen HJ, Meyer J, Effert S. Effects of heart rate changes on left ventricular volume and ejection fraction: A 2-dimensional echocardiographic study. Am J Cardiol 1984;53:590-7.
30. Iskandrian AS, Mintz GS. Pacemaker therapy in congestive heart failure: A new concept based on excessive utilization of the Frank-Starling mechanism. Am Heart J 1986;112:867-70.
31. Hochleitner M, Hörtnagl H, Ng C-K, Hörtnagl H, Gschnitzer F, Zechmann W. Usefulness of physiologic dual-chamber pacing in drug-resistant idiopathic dilated cardiomyopathy. Am J Cardiol 1990;66:198-202.
32. Karpawich P, Justice C, Chang C-H. Septal ventricular pacing in the immature canine heart: A new perspective. Am Heart J 1991;121:827-33.
33. Hochleitner M, Hörtnagl H, Hörtnagl H, Fridrich L, Gschnitzer F. Long-term efficacy of physiologic dual-chamber pacing in the treatment of end-stage idiopathic dilated cardiomyopathy. Am J Cardiol 1992;70:1320-5 .
34. Brecker SJD, Xiao HB, Sparrow J, Gibson DG. Effects of dual-chamber pacing with short atrioventricular delay in dilated cardiomyopathy. Lancet 1992;340:1308-12.
35. Auricchio A, Sommariva L, Salo RW, Scafuri A, Chiariello L. Improvement of cardiac function in patients with severe congestive heart failure and coronary artery disease by dual-chamber pacing with shortened AV delay. PACE 1993;16:2034-42.
36. Linde C, Gadler F, Edner M, Nordlander R, Rosenqvist M, Ryden L. Is DDD-pacing with a short AV delay a beneficial treatment in patients with severe heart failure? PACE 1993;16:1924 (abstract).
37. Feliciano Z, Fisher ML, Patten RD, Gottlieb SS, Gold MR. The optimal AV delay in heart failure patients. PACE 1993;16 (Pt II):884 (abstract).
38. Cowell R, Morris-Thurgood J, Ilsley C, Paul V. Septal short atrioventricular delay pacing: additional hemodynamic improvements in heart failure. PACE 1994;17(Pt II):1980-3.
39. Rosenqvist M, Isaaz K, Botvinick EH, Dae MW, Cockrell J, Abbott JA, Schiller NB, Griffin JC. Relative importance of activation sequence compared to atrioventricular synchrony in left ventricular function. Am J Cardiol 1991;67:148-56.
40. Bakker P, Jonge N de, Klöpping C, Meijburg H, BarmentLoo C, Wittkampf F, Mechelen R van, Mower M, Thomas A. Biventricular pacing in congestive heart failure. Clinical Research 1994;42:327A (abstract).
41. Bakker PF, Meijburg H, Jonge N de, Mechelen R van, Wittkampf F, Mower M, Thomas A. Beneficial effects of biventricular pacing in congestive heart failure. PACE 1994;17(Pt II):318 (abstract).
42. Bakker P, Chin A Sen K, Jonge N de, Klöpping, Algra A, Robles de Medina E, Bredée J. Biventricular Pacing improves functional capacity in patients with end-stage congestive heart failure. PACE 1995;18(Pt II):825 (abstract).

4 MISCELLANEOUS ASPECTS

Chapter 11

The Interplay Between Radiofrequency Catheter Ablation of Arrhythmias and Cardiac Pacing

Norbert M. van Hemel

Introduction

In contrast to direct current catheter ablation, the curative amount of energy of radiofrequency (RF) catheter ablation can be better dosed and located. General anesthesia is usually not required.[1-5] This is the reason why the advent of RF catheter ablation for selective elimination of tissue responsible for clinical arrhythmias has greatly widened the therapeutical scope of clinical arrhythmias in the past five years.

RF catheter ablation was originally applied for reentrant supraventricular tachycardia arising in the atrioventricular (AV) node area[1-3] or using accessory AV pathways.[1] Drug refractory atrial fibrillation and atrial flutter type 2 are currently treated indirectly by interruption of the AV conduction followed by cardiac pacing, in order to obtain rate control of these arrhythmias.[6,7] Very recently, recurrent monomorphic ventricular tachycardia[8,9], classic atrial flutter type 1[10] as well as modification of the AV node for rate control of atrial fibrillation[11] have become new areas of catheter therapy. These methods however, wait for validation by long-term follow-up studies of treated patients.

This study aims to evoke the awareness of the pacemaker clinic for hazardous conditions during and after RF catheter ablation of the AV node area in regard to impulse generation and conduction propagation. Secondly, because the applied RF energy may be of potential harm to pacemaker components, the risk of pacemaker damage or temporary malfunction of the pacing program should be clarified. Finally, after desired or undesired partly or total AV block, the question arises which pacing modality should be selected. The choice is essential in view of life-long pacemaker dependency and preservation of the quality of life.

The Escape Rhythm After AV Node Ablation for Atrial Fibrillation and Atrial Flutter

In spontaneously developed complete AV block, artificial cardiac pacing continuously suppresses the underlying escape rhythm. After inhibiton of the pacemaker by chest wall stimulation, recovery of the escape rhythm occurs gradually with irregular intervals due to interfering escape foci from different site in the heart and inherent rate.[12] In the majority of paced patients the first escape interval will not exceed 4 seconds, and the escape rhythm will stabilize within 3 minutes with cycle lengths varying from 1500 to 2000 ms after interruption of cardiac pacing.[12,13] Absence of a reliable escape rhythm indicating pacemaker dependency, appears not to be related to age, gender, prevalence of coronary heart disease, previous cardiac surgery or presumed etiology of the conduction disorder. However, the duration of the conduction disorder, use of antiarrhythmic drugs and a paced QRS complex wider than 180 ms can be identified as predictors for an unreliable escape rhythm associated with symptoms.[13] Furthermore, it should be emphasized that the escape rhythm can behave differently[14] during successive tests. In conclusion, one should bear in mind that in natural total AV block the escape rhythm occurs within 6 seconds after interruption of pacing in 100% of patients.[12]

Opposite to spontaneous AV block that usually develops gradually and permits escape rhythm to develop, RF energy induced AV block is instanteneously created, which inhibits the development of a prompt and stable escape rhythm. Moreover, potential escape foci arising in the common His bundle, bundle branches or in the ventricular myocardium may have been continuously suppressed by fast or irregular supraventricular impulses resulting from atrial fibrillation or by antiarrhythmic drugs prescribed in the treatment of these arrhythmias. Life-threatening ventricular arrhythmias have been reported following RF catheter ablation of the AV node area, which were ascribed to bradycardia-dependent QT_c prolongation of the escape rhythm, inducing polymorphic ventricular tachycardia and torsades de pointes.[15]

Between 1991 and 1994, in our institution RF catheter ablation of the AV node for rate control of drug refractory atrial fibrillation was undertaken in 96 successive patients. All patients with successful interruption of AV conduction received VVI pacing with minute ventilation rate responsive pacing. After ablation all antiarrhythmic drugs were withdrawn. Within one month after implantation, five patients had lead dislodgement and one showed loss of capture by excessive rise of threshold. In 4 of these 6 patients intermittent severe dizziness or near syncope occurred (figure 1 and 2).

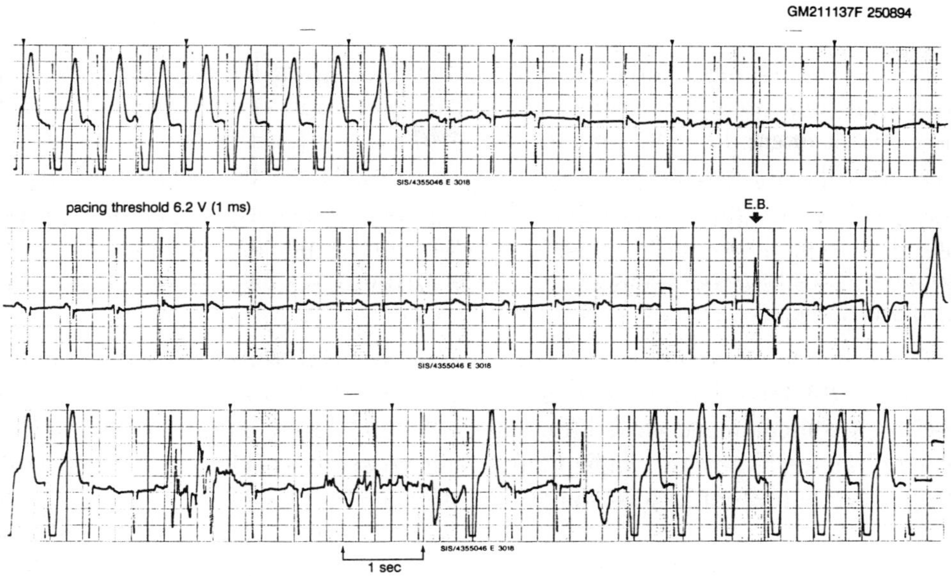

Figure 1. *One lead continued ECG recording of a 46-year-old female patient, recorded 23 days after VVIR implantation, following RF catheter ablation of the AV junction for drug refractory atrial fibrillation. Intermittent loss of pacemaker capture was observed due to lead dislodgement. The ECG recording shows total AV block and ventricular asystole during almost 17 sec until finally the first escape beat (EB) emerged. This insufficient escape rhythm was associated with episodes of severe dizziness and near syncope.*

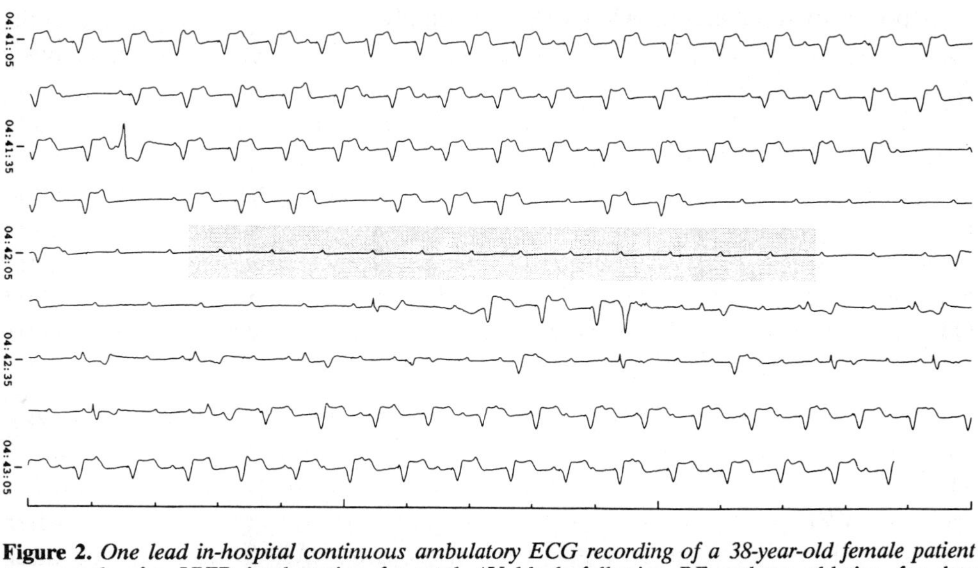

Figure 2. *One lead in-hospital continuous ambulatory ECG recording of a 38-year-old female patient one month after VVIR implantation for total AV block following RF catheter ablation for drug refractory symptomatic atrial fibrillation. In the upper part of the strip, total AV block and adequate ventricular pacing is observed whereas later intermittent loss of pacemaker capture arose due to an excessive rise of pacing threshold. Note the very long period of absent escape rhythm until finally an escape beat emerged. These episodes were frequently observed and caused severe dizziness and near syncope.*

The reason for this insufficient escape mechanism after RF catheter ablation is today still unknown. Lacombe *et al* studied the escape rhythm during transient heart block induced by DC catheter shocks of the AV junction for rate control of atrial fibrillation, and noticed that the site of origin of the escape rhythm was close to the area of damage of the AV node area.[14] It might be hypothesized that the most appropriate area of escape rhythm has been injured by RF catheter ablation but prospective studies on escape rhythms are needed to elucidate the true mechanism.

In conclusion, although our experience with an insufficient escape rhythm after RF catheter ablation of the AV junction for atrial fibrillation is preliminary and limited, we recommend close observation of temporarely paced patients waiting for definitive pacemaker implantation, and frequent checks of the implanted pacemaker to prevent serious complications.

High Risk Catheter Ablation Regarding Atrioventricular Conduction

Atrioventricular Nodal Reentry Tachycardia

Very recently RF catheter ablation of atrioventricular nodal reentry tachycardia (AVNRT) has been developed in several centers.[16,17] Ablation of the retrograde fast limb of the reentrant circuit of AVNRT can be achieved by lesions at the site that records the earliest retrograde atrial potential during AVNRT or during sinus rhythm by lesions of the AV junction resulting in a prolongation of the anterograde AV conduction.[18] Current results show successful treatment of 95% of the patients and an incidence of AV block by 2% to 8% of the ablated patients.[3,19,20]

Treatment of AVNRT can also be achieved by RF energy application to the atrial insertion of the slow pathway of the AVNRT circuit in the posterior septum remote of the AV node and the atrial insertion of the fast pathway. Positioning of the ablating catheter is guided by specific potentials.[16,21] When those signals cannot be detected, the anatomical approach is performed, referred to as aspecific ablation of the posterior perinodal atrium between the os of the coronary sinus and the tricuspid valve.[22] Absence of inducibility of AVNRT is also the endpoint of slow pathway ablation. Success rates of 95% in patients with AVNRT have been reported, witj an extremely low indidence of AV block.[3,19,20]

Although RF energy application for modification of the atrial insertions of the fast pathway is usually done with limited power output, the incidence of AV block is higher than in slow pathway ablation. However, unexpected partial or complete AV block may also occur during slow pathway approach due to instability or sudden moving of the ablating catheter into vulnerable AV junction tissue or due to anatomical variations of the AV compact node and its atrial insertions. Delayed development of AV conduction disturbances after RF ablation, sometimes arising more than 24 hours after the procedure, should also be taken into account and requires close rhythm monitoring in patients with extremely long AV conduction intervals or transient complete AV block during the ablation session.[20]

Finally, persistent or transient inappropriate sinus tachycardia can be observed in patients after fast pathway ablation, suggesting an altered autonomic state. This is probably due to a temporary parasympathetic denervation caused by ablation of afferent fibres of the vagal nerve, located in the area of the fast pathway (figure 3).[23] In cases of synchronized ventricular pacing for undesired postablation AV block, occurrence of this paroxysmal sinus tachycardia with rates up to 150 bpm can result in palpitations and other symptoms, mimicking an unsuccessfully ablated AVNRT, requiring new therapeutical measures and patient reassurance.

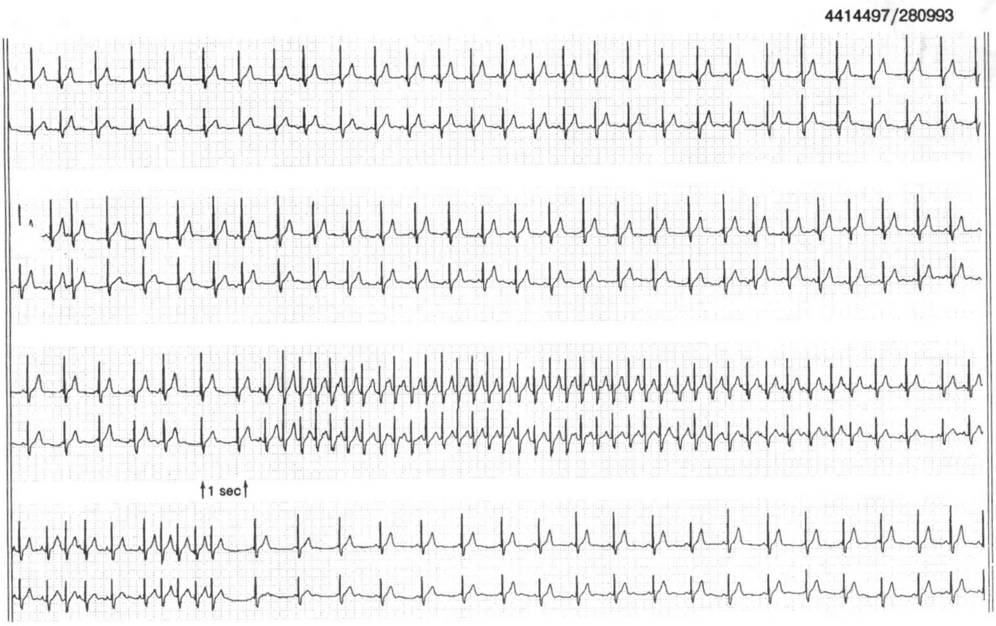

Figure 3. *Two-channel Holter recording of a sixty-years-old female patient, made one month after successful fast pathway ablation of atrioventricular nodal reentry tachycardia. The recording shows sudden increase in heart rate up to 150 bpm. This patient was free of any drug therapy.*

Septal Accessory Atrioventricular Pathways

Accessory AV pathways running in the atrial septum are subdivided into three different categories according to their ventricular insertion. Junctions with the lateral-superior right ventricular and conus region constitute anteroseptal accessory pathways, whereas junctions with the right posterior ventricular septum and the posteroinferior right ventricle compose the posteroseptal accessory pathway.[24] However, the ECG pattern, is determined by the timing and balance of the excitation wave running simultaneously through the specific AV conduction system and the accessory pathway. Anatomic variations such as the 'atypical' posteroseptal accessory pathway[25] and functional changes with or without anatomical variations, referred to as 'intermediate septal' accessory pathways[26], complicate the interpretation of the ECG pattern and the localization of the bundle during catheter mapping.

Previous surgical ablation results of anteroseptal, intermediate and posteroseptal accessory AV pathways have shown an increased risk for inadvertent interruption of AV conduction. This is understandable in view of the close anatomical proximity of the specific AV conduction system to the ventricular insertion of the accessory AV pathways.[25,26] Atrioventricular block is also the most frequent complication of RF catheter ablation of septal pathways, varying from 2% to 5%, and from 2% to 8.3% with catheter therapy using direct current shock.[27] However, more recent results show a lower risk, probably because of increased experience and more refined catheter mapping of the accessory pathways.[27,28]

One may conclude that patients in whom RF catheter ablation of septal accessory pathways will be undertaken, an increased risk for transient or permanent interruption of AV conduction should be anticipated. This risk greatly exceeds that of AV conduction interruption in patients with other types of accessory AV pathways. Because both the success rate of RF catheter ablation of septal AV pathways is lower and the recurrence rate is higher when compared to ablation of other accessory pathways[27], multiple ablation sessions are usually required. The risk of loss of AV conduction appears to be higher in this population.

Modification of AV Conduction to Control Ventricular Rate During Atrial Fibrillation

In some patients with chronic paroxysmal atrial fibrillation, control of the ventricular rate with antiarrhythmic drugs can be very difficult. Longstanding high ventricular rates may result in severe symptoms forcing some patients to stop daily duties and activities. Sometimes the uncontrollable high heart rates lead to cardiomyopathy. Although catheter ablation of AV conduction appears to be safe and efficacious, interruption of mechanical AV synchrony can be disadvantageous when sinus rhythm resumes after episodes of atrial fibrillation. Modification of AV conduction, using RF energy to slow the ventricular rate during atrial fibrillation, has recently been published.[29] Morady *et al* delivered RF energy to the posterior septal or midseptal right atrium in proximity to the os of the coronary sinus in 19 patients with drug refractory fast rates in atrial fibrilla-tion.[11] In 74% of the patients successful modification was achieved, showing a persistent lengthening of RR intervals during atrial fibrillation, and in 21% of the patients a third degree AV block occurred requiring permanent pacing.[11] The site of modification corresponded to the location of the posterior ablation for AVNRT (see above), but partial damage of the compact atrioventricular node could not be excluded.[29,30] This new approach to controlling heart rate during atrial fibrillation appears to be promising, but further experience and refinement are required due to the high risk of inadvertent AV block requiring lifelong pacemaker therapy.

Effects of RF Ablation on Implanted Pacemakers

Many endogenous and exogenous sources can inhibit or trigger implanted pacemakers inappropriately. RF catheter ablation involving application of RF power at frequencies between 0.5 and 1 MHz and with a range of 5 to 30 Watt should be considered a serious electromagnetic interference with pacemaker functioning.

Application of RF catheter ablation raises two questions:

1. Is it sensible to postpone pacemaker implantation until successful RF ablation of the AV node is obtained in order to prevent transient or permanent pacemaker damage?
2. Which measures are recommended when RF catheter ablation is applied after previous pacemaker implantation?

Question 1. Pacemaker implantation prior to RF ablation

In an experimental study, Chin *et al*[31] examined 16 different pacemaker models from seven manufacturers, implanted in dogs to assess their functioning during and after RF energy delivered between the distal electrode of an ablation catheter and a large diameter skin electrode, comparable to human catheter ablation. When RF energy was delivered with the catheter tip positioned within 4 to 5 cm from the implanted pacing lead, with 15 Watt for maximal 30 seconds at three successive ablations, only 3 of 19 pacemakers remained unaffected. Inappropriate inhibition (even when pacemakers were programmed to VOO or DOO) or abnormal rate pacing or noice mode behaviour and runaway pacing resulting in ventricular fibrillation, was observed in 13 of 19 pacemakers. However, all pacemaker changes were transient and could not be induced when the distance between the tip of the ablation catheter and the implanted lead exceeded 4 cm.

The experience of Pfeiffer *et al*[32] demonstrated an unfavourable influence of RF catheter ablation of the AV node on antitachycardia devices (N=4) and antibradycardia pacemakers (N=9). In one of the former types the antitachycardia mode was activated and in another one the magnet rate became manifest whereas all bradycardia pacemakers started pacing with programmed or magnet rates. One pacemaker temporarily showed exit block and another one changed its program from DDD to VVI after repeated RF ablation.

However, in a prospective study on the influence of RF catheter ablation of the AV node in patients with drug refractory atrial fibrillation (N=24) and septal AV bypasses (N=3) Chang *et al* observed only two cases of pacemaker malfunctioning.[33] All pacemakers were programmed to VVI at 50 bpm prior to the ablation session. RF ablation caused reproducibly persistent reversion to the magnet rate in one case, and inhibited pacemaker discharge in the second case whereas all other pacemakers functioned appropriately throughout the procedure. At follow-up of three to six months, all implanted DDD and VVI pacers showed unaltered pacing and sensing characteristics.

During RF catheter ablation, Ellenbogen *et al* monitored the function of implanted systems with telemetry, intracardiac electrograms and surface ECG. Extension of programmed refractory periods of the pacemaker and asynchronous pacing was temporarily seen whereas only one of 17 pacemakers reverted transiently to 'end of life' behaviour after RF ablation. In another patient permanent loss of atrial sensing of the DDDR system with decrease in atrial lead impedance was observed.

These findings show that RF catheter ablation of the AV node is feasible in patients with permanent pacing, but unpredictable changes of pacing mode and exit block during RF energy may occur. Furthermore, untoward effects of RF energy on sensors for rate adaptive pacing must also be taken into account. Van Gelder *et al* reported upper rate pacing following RF ablation in a minute ventilation DDDR pacemaker, which could be avoided by programming the pacemaker in DDD mode.[35] An identical behaviour of a minute ventilation

VVIR pacemaker during electrocautery was demonstrated, resulting in a serious clinical complication.[36] When these uncontrolled and unpredictable influences of RF catheter ablation are added to the potential risk of damage or dislodgement of already implanted leads[34] due to manipulation of the ablating catheter in the right atrium and/or ventricle, we strongly recommend to wait for pacemaker implantation until after the RF ablation session.

Question 2. Measures to be taken in presence of an implanted pacemaker.

1. Today no common opinion exists on the necessity of temporary demand pacing during the RF catheter session in case of already implanted pacemakers.[32,33] We strongly advise the availability of back-up ventricular pacing in **all** patients with implanted pacemakers, unless complete protection of the implanted pacemaker from RF energy is guaranteed by the manufacturer. In our series of five patients with implanted pacemaker, two Medtronics pacemakers, type Activitrac 8423, showed sudden 'end of life' after the first RF energy application. This complication can be solved with reprogramming ('power on reset').
2. All reports advise to switch the program to VVI or DDD mode, and disabling of sensors for rate adapted pacing[35,36], as well as antitachycardia programs prior to the catheter ablation. Programming to maximal pacemaker output values should be seriously considered to avoid transient loss of pacemaker capture during RF ablation.
3. Immediately after RF energy application, pacing thresholds, lead impedance and sensors for rate adaptive pacing should be tested, as well as all other program variables.
4. Finally, to unmask short- or long-term untoward effects of RF energy on the implanted pacemaker, it is recommended to repeat these measurements in the first month following RF catheter ablation. Patients with unsuccessful interruption of the AV node should also be followed extensively.

Pacing Mode After Atrioventricular Ablation for Atrial Fibrillation or Flutter

In atrial fibrillation the etiology and clinical manifestation in terms of incidence and duration of the arrhythmia can widely vary, which demands a clear vocabulary. For this reason we designed terminology for incidence of attacks, mode of onset and duration of atrial fibrillation[27] (Table 1). The underlying causes of the arrhythmia frequently remain obscure ('lone atrial fibrillation') and it is uncertain whether the enlargement of the left, right, or both atria is a consequence or the cause of atrial fibrillation. We have to admit that our current clinical tools for assessment of the etiology of atrial fibrillation are too limited to unmask the primary structural or electrophysiological changes of the atria attributing to paroxysmal or chronic atrial fibrillation. For example, Collette Guiraudon noticed a striking loss of nerve and ganglion cells of the autonomic nervous system in patients with paroxysmal atrial fibrillation, in whom the 'corridor' operation was undertaken.[38] Unfortunately, biopsies of the atrial tissue are only feasible during open-heart surgery, and the reason why we have such a limited insight in the histological changes and development of atrial fibrillation.

Table 1. **Types and Frequency of Attacks of Atrial Fibrillation or Atrial Flutter** [37]

Types	Mode of Onset and Duration
Paroxysmal AF or AFl	Sporadic, recurrent or frequent
Recent onset	lasting ≤24 hours
Long-standing	lasting >24 hours - 6 months
Transient AF or AFl	Acute, during intercurrent trigger/disease
Chronic AF or AFl	Sustained, frequently permanent lasting >6 months
Frequency	
Sporadic (infrequent)	Monthly or less
Recurrent	Weekly
Frequent	Almost daily, up to weekly
Incessant	Daily, covering >12 hours/day

Abbreviations: AF = atrial fibrillation; AFl = atrial flutter

In case of atrial fibrillation, it is worthwhile to determine the position of the patient in the natural course of this arrhythmia. Figure 4 shows a descriptive three-dimensional model, representing the relationship between the incidence and duration of the attacks of atrial fibrillation over the years following the first attack. Starting with a single attack, atrial fibrillation will occur more frequently and with a longer duration, and will finally end in chronic atrial fibrillation when adequate treatment is omitted. Actually, this three-dimensional model is much more complex because other clinical variables, such as age, etiology, patient compliance, number of antiarrhythmic drug failures[39], side-effects of anti-arrhythmic and concomitant heart diseases have to be added, resulting in an *N*th-dimensional model. Furthermore, preservation of sinus node function, characteristics of AV conduction, and possible deterioration of ventricular function (tachycardiomyopathy)[40] must be taken into account in this model.

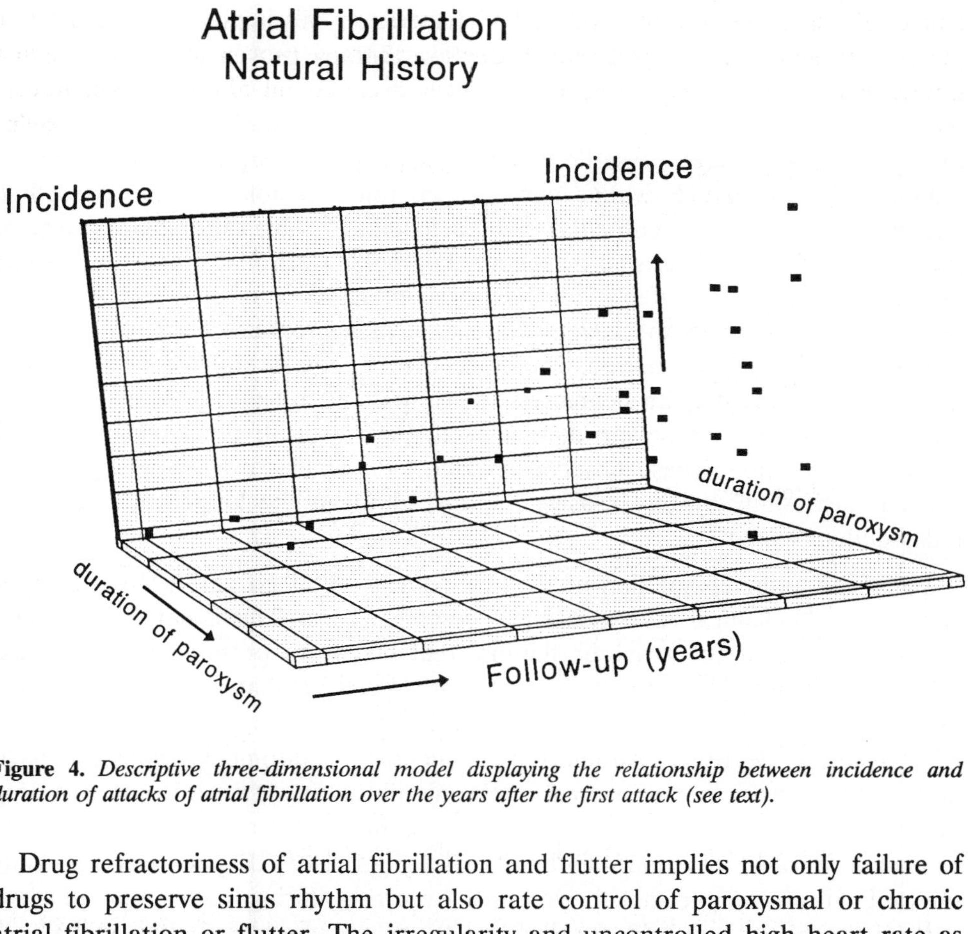

Figure 4. *Descriptive three-dimensional model displaying the relationship between incidence and duration of attacks of atrial fibrillation over the years after the first attack (see text).*

Drug refractoriness of atrial fibrillation and flutter implies not only failure of drugs to preserve sinus rhythm but also rate control of paroxysmal or chronic atrial fibrillation or flutter. The irregularity and uncontrolled high heart rate as well as absence of mechanical AV synchrony during atrial fibrillation and flutter cause symptoms such as palpitations, depressed functional capacity, heart failure and tachycardiomyopathy.[40] Under these conditions, invasive therapies such as the aselective catheter ablation of the AV area, selective surgical therapies for atrial fibrillation[41-43] and the very recent and experimental selective catheter modification of the AV node for rate control of atrial fibrillation[11] constitute alternative therapies.

In recent years, thousands of patients worldwide with drug refractory atrial fibrillation and flutter underwent DC or RF catheter ablation of the AV junction followed by pacemaker implantation. In a short-term randomized study Brignole *et al*[44] showed that AV ablation therapy with VVIR pacing increased significantly the functional capacity of patients measured both at 15 days and 3 months after the intervention, but an improvement of 9% to 40% was also observed in comparable patients in whom only a VVI pacemaker was implanted. Therefore, a placebo effect cannot be excluded. Ablation therapy proves to be particularly efficacious in controlling palpitations, which disappeared almost completely in most patients of various studies.[45,46] In addition, after ablation followed by pacing therapy, left ventricular systolic function appears to improve particularly in patients with depressed cardiac performance prior to ablation, as opposed to patients with a normal ventricular systolic function.[44] This different response to the invasive therapy, measured by echocardiographic fractional shortening, can be explained by opposite effects: the beneficial effect of control of heart rate in atrial fibrillation versus the adversed effect of asynchronous ventricular contraction due to ventricular pacing. Probably, the beneficial effect of rate control dominates in patients with depressed left ventricular function and the untoward effect of asynchronous pacing dominates in patients with previous normal left ventricular function. These observations show that tachycardiomyopathy can be treated successfully by the invasive therapy, although the long-term effects are today undetermined.[40]

When RF catheter ablation of the AV node is obtained and VVIR pacing is permanent, mechanical AV synchrony is completely lost. This is not the case with the 'maze' surgery for atrial fibrillation, that claims to preserve left and right sided AV synchrony[42], or with the 'corridor' operation that precludes left-sided mechanical AV synchrony but preserves the right-sided one.[41-43] In view of lost AV synchrony, depressed cardiac output and risk of thromboembolic complications resulting from the paroxysmal or chronic fibrillating atria, it is not surprising that the selection of pacing mode after ablation of the AV node is today a matter of debate. Because of the instability of atrial rhythms VVIR pacing is frequently selected. However, pacemaker syndrome occurring during resumption of sinus rhythm can be a draw-back for this choice, as observed by Sadoul in 33% of patients with VVIR following AV ablation.[47] For patients with paroxysmal atrial fibrillation, DDDR pacing is recommended because this pacing mode offers the greatest flexibility. DDDR pacing widely promotes the preservation of sinus rhythm and mechanical AV synchrony in patients with paroxysmal atrial fibrillation whereas in case of accepted chronic atrial fibrillation, reprogramming to VVIR is easily done, as occurred in 11% of paced patients reported by Rajamannan *et al.*[48] Gross *et al* reviewed the data of 17 DDD patients with a mean age of 59 years, predominant atrial fibrillation and normal left ventricular function, and observed a sinus rhythm in 60% of the outpatient's visits during a mean follow-up of 12.5 months.[33] However, after extensive follow-up, the incidence of preserved sinus rhythm and adequate DDDR pacing has substantially diminished. Wolfe *et al* followed 78 patients with ablation of the AV junction for paroxysmal atrial fibrillation, who had permanent DDD pacing (mean age 65±12 years).[50] All patients were anticoagulated and antiarrhythmic agents were discontinued. Kaplan Meier curves showed that maintained DDD pacing was 85% at one year and 77% at two years after implantation, showing a progressive increase in the number of patients who develop chronic atrial fibrillation. Therefore, DDD pacing may have limited long-term efficacy in the management of paroxysmal atrial fibrillation after AV nodal ablation, at least when antiarrhythmic drugs are withdrawn.

From these studies it can be concluded that RF ablation of the AV junction for drug refractory atrial fibrillation appears beneficial for the symptomatic patient in terms of increased exercise capacity and disappearance of palpitations. However, the long-term behaviour of the ventricular function after this intervention has not been sufficiently studied. Because randomized studies on the most favourable pacing mode after AV node ablation are today lacking, it is advised to select VVIR pacing when chronic atrial fibrillation is present prior to the intervention and DDDR or VDDR pacing in patients with paroxysmal atrial fibrillation, although the risk for development of chronic atrial fibrillation in patients with paroxysmal atrial fibrillation increases substantially over time. When preservation of mechanical AV synchrony after AV ablation is an important clinical target, automatic mode switch to VVIR for rate control of paroxysmal atrial arrhythmias is a prerequisite.[51] Whether DDDR or VDDR pacing modes are useful to diminish the incidence of atrial arrhythmias after ablation of the AV junction, must still be evaluated. Extensive prospective randomized studies are required to make reliable evaluation because atrial fibrillation is a disease with many clinical profiles.

Conclusions

This study describes the side-effects of RF catheter ablation of arrhythmogenic sites with emphasis on inadvertent interruption of AV conduction or insufficient escape rhythm after intended or undesired AV block. Although the beneficial results of modification of the AV node for the treatment of atrioventricular nodal reentry tachycardia or interruption of the symptomatic septal AV accessory pathways are fully recognized, a considerable risk for AV block should be anticipated. This risk is even greater when modification of the AV node for controlling the heart rate during atrial fibrillation is applied. We are convinced that with growing experience and improved catheter techniques, this risk gradually diminishes to an incidential case. However, when AV block occurs inadvertently or intentionally, the optimal pacing mode is still unclear today, at least in patients with frequent or chronic atrial tachyarrhythmias.

References

1. Jackman WM, Friday KJ, Yeung-Lai-Wah JA, Fitzgerald DM, Beck B, Bowman AJ, Stelzer P, Harrison L, Lazzara R. New catheter technique for recording left free-wall accessory atrioventricular pathway activation. Identification of pathway fiber orientation. Circulation 1988;78:598-611.
2. Haissaguerre M, Gaita F, Fischer B, Commenges D, Montserrat P, d'Ivernois C, Lemetayer P, Warin J-F. Elemination of atrioventricular nodal reentrant tachycardia using discrete slow potentials to guide application of radiofrequency energy. Circulation 1992;85:2162-75.
3. Jazayeri MR, Hempe SL, Sra JS, Dhala AA, Blanck Z, Deshpande SS, Avitall B, Krum DP, Gilbert CJ, Akhtar M. Selective transcatheter ablation of the fast and slow pathway using radiofrequency energy in patients with atrioventricular nodal reentrant tachycardia. Circulation 1992;85;1318-28.
4. Wittkampf FHM, Hauer RNW, Robles de Medina EO. Control of radiofrequency lesion size by power regulation. Circulation 1989;4:962-8.
5. Avitall B, Khan M, Krum D, Hare J, Lessila C, Dhala A, Deshpande S, Jazayeri M, Sra J, Akhtar M. Physics and engineering of transcatheter cardiac tissue ablation. J Am Coll Cardiol 1993;22:921-32.
6. Huang SK, Bharati S, Lev M, Marcus FI. Electrophysiologic and histologic observations of chronic atrioventricular block induced by closed-chest catheter desiccation with radiofre-quency energy. PACE 1987;10:805-16.
7. Langberg JJ, Chin MC, Rosenquist M, et al. Catheter ablation of atrioventricular junction with radiofrequency energy. Circulation 1991;83:1562-76.
8. Kuck KH, Schlüter M, Geiger M, Siebels J. Successful catheter ablation of human ventricular tachycardia with rediofrequency current guided by an endocardial map of the area of slow conduction. PACE 1991;14:1060-71.
9. Gonska B-D, Cao K, Schaumann A, Dorszewski A, Mühlen F von zur, Kreuzer H. Catheter ablation of ventricular tachycardia in 136 patients with coronary artery disease: results and long-term follow-up. J Am Coll Cardiol 1994;24:1506-14.
10. Cosio FG, Lopez GM, Goiocolea A, Arribas B, Barroso JL. Radiofrequency ablation of the inferior vena cava - tricuspid valve isthmus in common atrial flutter. Am J Cardiol 1993;71: 705-9.
11. Williamson B, Ching Man K, Daoud E, Niebauer M, Strickberger SA, Morady F. Radiofrequency cathter modification of atrioventricular conduction to control the ventricular rate during atrial fibrillation. N Engl J Med 1994;331:910-7.
12. Grendahl H, Kjekshus J, Soyland E, Sivertssen E. Escape rhythm in complete A-V block. The recovery phase after overdrive suppression from artificial ventricular pacing. PACE 1979;2:455-61.

13. Rosenheck S, Bondy C, Weiss AT, Gotsman MS. Comparison between patients with and without reliable ventricular escape rhythm in the presence of long-standing complete atrioventricular block. PACE 1993;16:272-6.
14. Lacombe P, Lévy S, Metge M, Cointe R, Bru P, Gérard R. Electrocardiographic character-istics of the escape rhythm in transient complete atrioventricular block induced by trans-catheter electrical ablation of the atrioventricular junction. PACE 1988;11:151-57.
15. Peters RHJ, Wever EFD, Hauer RNW, Wittkampf FHM, Robles de Medina E.O. Bradycardia dependent QT prolongation and ventricular fibrillation following catheter ablation of the atrioventricular junction with radiofrequency energy. PACE 1994;17:108-12.
16. Jackman WM, Beckman KJ, McClelland JH, Wand X, Friday KJ, Roman CA, Moulton KP, Twidale N, Hazlitt HA, Prior MI, Oren J, Overholt ED, Lazzara R. Treatment of supraventricular tachycardia due to atrioventricular nodal reentry by radiofrequency catheter ablation of slow-pathway conduction. N Engl J Med 1992;327:313-8.
17. Langberg JL, Harvey M, Calkins H, El-Atassi R, Kalbfleisch SJ, Morady F. Titration of power output during radiofrequency catheter ablation of atrioventricular nodal reentrant tachycardia. PACE 1993;16:465-70.
18. Langberg JJ. Radiofrequency catheter ablation of AV nodal reentry: the anterior approach. PACE 1993;16:615-22.
19. Kalbfleisch SJ, Strickberger A, Williamson B, Vorderian VR, Man CH, Hummel JD, Langberg JJ, Morady F. Randomized comparison of anatomic and electrogram mapping approaches to abaltion of the slow pathway of atrioventricular node reentrant tachycardia. JACC 1994;23:716-23.
20. Ching Man K, Kalbfleisch J, Hummel JD, Williamson BD, Vorperian VR, Strickberger SA, Langberg JJ, Morady F. Safety and cost of outpatients radiofrequency ablation of the slow pathway in patients with atrioventricular nodal reentrant yachycardia. Am J Cardiol 1993;72: 1323-4.
21. Haissaguerre M, Gaita F, Fischer B, Commenges D, Montserrat P, d'Ivernois C, Lemetayer P, Warin J-F. Elimination of atrioventricular nodal reentrant tachycardia using discrete slow potentials to guide application of radiofrequency energy. Circulation 1992;85:2162-2175.
22. Wathan M, Natale A, Wolfe K, Yee R, Newman D, Klein G. An anatomically-guided approach to atrioventricular node slow pathway ablation. Am J Cardiol 1992;70:886-9.
23. Kocovic D, Shea J, Friedman P. Evidence for parasympthetic denervation of the sinus node after radiofrequency modification of the AV node in patients with AV nodal reentry. JACC 1993;21:50A.
24. Boineau JP. Intermediate septal accessory pathways: electrocardiographic localization of pre-excitation. J Am Coll Cardiol 1991:17:1579-80.
25. Guiraudon GM, Klein GJ, Sharma AD, Yee R, Pineda EA. 'Atypical' posteroseptal accessory pathway in Wolff-Parkinson-White syndrome. J Am Coll Cardiol 1988;12:1605-8.
26. Epstein AE, Kirklin JK, Holman WL, Plumb VJ, Kay GN. Intermediate septal accessory pathways: electrocardiographic characteristics, electrophysiologic observations and their surgical implicatins. J Am Coll Cardiol 1991;17:1570-8.
27. Xie B, Heald SC, Bashir Y, Camm AJ, Ward DE. Radiofrequency catheter ablation of septal accessory atrioventricular pathways. Br Heart J 1994;72:281-4.
28. Schlüter M, Kuck K-H. Catheter ablation from right atrium of anteroseptal accessory pathways using radiofrequency current. J Am Coll Cardiol 1992;19:663-70.
29. Fleck RP, Chen PS, Boyce K, Ross R, Dittrich HC, Feld GK. Radiofrequency modification of atrioventricular conduction by selctive ablation of the low posterior septal, right atrium in a patient with atrial fibrillation and a rapid ventricular response. PACE 1993;16:377-81.
30. Kunze KP, Schluter M, Geiger M, Kuck KH. Modulation of atrioventricular nodal conduction using radiofrequency current. Am J Cardiol 1988;61:657-8.
31. Chin MC, Rosenqvist M, Lee MA, Griffin JC, Langberg JJ. The effect of radiofrequency

catheter ablation on permanent pacemakers: an experimental study. PACE 1990;13:23-9.
32. Pfeiffer D, Tebbenjohanns J, Jung W, Manz M, Lüderitz B. Pacemaker function during radiofrequency ablation. PACE 1993;16[Pt II]:882.
33. Chang AC, McAreavey D, Tripodi D, Fananapazir L. Radiofrequency catheter atrioventricular node ablation in patients with permanent cardiac pacing systems. PACE 1994;17:65-9.
34. Ellenbogen KA, Wood MA, Stambler BS, Fields III EM, BSE and co-investigators. Effects of radiofrequency ablation on implanted pacing systems. PACE 1994;17[Pt II]:770.
35. Gelder BM van, Bracke FALE, El Gamal M. Upper rate pacing after radiofrequency catheter ablation in a minute venticlation rate adaptive DDD pacemaker. PACE 1994;17:1437-40.
36. Hemel NM van, Hamerlijnck RPHM, Pronk KJ, Veen EP van der. Upper Limit Ventricular Stimulation in Respiratory Rate Responsive Pacing due to Electrocautery. PACE 1989;12:1720-3.
37. Suttorp MJ. Paroxysmal atrial fibrillation and atrial flutter: current concepts and new strategies. Thesis. State University Groningen, The Netherlands, p 7.
38. Guiraudon CM, Ernst NM, Guiraudon GM, Yee R, Klein GJ. The pathology of drug resistant lone atrial fibrillation in eleven surgically treated patients. In: Kingma JH, Hemel NM van, Lie KI (eds), Atrial Fibrillation, a treatable disease? Kluwer Academic Publishers, 1992, pp 41-58.
39. Kingma JH, Verrostte J, Tiessen G, Hemel NM van. Sequence of anti-arrhythmic intervention related to efficacy in sustained ventricular tachycardia late after myocardial infarction. Eur Heart J 1988;9:66.
40. Lemery R, Brugada P, Cheriex E, Wellens H. Reversibility of tachycardia-induced left ventricular dysfunction after closed-chest catheter ablation of the atrioventricular junction for intractable atrial fibrillation. Am J Cardiol 1987;60:1406-8.
41. Guiraudon GM , Pineda EA, Klein GJ, Sharma AD, Yee R. Early clinical results of corridor surgery for treatment of chronic atrial fibrillation. J Am Coll Cardiol 1988;11:IIIA.
42. Cox JL, Bioneau JL, Schuessler RB, Kater KM, Lappas DG. Five year experience with the maze procedure for atrial fibrillation. Ann Thorac Surg 1993;56:814-24.
43. Hemel NM van, Defauw JJAM, Kingma JH, Jaarsma W, Vermeulen FEE, Bakker JMT de, Guiraudon GM. Long-term results of the corridor operation for atrial fibrillation. Br Heart J 1994;71:170-76.
44. Brignole M, Gianfranchi L, Menozzi C, Bottoni N, Bollini R, Lolli G, Oddone D, Gaggioli G. Influence of atrioventricular junction radiofrequency ablation in patients with chronic atrial fibrillation and flutter on quality of life and cardiac performance. Am J Cardiol 1994;74:242-6.
45. Kay GN, Bubien R, Epstein A, Plumb V. Effect of catheter ablation of the atrioventricular junction on quality of life and exercise tolerance in paroxysmal atrial fibrillation. Am J Cardiol 1988;62:741-4.
46. Rosenqvist M, Lee M, Mouliner L, Springer M, Abbott J, Wu J, Langberg J, Griffin J, Scheinman M. Long-term follow-up of patients after transcatheter direct current ablation of the atrioventricular junction. J Am Coll Cardiol 1990;16:1467-74.
47. Sadoul N, Dodinot B, Chillou C de, Lamouri N, Reeb T, Simon JP, Pescariu S, Aliot E. Pacemaker selection after atrioventricular node abaltion. PACE 1994;17[PtII]:770.
48. Rajamannan NM, Neubauer SA, Hayes DL. Permanent pacing following AV nodal ablation. PACE 1994;17[Pt II]:770.
49. Gross JN, Roth JA, Ben-Zur UM, Ferrick KJ, Kim SG, Andrews C, Ritacco R, Benedek M, Sisher JD, Furman S. DDDR pacing post AV node ablation: a reasonable strategy or an exercise in futility? PACE 1994;17[Pt II]:769.
50. Wolfe DA, McLaughlin S, Windecker S, Epstein AE, Plumb VJ, Kay GN. DDDR pacing following AV nodal ablation: long-term outcome in patients with paroxysmal atrial fibrillation. PACE 1994;17[Pt II]:862.
51. Mond HG, Barold SS. Dual chamber, rate adaptive pacing in patients with paroxysmal supraventricular tachyarrhythmias: protective measures for rate control. PACE 1993;16:2168-85.

4 MISCELLANEOUS ASPECTS

Chapter 12

Cardiac Pacing in Children, Special Skills Needed?

Margreet Th.E. Bink-Boelkens and Gertie C.M. Beaufort-Krol

Introduction

The difference between pacing children and adults is not just a question of patient size. Pacing children means an expected period of pacing of 70-80 years, in which children grow to adult size, are very active and participate in sports. This requires a great deal more of the pacemaker system than when used in the elderly. Moreover, the major indication for pacing in children is injury to the conduction system by cardiac surgery. This implies pacemaker implantation in anatomical abnormal hearts with e.g., abnormal connections of the systemic veins, discordant atrioventricular (AV) connections, AV valve atresia, or myocardial scarring. Therefore, pediatric pacing requires specific knowledge to cope with the potential problems in pacing congenitally abnormal hearts.

The challenge of pacing children is to provide for adequate pacing during this long period, with the smallest number of surgical interventions. The goal should be, to give these children a quality of life that is as normal as possible. This means, among other things, that the implantation technique and the mode of pacing should allow participation in sports. Therefore, rate-responsive and physiologic pacing is, even more so than in adults, the rule and not the exception. The degree of psychological acceptance of the pacemaker also influences the quality of life. Especially teenagers find it difficult to accept the electronic instrument in their body and the resulting scar. Therefore, counselling and support of child and parents before and after implantation is essential and worthwhile.

Table 1. **Indications for Permanent Pacing in Children**[1]

Class I

A. Second or third degree AV block with symptomatic bradycardia.
B. Advanced second or third degree AV block with moderate to marked exercise intolerance.
C. External ophthalmoplegia with bifascicular block.
D. Sinus node dysfunction with symptomatic bradycardia.
E. Congenital AV block with wide QRS escape rhythm or with block below the His bundle.
F. Advanced second or third degree AV block persisting 10-14 days after cardiac surgery.

Class II

A. Bradycardia-tachycardia syndrome with need for an antiarrhythmic drug other than digitalis or phenytoin.
B. Second or third degree AV block within the bundle of His in an asymptomatic patient.
C. Prolonged subsidiary pacemaker recovery time.
D. Transient surgical second or third degree AV block that reverts to bifascicular block.
E. Asymptomatic second or third degree AV block and a ventricular rate <45 beats when awake. Complete AV block when awake, with an average ventricular rate <50 beats/min.
F. Complete AV block with double or triple rest cycle length pauses or minimal heart rate variability.
G. Asymptomatic neonate with congenital complete heart block and bradycardia in relation to age.
H. Complex ventricular arrhythmias associated with second or third degree AV block or sinusbradycardia.
I. Long QT syndrome.

Class III

A. Asymptomatic postoperative bifascicular block.
B. Asymptomatic postoperative bifascicular block with first degree AV block.
C. Transient surgical AV block that returns to normal conduction <1 week.
D. Asymptomatic type I second degree AV block.
E. Asymptomatic congenital heart block without profound bradycardia in relation to age.

Table 2. **Asymptomatic Bradycardia in Complete AV Block: Pacemaker Implantation Guidelines.**[2] **(>6 sec ECG recording while awake)**

	Normal heart Rate (bpm)	Structural heart defect Rate (bpm)
Infants	< 55	< 65
Children	< 45 – 50	< 55 – 60
Adolescents	<40	< 50

Indications

Only one percent of pacemakers is implanted in infants and children. In 1991 the American College of Cardiology and the American Heart Association published their guidelines for implantation of cardiac pacemakers in children and adults (Table 1).[1] Class I indications are those conditions for which there is general agreement that permanent pacemakers should be implanted. Class II contains conditions for which pacemakers are frequently used, but there is divergence of opinion with respect to the necessity of their insertion. Class III holds conditions for which there is general agreement that pacemakers or antitachycardia devices are unnecessary. Symptomatic bradycardia refers to clinical manifestations that are directly attributable to the slow heart rate. This is often difficult to prove, especially in children, and requires frequent Holter monitoring or event recording. Asymptomatic bradycardia should always be related to the age of the patient and the presence or absence of heart disease. The lower limits for an acceptable heart rate are given in Table 2.[2]

Reviewing the literature, surgical complete AV block is the indication for pediatric pacing in 50-60% of patients, congenital complete AV block in 20-30% and surgical sick sinus syndrome in 5-20%.[3,4,5] Therefore, the indication for pacing in ±75% of the children is injury of the conduction system after surgery for congenital heart disease.

In complete AV block after surgery, the risk of sudden death is 35%. Therefore, if the AV conduction does not recover within two weeks of temporary pacing, this is a class I indication. Surgical AV block is mainly seen after repair of atrioventricular septal defect, ventricular septal defect, tetralogy of Fallot, congenitally corrected transposition with additional abnormalities or after AV valve surgery. Increased knowledge of the position of the conduction system and its blood supply in the different cardiac defects, has led to a substantial decrease in the incidence of surgical damage to the conduction system over the last 5-10 years.[6]

In 30% of patients, congenital complete AV block is accompanied by congenital heart disease, sometimes by very complicated forms, such as left isomerism. The main cause of congenital AV block without heart disease is the transplacental transport of anti-RO(SS-A) antibodies to the child, in mothers with often still asymptomatic connective tissue disease. Sometimes these children are already symptomatic before birth. Hydrops fetalis, often caused by a heart rate of 50 b.p.m. or lower, is an indication for premature delivery and neonatal pacemaker implantation (figure 1). The main clinical indications for pacing in congenital

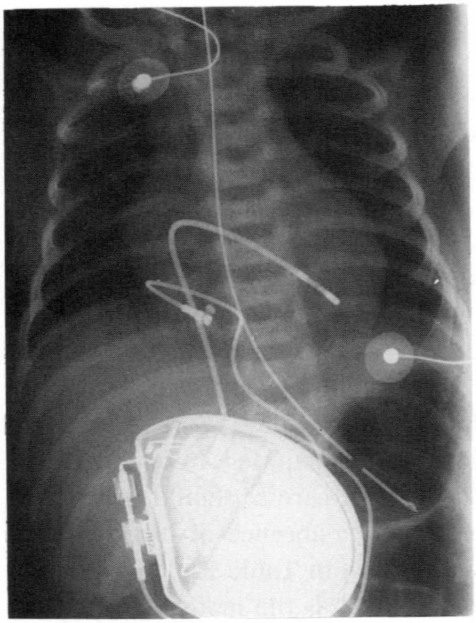

Figure 1. *Chest X ray of a newborn with congenital complete AV block immediately after implantation of a WIR pacemaker with an epicardial electrode. The temporary pacing catheter is still in the right ventricle.*

complete block are symptomatic bradycardia (Table 2), syncope, diminished exercise capacity, progressive dilatation of the heart, or bradycardia-dependent ventricular arrhythmias.

Sick sinus syndrome is especially seen after atrial surgery, e.g., after the Mustard or Senning operation for transposition of the great arteries, or atrial septal defect repair with or without partial or total anomalous pulmonary venous drainage. It also frequently develops after the Fontan operation or 'Fontan-like' operations for univentricular heart. Sick sinus syndrome after cardiac surgery often consists of bradycardia in rest, a decreased heart rate response during exercise and tachy-arrhythmias, especially atrial flutter. Atrial flutter carries a high risk of sudden death, particularly after the Mustard or Senning operation.[7] The prevention and treatment of atrial flutter often consists of drug treatment combined with pacemaker implantation. The pacing mode should be AAIR or anti-tachycardia pacing. In practice the main indication for pacing in sick sinus syndrome is first, the necessity of drug treatment in the brady-tachy syndrome, and further, impaired exercise tolerance due to an insufficient heart rate response and symptomatic bradycardia.

Pulse Generator

Size and Shape

During the last years pulse generators have become considerably smaller. Nowadays it is possible to find a VVI, DDD or rate-responsive pacemaker that can be implanted in a neonate. Especially if the shape of the connector block is rounded, the pacemaker can fit well between the posterior fascia of the rectus abdominis muscle and the muscle itself. Smaller dimensions are not necessary and desirable, if this implies decreased battery capacity. Epicardial pacing and high pacing rates in children make heavy demands on the battery, so smaller pacemakers then will result in an unacceptable short life of the pacemaker and an increase in the number of surgical interventions in children.

Mode of Pacing

In active young children the pacing mode should be as physiologic as possible; DDD or VDD in complete AV block, AAIR in sick sinus syndrome, DDDR in postoperative bi-nodal disease. In children that are too small for two endocardial leads, VVIR pacing is a good alternative. An activity sensor performs well in the active child, and results in an almost normal exercise capacity.[8,9] Surprisingly, the pacemaker syndrome caused by VVI pacing is seldom seen in children.

Single lead atrial synchronous ventricular pacing is a fascinating new development in pacing.[10] It will probably reduce the number of electrodes required during a lifetime of pacing. Children with congenital AV block, who nearly always have normal sinus node function and no supraventricular tachycardias, are good candidates. Experience with this special electrode is still limited, but our first impression and that of others is favorable. It is possible to use an adult length of the electrode; a loop, made in the atrium, will allow growth.

Programmability

Pacemakers should be highly programmable, if they are used in children: e.g., high rates for infants, small steps in sensitivity and output to solve problems of muscle sensing and stimulation in the children, who often are stimulated unipolarly and circadian rhythm to save the battery during the night. More so than in older people, it is important to have the possibility of increasing the output with small quantities to save energy and prolong the longevity of the pacemaker. The output of the battery should be at least 8V if epicardial leads are used, because epicardial thresholds are many times higher than endocardial thresholds and can sometimes rise progressively in the first months.[5]

Electrodes

Endocardial versus Epicardial

For a long time epicardial leads were used in most children, because they could be used at all ages and weights. However, epicardial leads have many disadvantages: extensive surgery is necessary for implantation and the stimulation thresholds are often high and increase progressively with time. Together with the high pacing rate in children this leads to a substantial decrease in longevity of the battery. In our own experience in 50 children followed for 5.3±3.7 years (mean ±SD), epicardial lead problems caused 47% of the surgical interventions.[5] These problems consisted of fractures mainly of the older 'sutured' leads and exit block of the 'screw-in' and 'stab-on' leads. After we started using the new steroid-eluting epicardial leads, the incidence of fractures and exit block, has decreased considerably. Clinical research showed a marked improvement of the acute and chronic thresholds during the follow-up of one year.[11] A new design of a bipolar epimyocardial steroid-eluting electrode is already being developed.[12]

In view of their low thresholds, endocardial leads are more and more used in young children. This is technically feasible even in children below the weight of 15 kg.[13] Growth-related problems can be solved by intracardial loops of the leads, and occlusion of the systemic veins was not found after endocardial pacing in children.[14] Moreover, in our experience the 5-year survival of endocardial leads is 87±7%, compared with 71±10% in epicardial leads.[5] However, with the use of steroid-eluting epicardial electrodes the 5-year survival will probably improve. In addition, Lau *et al*[15] reported a lower 5-year survival of 76% in a large series of endocardial leads. Therefore, it could well be that nowadays the 5-year survival is about equal for epi- and endocardial electrodes. Still the number of endocardial leads a child will need during the rest of its life and the resulting problems, remain a cause for concern. Would it perhaps be wiser to keep the veins unused in smaller children, particularly now that there seems to be a good epicardial alternative?

Active or Passive Fixation

The choice between active and passive fixation of endocardial leads depends mainly on the often abnormal anatomy of the heart. An argument in favor of active fixation is that these leads can be brought into a stable position in abnormal and operated hearts, but also that they can be removed more easily in case of lead failure.[16] This is of great benefit in view of the long pacing period in children.

Unipolar or Bipolar

The advantages and disadvantages of uni- or bipolar pacing and sensing are well known. Bipolar pacing solves the problem of muscle sensing and stimulation in small children in whom a subpectoral pocket is necessary. On the other hand, bipolar electrodes are thicker, more vulnerable and less flexible, which is a disadvantage in this age group. Until bipolar leads become thinner and easier to handle in a small heart, endocardial bipolar pacing will only be possible in older children. Bipolar epicardial pacing will mostly be possible, especially when the new design of the steroid-eluting lead becomes clinically available.[12]

Growth

There are three possible ways of dealing with growth of a child with a pacemaker. Firstly, it is possible to leave a loop in the right atrium. The length of the loop can be calculated from a table that combines height versus intravascular lead length.[17] Secondly, by fastening the electrode with dissolvable sutures, extra length of the electrode can be drawn in the vessel during growth.[18] Thirdly, during pacemaker replacement the electrode can be pushed in the subclavian vein to allow further growth.

Implantation Technique

As in adults, the endocardial leads are mostly inserted through a medial subclavian puncture. This method, however, carries an increased risk of compression and fracture of the lead. The medially inserted lead will be compressed in the costo-clavicular angle and will be easily damaged in active persons.[19,20] Therefore, it is better to insert the electrode either through the cephalic vein or through a more lateral subclavian puncture. This puncture could be guided by a catheter positioned in the subclavian vein from the femoral vein.[18] In addition, the pacemaker should be implanted at the contralateral side to the dominant upper extremity.

Epicardial atrial leads can only be implanted by a sternotomy or a lateral thoracotomy. Ventricular leads can be placed epicardially by a Sauerbruch incision.

In view of the small number of pediatric implantations, we recommend that the implantation be performed by a thoracic surgeon in cooperation with a pediatric cardiologist. We use general anaesthesia and give prophylactic antibiotics for 48 hours.

Pocket

In older children, the pacemaker can be placed subcutaneously in the pectoral region, as is done in adults. In smaller and thinner children with less subcutaneous fat, the pacemaker has to be placed in a subpectoral position. This improves the cosmetic aspect and reduces the risk of skin erosion and trauma. It could be argued that pacemakers should be placed subpectorally in all children and young adults to diminish the incidence of trauma of the pacemaker system.[18] In infants, and if epicardial leads are used, the pocket is made between the rectus abdominis muscle and its posterior fascia. In neonates both rectus sheaths should be used, even for the smallest pacemaker, in view of the required space. If a subpectoral or subrectus pocket is made, attention should be paid to a good postoperative analgesia.

Gongenital Heart Disease and Pacing

Many difficulties may be encountered in children with (operated) congenital heart disease. In the past this was a problem for the pediatric cardiologist only. However, these children are becoming adults now, and therefore the adult cardiologist is confronted with the problem of pacing in anatomical abnormal hearts.

In these patients, the stimulation threshold is generally higher than in normal hearts, due to post-surgical scarring or to fibrosis as a result of prolonged cyanosis or pressure overload. Furthermore, there can be abnormal venous connections or even no venous access to the heart. Anatomically systemic venous atrium or systemic venous ventricle are sometimes left atrium or left ventricle. After cardiac surgery there is no normal right atrial appendage, so in case of atrial pacing an electrode with active fixation has to be used. The main anatomical problems that require special techniques or precautions are summarized below.

Left Superior Vena Cava

Some patients with or without congenital heart disease have a single or additional left SVC that drains in the coronary sinus. Transvenous pacing is possible, but requires a lead with active fixation that makes a 180° clockwise loop in the frontal plane in the atrium before entering the ventricle.[21] Persistent left superior vena cava can be diagnosed by echocardiography.

Right to Left or Left to Right Intracardiac Shunts

The presence of a right to left intracardiac shunt is an absolute contraindication for endocardial pacing because of the risk of systemic emboli. Doppler echocardiography shows that also in left to right shunts there is the possibility of incidental right to left shunting. Therefore, an intracardiac left to right shunt is a relative contraindication for endocardial pacing.

Congenitally Corrected Transposition

In congenitally corrected transposition, the right atrium is connected through a mitral valve with the anatomical left ventricle. This anatomical left ventricle is connected with the pulmonary artery, so the circulation itself is normal. The congenitally corrected transposition may be accompanied by other malformations, such as VSD or pulmonary stenosis. There is a high incidence of spontaneous or post-operative complete AV block. The ventricle to be paced is the smooth anatomical left ventricle, so active fixation should be used for the endocardial lead.

Mustard and Senning Operation for Transposition of the Great Arteries

Until recently, the transposition of the great arteries was repaired by an atrial tunnel that connected the systemic veins with the left ventricle and the pulmonary artery to normalize the circulation. The main difference between the Mustard and the Senning operation is that in the former operation prosthetic material is used. The incidence of sinus node dysfunction is very high after these operations. The patients mainly show bradycardia alternating with atrial flutter. If pacing is indicated there are three problems. Firstly, the superior vena cava may be narrowed at the entrance of the tunnel. Therefore, a normal blood flow has to be ascertained by echocardiography or digital subtraction angiography before electrode implantation. Secondly, it is difficult to find a place for pacing in the atrium. In most cases the roof of the anatomical left atrium is the best place for the electrode with active fixation. Thirdly, the ventricular electrode has to be placed in the left ventricle, so again active fixation is necessary (figure 2). The best treatment of the arrhythmias in these patients is often a combination of AAIR pacing and drugs that prevent the development of atrial flutter (e.g., sotalol).

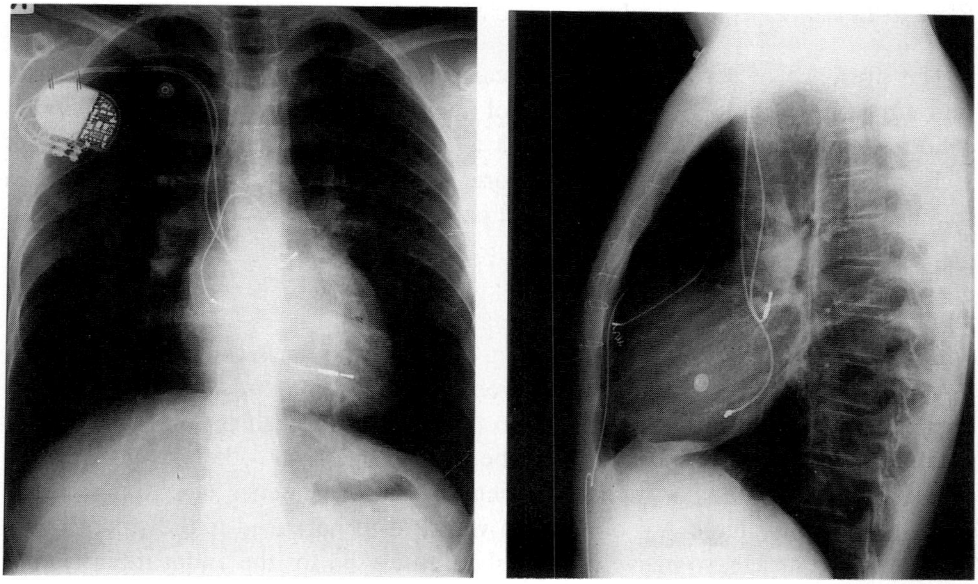

Figure 2. *Anterior-posterior and lateral chest X ray of a child, who underwent a Mustard operation for transposition of the great arteries. A DDDR pacemaker is implanted with a bipolar electrode in the anatomical left atrium and a bipolar electrode in the anatomical left ventricle (viz. systemic venous ventricle). The former epicardial ventricular 'screw-in' lead is fractured.*

Fontan Operation and Total Cavo-Pulmonary Connection for Univentricular Heart

In the Fontan operation, the right atrium is directly connected to the pulmonary artery, so there is no access to the ventricle for endocardial pacing. In the total cavo-pulmonary connection, both caval veins are directly connected to the pulmonary artery, so neither the atrium nor the ventricle can be paced endocardially. As after the Mustard and the Senning operation, the incidence of sinus node dysfunction and atrial flutter is high after the Fontan operation. This incidence seems to be slightly lower after the cavo-pulmonary connection. If there already is an arrhythmia problem immediately after operation, epicardial electrodes are recommended. This makes a second thoracotomy, only for pacing, unnecessary. For cases in which epicardial thresholds are high, special techniques have been developed to place endocardial leads transmurally at operation, e.g., transatrial, transventricular or periprosthetic valvular.[22,23]

Morbidity of Pacing

Pacing is generally well-tolerated in children. Most children have a normal exercise capacity and participate in gymnastics and sports. At the same time this activity increases the risk of injury to the pacemaker system, above all the risk of fractures of epicardial, but also of endocardial leads and connectors. Physiologic and rate-responsive pacing makes normal activity possible, but in the meantime it decreases the longevity of the battery. The five-year survival of the total pacing system in children is only 50-75%.[3,5,13] The reasons for surgical interventions are lead complications in 70%, and end of life criteria of the pulse generator in only 30%.[5] In our first 50 patients, surgical interventions were necessary every 4.9 patient-years. This is much too frequent, if a 70-80 years period of pacing lies ahead.

In order to lower morbidity in lifelong pacing, special care should be taken during implantation to prevent trauma during exercise. Programming should be done carefully, to allow activity on the one hand but to save the battery on the other hand. To increase the longevity of their electrodes and pacemakers, and in the meantime to develop new electronic possibilities, is a challenge for pacemaker manufacturers.

Conclusions

- Special skills are needed for pacing children and for pacing adults with (operated) congenital heart disease.
- The goal of pacing children and young adults should be to allow a normal active life with the least number of surgical interventions during their lifetime.
- This should be taken into account by the manufacturer, the implanting physician, the programming technician and the (pediatric) cardiologist.
- Good counselling and support of the patient will help to overcome the acceptance problems of the teenager and the young adult.
- Some adult cardiologists should specialize in pacing adult patients with (operated) congenital heart disease.

References

1. American College of Cardiology/American Heart Association Task Force Report. Guidelines for implantation of cardiac pacemakers and antiarrhythmia devices. J Am Coll Cardiol 1991;18: 1-13.

2. Smith RT Jr. Pacemakers for children. In: Gillette PC, Garson A Jr (eds), Pediatric arrhythmias: Electrophysiology and pacing. Saunders, Philadelphia, 1990, pp 533-4.
3. Smith RT Jr. Ppacemakers for children. In: Gillette PC, Garson A Jr (eds), Pediatric arrhythmias: Electrophysiology and pacing. Saunders, Philadelphia, 1990, pp 553-5.
4. Williams WG, Izukawa T, Olley PM, Trusler GA, Rowe RD. Permanent cardiac pacing in infants and children. PACE 1978;1:439-47.
5. Kerstjens-Frederikse WS, Bink-Boelkens MTE, Jongste MJL de, Homan van der Heide J. Permanent cardiac pacing in children: Morbidity and efficacy of follow-up. Int J Cardiol 1991;33:207-14.
6. Anderson RH, Ho SY, Becker AE. The surgical anatomy of the conduction tissues. Thorax 1983;38:408-20.
7. Garson A Jr, Bink-Boelkens MTE, Hesslein P, Hordof AJ, Keane JF, Neches WH, Porter C-BJ. Atrial flutter in the young: A collaborative of 380 cases. J Am Coll Cardiol 1985;6:871-8.
8. Zeigler VL, Gillette PC, Kratz J. Is activity sensored pacing in children and young adults a feasible option? PACE 1990;13:2104-7.
9. Paridon SM, Karpawich PP, Pinsky WW. Exercise performance with single chamber rate responsive pacing in congenital heart defects after operation. Am J Cardiol 1991;68:1231-3.
10. Antonioli GE. Single lead atrial synchronous ventricular pacing: A dream come true. PACE 1994;17:1531-47.
11. Hamilton R, Gow R, Bahoric B, Griffiths J, Freedom R, Williams W. Steroid-eluting epicardial leads in pediatrics: Improved epicardial thresholds in the first year. PACE 1991;14:2066-72.
12. Karpawich PP, Stokes KB, Proctor K, Schallhorn R, McVenes R, Factkor M. Improved epimyocardial pacing: Initial experience with a new bipolar steroid-eluting, high irnpedance lead design. PACE 1994;17:2032-7.
13. Till JA, Jones S, Rowland E, Shinebourne EA, Ward DE. Endocardial pacing in infants and children 15 kg or less in weight: Medium-term follow-up. PACE 1990;13:1385-92.
14. Gillette PC, Zeigler V, Bradham GB, Kinsella P. Pediatric transvenous pacing: A concern for venous thrombosis? PACE 1988;11:1935-9.
15. Lau YR, Gillette PC, Buckles DS, Zeigler VL. Actuarial survival of transvenous pacing leads in a pediatric population. PACE 1993;16:1363-7.
16. Friedman RA, Moak JP, Garson A Jr. Active fixation of endocardial leads: The preferred method of pediatric pacing. PACE 1991;14:1213-6.
17. O'Sullivan JJ, Jameson S, Gold RG, Wren C. Endocardial pacemakers in children: Lead length and allowance for growth. PACE 1993;16:267-71.
18. Gillette PC, Zeigler VL. Pacemakers in children. Cardiol Rev 1994;2:267-71.
19. Jacobs DM, Fink AS, Miller RP, Anderson WR, McVenes RD, Lessar JF, Cobian KE, Staffanson DB, Upton JE, Bubrick MP. Anatomical and morphological evaluation of pacemaker lead compression. PACE 1993;16:434-44.
20. Magney JE, Flynn DM, Parsons JA, Staplin DH, Chin-Purcell MV, Milstein S, Hunter DW. Anatomical mechanisms explaining damage to pacemaker leads, defibrillator leads and failure of central venous catheters adjacent to the sternoclavicular joint. PACE 1993;16:445-57.
21. Westerman GR, van Devanter SH. Surgical management of difficult pacing problems in patients with congenital heart disease. J Cardiac Surg 1987;2:351-60.
22. Byrd CL, Schwartz SJ. Transatrial implantation of transvenous pacing leads as an alternative to implantation of epicardial leads. PACE 1990;13:1856-9.
23. McCallister BD, Vlietstra RE, Westbrook BM, Hayes DL. A transmural approach for endocardial ventricular pacing. Am J Cardiol 1990;65:263-4.

4 MISCELLANEOUS ASPECTS

Chapter 13

Cardiac Pacing in Europe: Anno 1993

Hugo Ector and Giorgio A. Feruglio

Introduction

The European pacemaker registration has a long tradition and was an early research topic, promoted by the Working Group on Cardiac Pacing[1-3]. Pacing surveys are on the program of all World and European symposia on cardiac pacing. A list of surveys has been published recently[4].

The European Pacemaker Registration System is based on the use of the European Pacemaker Registration Card. It is now operating in 18 countries and has a database of over 800,000 registered pacemakers: the world's largest collection of patient-related pacing information!

In 1993, an estimate of 169,342 pacemakers were used in 2,758 implanting hospitals of 21 European countries. We have obtained information on 112,710 implanted units. Data include demographics, indications for pacing and pacemaker replacement, hardware and pacing modes, complications and causes for file closure.

Implantation Rate, Demographic Data

In Europe, the average continental implantation rate is still increasing. In 1993, it has reached a rate of 306 new implants per million population. Such a rate, still lower than in North America, varies considerably from country to country, being over 600/M in Belgium, close to 500 in France and Germany but as low as 127/M in Poland and less than 100/M in Yugoslavia (figure 1).

The ratio first implants/replacements was 4.2. Men were paced more frequently than females (54% vs 46%); the mean age was 74 ys for males and 76 ys for females. Patients over 80 years of age, at first implant, accounted for over 30% of the cases in 10 countries; while patients under 40 years of age were less than 3%. Patients paced at the age of 100 years or more were rare but not exceptional

Figure 1. **Pacemaker Implantations in Europe Anno 1993 number per million population**

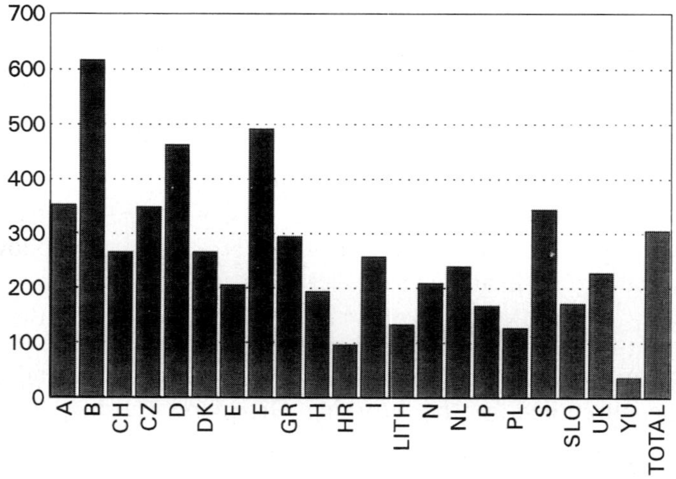

Figure 2. **Europe Anno 1992: Correlation Between PM implantation Rate (number per Million per Year) and Number of Implanting Centers per Million Inhabitants**

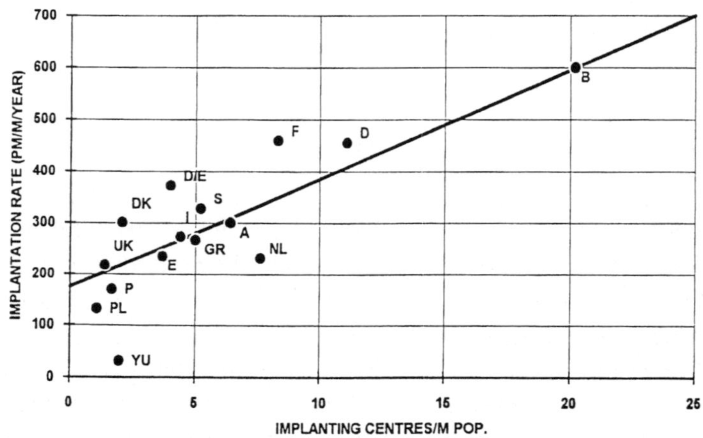

r = 0.804
p 0.001

(0.1% - 03%). The prevalence of elderly in the various countries does not seem to affect implantation rates to any extent. When comparing different European countries we have found a significant correlation between the number of implanting hospitals and the rate of new implants (figure 2). In Belgium we have 19.7 pacemaker centers/M, largely the highest figure in Europe.

Indications

Among clinical indications for pacing, syncope was the leading cause (up to 47.3% of cases in the United Kingdom and 51% in Greece) followed by dizzy spells, bradycardia and heart failure - in that order. Prophylactic pacing was performed in up to 4.7% of cases in France and 4.95 in Italy. With regard to the pre-pacing ECG, AV block of all degrees was the major indication (over 50% of cases in one third of the countries), followed by atrial rhythm disturbances (over 50% in one fourth of the countries). Atrial and ventricular tachycardias as indications for pacing, remained below or about 1% in most countries, with the exception of Norway 1.5% and Denmark 1.7% of cases.

Electrophysiologic studies were performed in up to 15% of pacemaker patients in Greece and Italy, and as low as 2% in the United Kingdom and 1% in Norway.

According to etiology, fibrosis and ischemic damage of the conducting tissue resulted as the most frequent causes; among others, carotid sinus syndrome (up to 11.6% of cases in Austria and Switzerland), post-AMI AV block (4% of cases in France and 5.6% in Germany), congenital and post-surgery AV block (0.5% and 1.8% of cases respectively) were reported in Germany.

Pacing Modes

With regard to pacing modes and device types (figures 3 and 4), single-chamber pacing and standard programmable generators were the most used (in 50.6% of cases in Italy; 53.8% in Germany and 57.4% in the United Kingdom); single-chamber rate adaptive pacing was reported in up to 29% of cases (Sweden); VDD pacing with a single-pass lead was used in up to 7% of cases in Italy, dual-chamber pacing with a standard programmable generator was used in up to 31.3% of cases in France and dual-chamber rate adaptive pacing in up to 32.3% of cases in Belgium. Activity sensors were most commonly utilized (in up to 83.6% of cases in Sweden) followed by breathing (31.8% in the United Kingdom) and combined sensors (up to 20.9% of cases in The Netherlands).

Figure 3. EUROPE ANNO 1993: PACING MODES

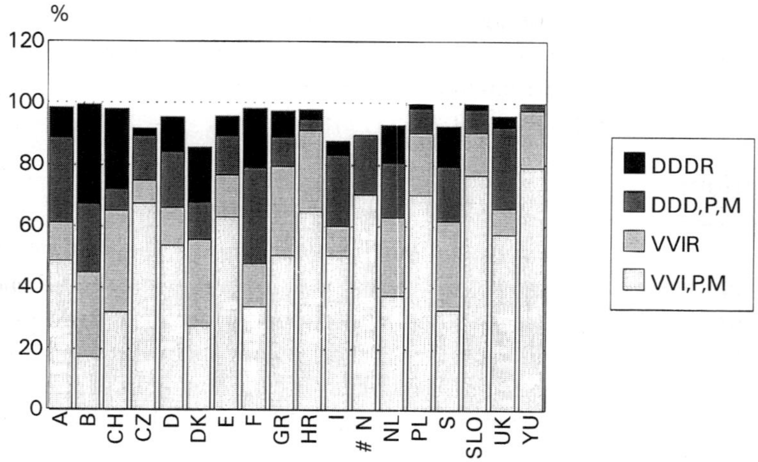

Total % of all VVI generators

Figure 4. EUROPE ANNO 1993
AAI VDD ANTITACHY PACING
% OF TOTAL NUMBER OF IMPLANTATIONS

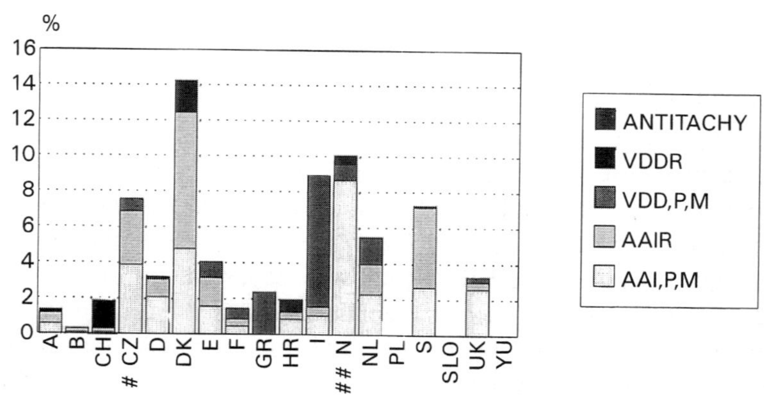

Total % of all VDD pacers ## Total % of all AAI pacers

Considering the pacing modes in AV block, single-chamber pacing was preferred in up to 42.6% of cases in the United Kingdom, while a dual-chamber mode was used in up to 59.2% and 66.9% of cases in Sweden and Belgium, respectively. In SSS, a single-chamber ventricular pacing mode was used in up to 67.5% in Germany; single-chamber pacing the atrium, in up to 71.3% in Sweden and a dual-chamber mode, in up to 62% in Belgium.

Pacing Leads

The transvenous approach for lead insertion was the method of choice througout Europe and, in up to 100% of cases in the United Kingdom. Venous cut-down was preferred in Sweden and Belgium (80% of cases) and percutaneous insertion (80% of cases) in the United Kingdom, Norway and Switzerland. With regard to the use of unipolar versus bipolar leads, no significant trends have emerged. While passive versus active fixation was definitely preferred for ventricular pacing (up to 95% and 97% of cases in Switzerland and Denmark respectively); an opposite trend was reported for pacing in the atrium.

Lead change was 'elective' in up to 1/5 of the cases of lead explantation; other indications for electrode removal were: infection (up to 26.5% of cases in Norway), displacement, exit block, insulation and connection break, in that order.

For lead removal, traction was the technique, most frequently used (over 90% in France); extraction was used in up to 9% of cases in Italy and the Czech Republic; open heart surgery was reported in up to 5% of cases in the United Kingdom.

Generators: Replacements, Cost

The most common cause of generator explantation was battery depletion: up to 52% and 59% of cases in Germany and Switzerland; premature battery depletion occurred in up to 3.7% and 4.2% of cases in the same countries. Major generator failures were reported in up to 7.5% of cases in Denmark. Local complications (infection, ulceration) occurred in up to 9.1% (Germany).

The average price of a single-chamber pacemaker varied from $1,600 to $5,600 (US dollars); dual-chamber units were priced $3,700 to $8,000 (US dollars) according to type and level of sophistication. Although all manufacturers were present on the European market, it appears that a single manufacturer occupied most of the pacemaker market in one fourth of the countries. Pacemaker reuse was reported in up to 4.3% of cases in Denmark.

File Closure

Among the indications for file closure, death related to pacemaker malfunction was reported in up to 1.6% of cases in Italy; other indications were: sudden death (up to 3% in Germany) and death cause unknown (up to 63.7% in Austria).

Failure Reporting

In Europe an on-line failure reporting system was started in the early 1970s by Prof. J.J. Welti.[5] In 1973, he was the founder of the Stimarec Association. Today his work is continued by J.F. Godin, J.C. Petitot, G. Pioger. The Stimarec Bulletin[6] continues to be published at regular intervals. It collects data on generator and lead failures from Austria, Belgium, Finland, France, Germany, Hungary, Italy, The Netherlands, Norway, Poland, Portugal, South Africa, Spain, United Kingdom, Yugoslavia. The particular value of this failure reporting system is, that it provides a fast response to new generator and lead failures. On appropriate forms, data are collected from the contributing pacing centers. Figure 5 gives an overview of pacemaker defects, as reported from 1981 to 1994. Special attention is given to dangerous cases.

Figure 5.

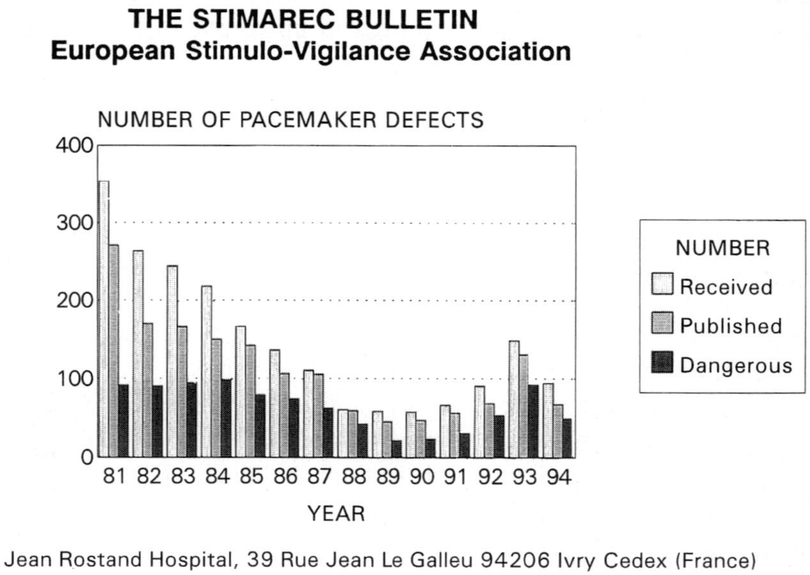

Too Many Pacemakers? Too Few?

This is an old recurrent question. Sick sinus syndrome and intraventricular conduction defects are suggested to be the major indications for unnecessary pacemaker implantations.[7,8] Reports suggested that 23% of pacemakers in the State of Maryland[9] were unnecessary, and that another 13% were questionably indicated. The Maryland Society of Cardiology in cooperation with 32 hospitals reviewed 610 of 817 patients so classified. A review of the complete medical record demonstrated valid indications in 95% of hospital records reviewed.
The clinical 'to pace or not to pace' decision is a daily challenge for the cardiologist. Although the use of pacemakers has grown rapidly, the indications have not changed a great deal. We still usually insert a pacemaker to relieve symptoms produced by bradyarrhythmias, that have been documented by a standard ECG, Holter recording, or occasionally by an electrophysiologic study. There is no need to modify this approach substantially. It is sometimes reasonable to advise that a pacemaker be inserted in a patient with bundle branch block and such symptoms as syncope or dizziness when no definite cause can be established despite exhaustive investigation.[10] The use of the 'Head-up tilt testing' adds to a more appropriate evaluation of unexplained recurrent syncope.[11-13] A clear differential diagnosis of neurocardiogenic syncope may prevent the insertion of a number of unnecessary pacemakers. This, in particular, applies to the vasodepressor type of syncope. In general, for neurocardiogenic syncope, a consensus is emerging to use pacing only in highly selected cases, not responding to medical treatment.

The European Pacing Survey illustrates how medical care is distributed in different countries. It proves also that not all European patients have the access to the medical care, they deserve. When envisaging the needs on a worldwide scale, Western cost benefit discussions, megatrials claiming for a small but important percent of benefit, may appear futile.

Pacing Groups and Guidelines

International and national registrations by pacing groups contribute to an objective survey of pacing work. With respect to controversial indications, a pacing group can offer peer review, improving appropriate patient selection. When guidelines are issued[14-15], and when they recommend the use of more sophisticated pacing units than previously prescribed, their implementation can have important financial implications both in the initial outlay for hardware and in increased costs of follow up.
The Working Group on Cardiac Pacing of the European Society of Cardiology

was always actively involved in implementing a pacemaker registration system throughout Europe. As early as in 1980, a European Centres Directory was issued.[16] To be mentioned as a pacemaker center, a minimum number of 50 pacemaker procedures per year was required (sum of first implants and repacements). With this guideline 50 procedures per year are assumed to be the minimum standard for maintaining a desirable quality of medical practice.

Belgium and Medical Care

With a stable population of 10 million people, there was an important increase in the implantation rate over the last 10 years (figure 6). Possible explanations are: (i) national health insurance system covering all costs of medical care; (ii) high number of practicing doctors; (iii) high number of hospitals; (iv) a countrywide completely free choice of doctor and hospital by the patient; (v) easy and prompt access to all medical facilities. Per million inhabitants, Belgium has the highest number of pacemaker centers (figure 2). For Europe, there is a significant correlation between the implantation rate and the number of centers/million people. In Belgium, an important part of implantation work is done by small centers (figures 7 and 8).

Figure 6. **Pacemaker Statistics Belgium Years 1984 - 1993**

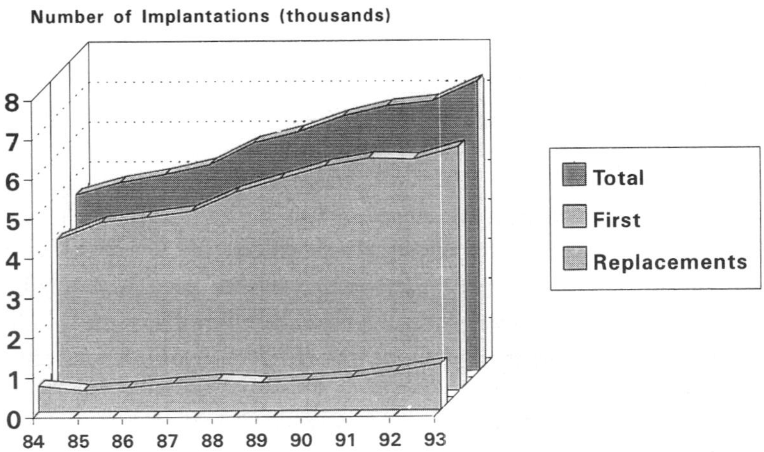

Table 7.

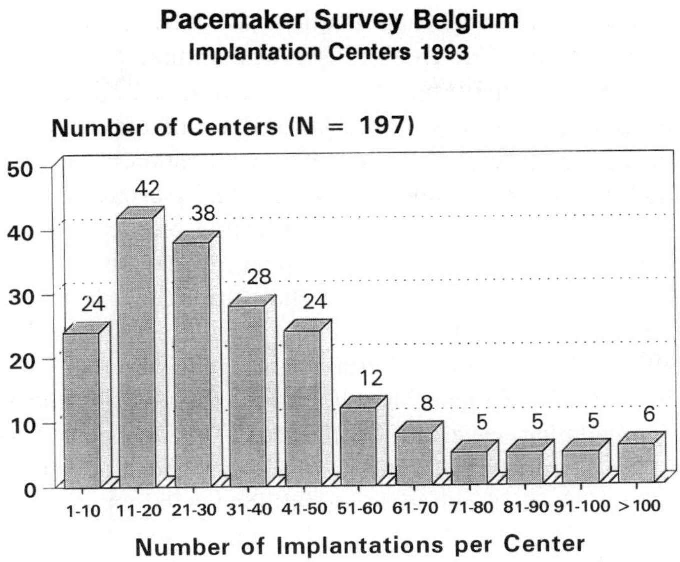

Table 8.

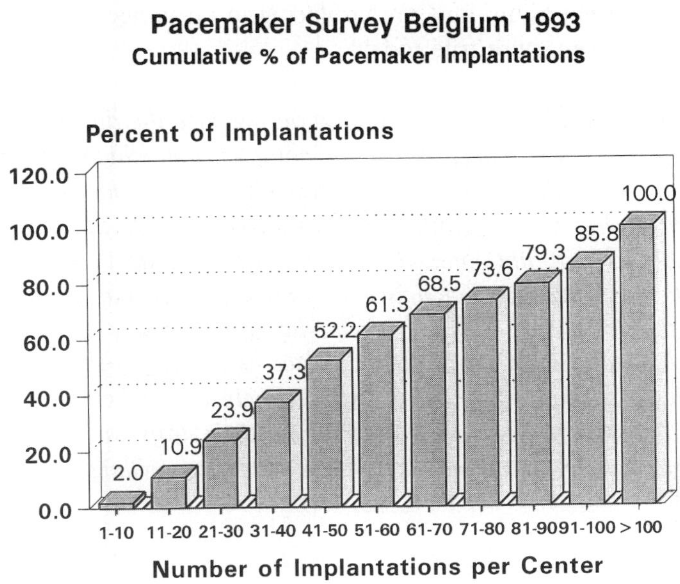

The experience with the high implantation rate is an incentive for organizing some form of peer review. The Health Insurance Authority is actually considering some initiative. The pacing experience also led to a continuous prospective monitoring of ICD implantations. The National Health Insurance Authority has introduced a convention system, where ICD implantations are restricted to a limited number of hospitals. A demand for covering the costs of an ICD implant must be submitted to a board of medical directors before the intervention. All implanting centers have agreed to accept peer review on their indications. In Belgium, medical care is based on a free choice principle. Every Belgian citizen is entitled to ask as many opinions he wants. He is free to enter any hospital in the country. When he is abroad, certainly in the European Union, there are agreements between the Belgian Health Insurance Authority and foreign health care systems, regulating coverage of the costs of unexpected or emergency medical care. The privileges of the so-called Belgian 'Social Security System' also apply to residents of other nationalities, fulfilling a minimum of legal requirements.

Conclusion

The dilemmas of modern medicine have been discussed in a straight forward style by HRH Prince Claus of The Netherlands[17], in his opening address at the 4th International Symposium on Cardiac Pacing in Groningen, 1973. His message of 20 years ago is even more true today:

> ' *As in other fields of scientific exploration, we face the dilemma that the more progress we make, the more complex the ethical implications become. As medical science advances, the demand for its services is also increasing. Consequently it is most regrettable that the medical skill available is still not enough to meet the demand, certainly where complicated medical techniques are involved. In the organizational sense the limits are set by the availability of equipment and manpower. A doctor sees his patient in the first place as a person instead of a case, as a human being whom he is trying to help to the best of his ability. The question is not only what doctors and their staffs can offer, but also what the people, that is we all, can afford and are willing to pay for.'*

European PM Registries:

Austria (A), K. Steinbach; Belgium (B), H. Ector; Croatia (HR), V. Goldner; Czech Rep. (CZ), J. Lukl; Denmark (DK), E. Simonson; France (F), M. Salvador-Mazenq, G. Pioger; Germany (D), W. Irnich; Greece (GR), P.E. Vardas; Hungary (H), F. Stolti; Italy (I), GA. Feruglio, L. Prelli; The Netherlands (NL), C. Hooijschuur; Norway (N), H. Grendahl; Poland (PL), G. Swiatecka; Portugal (P), J. Correia da Cunha; Slovenia (SLO), P. Rakovec; Spain (S), J. Silvestre; Sweden (S), R. Norlander; Switzerland (CH), H. Gloor, L. Kappenberger; UK, AF Rickards, D. Cunningham; Yugoslavia (YU), D. Velimirovic.

References

1. Shaudig A, Rickards AF, Thalen HJTh. Multi-purpose pacemaker registration card (PPRC). In: Meere C (ed.), Cardiac Pacing: State of the Art 1979; Proceedings of the VIth World Symposium on Cardiac Pacing. Montreal 1979, Section 26-4.
2. Feruglio GA, Steinbach K. Cardiac pacing in Europe after two decades: a comprehensive survey. In: Feruglio (ed.), Cardiac Pacing: Proceedings of the 2nd European Symposium on Cardiac Pacing. Piccin Medical Books, Padova 1982, pp 1-13.
3. Rickards AF. The European registration Card. Stimulation, June 6, 1988:7-10.
4. Feruglio GA. Cardiac pacing in Europe in 1992: a new survey. In: Aubert AE, Ector H, Stroobandt R (eds), Cardiac Pacing and Electrophysiology. A bridge to the 21st century. Kluwer Academic Publishers, Dordrecht, The Netherlands, 1994, pp 157-68.
5. Fontaine G, Furman S. Jean-Jacques Welti. PACE 1988;11:988.
6. Stimarec. Jean Rostand Hospital, 39 rue Jean Le Galleu, 94206 IVRY Cedex, France.
7. Friedman HS. Have pacemakers found their way into too many patients? JAMA 1980;243: 2371-2.
8. Friedman HS. Are too many permanent pacemakers being implanted? PACE 1981;4:232-4.
9. Scherlis L, Dembo DH. Excessive permanent pacemaker utilization in the state of Maryland. A fallacy of the hospital record face sheet. In: Steinbach K (ed.), Cardiac Pacing: Proceedings of the VIIth World Symposium on Cardiac Pacing. Steinkopff Verlag, Darmstadt 1983, p 981.
10. Kastor JA. Preventive pacemaking. N Eng J Med 1982;307:180-1.
11. Hargreaves AD, Hag OE, Boon NA. Head-up tilt testing. Br Heart J 1994;72: 216-7.
12. Fitzpatrick AP, Theodorakis G, Vardas P, Sutton R. Methodology of head-up tilt testing in patients with unexplained syncope. J Am Coll Cardiol 1991;17:125-30.
13. Sra JS, Jazayeri MR, Avitall B, Dhala A, Deshpande S, Blanck Z, Akhtar M. Comparison of cardiac pacing with drug therapy in the treatment of neurocardiogenic (vasovagal) syncope with bradycardia or asystole. N Engl J Med 1993;328:1085-90.
14. Recommendations for pacemaker prescription for symptomatic bradycardia. Report of a working party of the British Pacing and Electrophysiology Group. Br Heart J 1991;66:185-91.
15. Mounsey JP, Ray SG, Griffith MJ, Gold RG, Bexton RS. Impact of internal audit on pacemaker prescription and the immediate costs of pacing in the Northern Region: towards implementations of the British Pacing and Electrophysiology Group. Br Heart J 1994;71:395-8.
16. European Pacing Centres Directory: published by the British Pacing Group, London 1980.
17. HRH Prince Claus of The Netherlands. Opening Address. In: Thalen HJT (ed.), Cardiac Pacing: Proceedings of the IVth International Symposium on Cardiac Pacing, Groningen 1973. Van Gorcum, Assen, The Netherlands 1973, p XII.

4 MISCELLANEOUS ASPECTS

Chapter 14

The Safety and Medico-Legal Responsibilities of the Pacemaker Implantation Team

Bas A.J.M. de Mol

Introduction

There is no doubt that thanks to the large-scale availability of pacemakers and cardioverter-defibrillators, the life expectancy and quality of life of numerous patients has much improved. Pacemakers are used since a long time, they have proven their value, and they have become big business for the industry, scientists, and cardiologists.[1] Although technical innovation has resulted in safer and more effective pacemakers, thereby reducing the number of adverse effects and improving patient compliance, it has also created three areas of potential conflicts of interest:

1. Innovation may still have to prove its value for the patient. Extensive clinical testing and patient follow-up studies are then required, for which recognized end-points within the framework of evidence-based medicine are needed.[2]
2. As pacemakers are widely used, innovation may yield enormous financial rewards to the industry and cardiologists. This could interfere with safety priorities, the patient-doctor relation, and the cardiologists' independence of the industry.[3,4]
3. As pacemakers and cardioverter-defibrillators are potentially life-saving devices, cardiologists may adopt a liberal policy in terms of the indication for use. This might lead to technical and budgetary disputes on what should be considered an appropriate indication.[5]

Medico-Legal Responsibilities of the Cardiologist

A doctor's duty is characterized by his responsibility for medico-technical patient care within the constraints of the medical standards. These medical standards can be imposed by legislation or by a hospital, a medical profession, or an individual doctor.[6] So, medical standards are laid down in laws or regulatory directives and are present as unwritten medical practice codes based on bioethical and moral principles.

The purpose of this study is to provide information on the legal regulations that are important to those dealing with decision-making on pacemaker application and patient safety. It particularly focuses on the regulations and pre- and postimplant responsibilities of the cardiologist and the industry.

When we review the contents of these regulations, we will note that the regulations on the preimplant responsibilities are meant to ensure that the implant is safe and effective before it is used in patients, while those on the postimplant responsibilities underline the importance of consumer protection and civil litigation. (As criminal behaviour is hardly ever exposed, criminal litigation is rare).

Taking as our basic assumption that the use of a medical device presupposes the presence of a legitimate indication (medical diagnosis or treatment), it is important to recognize that the cardiologist can be put in a position where he has to act as his patient's representative (e.g. when selecting a device or when dealing with the industry).[7] His relation with the patient becomes even more complex when he has entered the patient in a clinical study. This forces the cardiologist not only to provide patient care but also to pursue scientific progress while remaining loyal to the sponsor. Whatever the circumstances may be, a cardiologist should, of course, always reserve his primary loyalty for his patient. Although one has to admit that there has not been much arguing about this yet, the proper sequence when serving various interests cannot be reiterated often enough.

For health administrators, this can be different, because the occasion may arise that the interest of an individual patient should become secondary to the interest of the general public. Interestingly enough, the industry, which likes to boast that its top priority is patient welfare whatever the circumstances may be, feels usually obliged to pursue a thriving business, the reasons for which are obvious.

Therefore, for the patient, the cardiologist is the first to rely on for effective and safe medical treatment. Second, via the cardiologist or hospital, the patient is exposed to subsets of rulings on product quality and safety, which are the aspects a manufacturer likes to emphasize most. Third, the framework of rules on standardization, certification, and product liability, which applies to most industrial and economic activities, provides an outer legal shell.

In this study, we will review three types of pacemaker problems to provide a cross-section of these three subsets of rules:

1. The failed pacemaker wire.
2. The large-scale implantation of cardioverter-defibrillators.
3. The reduced availability of pacemaker materials due to the so-called biomaterials crisis in the USA.

The Regulatory Framework

Regulation on how to prevent implant failure is essential, as an implant's function can rarely be adjusted once it is in situ. However, the pacemaker, which is an active electrical implant, is an exception. Once pacemaker generator and lead have been properly implanted, adjustments can still be made to achieve optimal pacemaker functioning. Although this offers advantages, it also introduces potential failure modes, especially where it relates to 'communicating' with the pacemaker. The industry will try to market a pacemaker of the highest quality. The options to achieve this are limited to improvements in product design, manufacturing, packing, and user's instructions.[8]

Premarket Regulations in the USA

In the US Medical Device Amendments of 1976, a class-III device is described as a device that 'supports or sustains human life or is of substantial importance in preventing impairment of human health or presents a potential, unreasonable risk of illness or injury'. The clinical testing of a class-III device is only allowed after one has obtained explicit permission of the Food and Drug Administration (FDA) (the so-called Investigational Device Exemption (IDE)). This permission will only be given when sufficient in-vitro and animal studies have been carried out. When the first clinical data are available, the so-called Pre-Market Approval (PMA) procedure is brought into effect. This permits the systemic collection of data by means of clinical trials with a focus on safety and efficacy. Regulations on other aspects, such as patient-tracking, adverse-effect-reporting, product recalls, and (some) civil penalties, can be found in the Safe Medical Device Act (SMDA) of 1990.

Premarket Regulations in Europe

Many European states have regulations equivalent to those of the US Medical Device Act. Because of Europe's many differences from country to country and the objective of the European Union to harmonize the regulations on medical products, a framework of directives has been set up by the European Committee for Standardization (CEN). Of relevance for pacemakers are the European Products Liability Directory and the Active Implantable Medical Device Directory (90/385/EEC), which became mandatory for all member states on January 1, 1995. The general objective of the latter directory is to ensure patient safety and a correct indication for device application. A product meets the official standards on product safety and product performance when it complies with the so-called 'Essential Requirements'. There are three classes of products, the pacemaker family belonging to class III (i.e. highest risk of death and/or serious damage). These standards were drafted according to the guidelines of the European Committee for Standardization. Under the supervision of a national normalization or standards body, working committees or so-called Technical Committees (TC) subsequently customize these standards for the specific products. In these TC's, one can find representatives of manufacturers, health authorities, medical professions, and other standardization institutes. Together, they review all aspects, leading to a draft proposal. Due to the Committee's diverse composition, however, it usually involves more than just one draft. Their final proposal will then be voted on for adoption by the Central Committee, which makes the standard official.

To have a product tested according to the official standards, the manufacturer can take the initiative to approach a so-called national notified body (e.g. TÜV in Germany, KEMA in The Netherlands, and DHSS in United Kingdom). When the test results meet the standard, the device will receive a CE-mark, containing the number of the testing authority or notifying body. Should a device not pass the test, then one is not allowed to submit it to another notifying body until relevant changes have been made.

A cardiologist is expected to thoroughly inspect the CE-mark. Although notifying bodies have to meet standards too, i.e. on test capabilities and test facilities, it is probable that they compete with one another, not just for the absolute minimum of the number of requirements, but also for the best equipped and most reliable test set-up. Especially when innovative products are involved, it is unlikely that the usual tests are sufficient to confirm an 'added value'. Because of this, the manufacturer is usually not able to use the test results to support his claims on improved performance.

As the CE-mark reflects the thoroughness of a test procedure, based on the reputation a test center may have, the cardiologist should certainly look at the CE-mark when selecting a pacemaker. The CE-mark also offers the cardiologist the option to retrieve additional test data. This is especially important as these data are obtained without the interference of the manufacturer. Although in principle all pacemakers and cardioverter-defibrillators have to have a CE-mark, niche products and developing products that are custom-made, may be exempted. These products remain, of course, subject to the law and the regulations on medical experiments and products liability, putting the burden of strict liability with the doctor or manufacturer or both.

The Relevance of Good Manufacturing and Clinical Practice

Good Manufacturing Practice Regulations

Obviously, not just the test samples but all devices must meet the requirements on manufacturing and testing. Therefore, controlling bodies scrutinize the manufacturing process and quality control procedures too.

In fact, the manufacturer has to meet the so-called Good Manufacturing Practice (GMP) Regulations for Medical Devices.[9] These regulations require the following:

1. A quality assurance programme, covering numerous matters, ranging from an adequate organization with properly trained personnel to periodic audits and corrective action.
2. An up-to-date device master record or device history record, in which all steps of the manufacturing process are documented. (Thanks to such records, the relation between a particular welder and a series of fractured Björk-Shiley convexo-concave valves could be established.[10])
3. Documented standard operating procedures and deviations of the normal procedures.
4. The checking of the used components and materials (specifications, sources, storage method).
5. Buildings and environment must provide a safe work area, allow proper cleaning, and pose minimal toxic danger. Sanitation and contamination control procedures must regularly be checked.
6. Equipment must be properly installed, maintained, and calibrated.
7. The requirements for packaging, labelling, and sterilization must be met.
8. Adequate control of changes in software, components, manufacturing process, labelling, etc. to prevent product liability actions.
9. Production and process control to ensure the accurate transfer of product design to written specifications of the device and the manufacturing process.
10. Complaints and failure investigation to provide feed-back on design and

manufacturing process. (A complaint is defined as an 'expression of dissatisfaction with the identity, quality, durability, reliability, safety, effectiveness, or performance of a device'.)

Good Clinical Practice Regulations

The purpose of good clinical research is to prove that the medical expectations in terms of device performance and effectiveness, are justified. The FDA has laid down some basic rules to this effect, e.g. on the lay-out of clinical research protocols, Medical Ethics Committee approval, patient information, informed consent, adverse-effect reporting, trial monitoring, and completing/processing case record forms.[11-13]

In 1993, the European Committee for Standardization approved the European Standard for Clinical Investigation of Medical Devices for Human Subjects (EN 540), which can be obtained from the national standards bodies. In the EN 540 Standard, terminology, clinical testing process, and role of sponsor, monitor, and clinical investigator are described in detail.

Pacemaker Implantation and Tort Law

Should a pacemaker fail, then the first to be responsible for the damage is the manufacturer, provided the damage is solely due to pacemaker failure beyond the normal expectations in terms of performance, durability, and use. This enables the patient to sue the manufacturer based on product liability. Doctors and hospitals are often able to transfer the risk of insurance claims to a third party. In fact, in many countries this option is provided by legislation and case law. The patient is considered to need extra legal protection in the setting of an experiment, as 'the patient should not suffer from dispute or doubt related to the medical treatment by his doctor'. (This is important to know, as the patient has the choice to participate in a trial, e.g. to study an innovated pacemaker or to opt for a regular state-of-the-art treatment.)

Negligence of the manufacturer or doctor does not have to be proven. What counts primarily is that the patient may not suffer damages from an innovated study device that proved to be harmful beyond his influence. This is called 'the strict liability of a doctor or hospital'. Whether or not the 'risk of innovation' or 'risk of development' should exclusively be carried by the manufacturer, is increasingly disputed. Implant failure may be exposed after a considerable amount of time only, as damage to the patient remains limited. Nevertheless, whether failure is considered an acceptable safety risk, generally depends on the type of flaw and state of the art of the device. Also the decision of many legislators and courts to accept corporate hospital liability in case of product failure or medical malpractice, was based on the reasoning that the patient should be maximally protected in situations beyond his control (as in a medical experiment).

When a device fails, the patient has the theoretical choice to sue either the hospital or the manufacturer. Often, the patient does not want put his relationship with the doctor and hospital at risk and will opt for suing the manufacturer. The latter might be just too eager to accept this burden, as it offers him the chance to preserve as much of his relationship with the hospital as possible. The bigger companies are usually well insured, enabling them to cope with the risk of litigation.

However, innovative medical devices are often spin-offs of small-company creativity and entrepreneurship. Even in the early days of medical devices, when the litigation climate in the USA was still 'mild', smaller companies put themselves up for sale, just because of the litigation risk. Despite changes in the FDA's approval procedures and serious efforts to restructure the US device industry such that it becomes similar to the pharmaceutical industry[14-16], many US medical device industries prefer to move to Europe to carry out the required clinical studies. Although the regulatory climate is still more hospitable in Europe than in the USA, the European litigation climate is becoming harsher by the year.

Apart from the fact that US manufacturers may have to face law suits by European citizens in US courts, the 'litigation awareness' of most urban Europeans is rapidly expanding and already almost equal to that of US citizens. The difference with the US system is that the European system lacks provisions for punitive damages, while the tort system is less expensive. However, the willingness of patients, doctors, and hospitals to embark on a clinical trial soon after a device failure due to design and manufacturing shortcomings, usually rapidly disappears.

Taking care of disappointed patients is a tremendous drain on doctors, requiring substantial medical resources (extra consultation time, extra tests), while doctors also have to face the additional burden of damaged patient confidence. Furthermore, the calling-off of a trial usually leads to all kinds of organizational trouble and can seriously damage the research reputation a hospital may have. The principal questions of patients and hospital managers to clinical investigators in these situations are basically always the same:

1. 'Why you did you decide to test that particular device?'
2. 'Could you reasonably have foreseen the problem?'

The doctor involved should always have his answer to these questions ready.

Safety and Risk Acceptance

Safety presupposes a consensus on an acceptable minimal risk for injury, which remains in spite of all possible efforts and precautions: the residual risk. The following test criteria should be applied to judge whether or not a risk of failure is acceptable[17]:

1. failure usually results either in avoidable death or in disability;
2. the manufacturing, user's instructions, or the use of the technology are substandard and/or the used technology is substandard according to the basic rules of good manufacturing/clinical practice;
3. the manufacturer and/or members of the medical profession are aware of the problem but neither willing nor able to solve the problem;
4. marketing and using the product in patients continues in spite of knowledge of the presence of deficiencies;
5. the failure rate of alternative procedures is low;
6. society's investments to save human lives in other areas, e.g. air traffic and chemical industry, are enormous and make carelessness and preventable loss of lives in a health care system unacceptable.

No definite answer can be given to the question whether a specific invasive treatment is safe enough. Circumstances of treatment, level of training, type of facility available, and applied assessment techniques that discriminate safe from unsafe institutions, all contribute to that judgement. From the results of the studies[1,18-25] and data on the risk control techniques, one may assume that invasive cardiovascular treatment should be made safer. There is no reason to wait for imposed legislation. It can be done on the basis of self-regulation, and hospitals may decide to compare results and embark on internal and external auditing. Should this reveal unsatisfactory performance, professorial knowledge and risk-management experience has to be made available to adjust medical practice.

Risk Disclosure Improves Safety

In surgery and invasive medicine, an adverse event is frequently labelled as an unexpected complication of surgical treatment. The use of this euphemism may be induced by fear of litigation. The negative effects of fear of litigation for patients and doctors are well described.[26,27] Also, a conflict of interest between doctor and patient, e.g. on financial matters or research participation, may blur the required candour of disclosure and the informed consent.[3] Additionally, doctors should be aware of the fact that for laymen information concerning prognosis and risks of surgery is often difficult to appreciate.[28] Sharing prognostic information appears to have a positive effect on the patient's willingness to participate in clinical research.[29]

However, it is virtually impossible to be complete when discussing the wide variety of risks related to invasive treatment.

Post Marketing Surveillance and Retrieval Analysis

Despite the quality standards, pre-market assessment procedures, and Good Manufacturing Practice, it has become quite common for patients, doctors, and industry to encounter reports on device deficiencies. To obtain feed-back on technical innovation and to control patient damage due to device failure, many US states demand that adverse events are officially reported.[30] However, even fatal failures do not always generate unequivocal and easy measures. Information on the extent of the problem is needed, not only about the number of patients at risk, but also about the damage-control measure (i.e. can it be applied without causing much harm?).

So, after one or two reports of failed pacemakers, the first action to be taken is to assess whether a structural phenomenon is involved or whether it is just a case of 'bad luck'. Therefore, 'Early-Warning and Quick-Rating Rules' for a variety of devices are now being developed. A common and harmless action is starting a 'recall procedure', i.e. all not-implanted devices should be returned to the manufacturer in order to be checked. When product failure is structural and potentially lethal, it can be wise to carry out elective implant explantation.[8] However, the hazards of this may outweigh the hazards of device failure. Patient-related circumstances may also have to be considered, e.g. a prolonged life expectancy constitutes a greater risk of exposure to implant failure. Younger patients are therefore usually more eligible for preventive implant explantation (an increased cumulative risk and relatively good physical condition).

When the tilted disk of a Björk-Shiley convexo-concave valve gives way, the patient dies within minutes or hours unless emergency surgery is carried out. Unfortunately, a diagnostic tool to screen patients for imminent valve fracture is still lacking. By contrast, the gradual depletion of a pacemaker generator or a fracture in a lead support wire can, in fact, be anticipated or diagnosed by screening. Even when this does not occur, patients still have a fair chance to reach a hospital to be adequately treated. We already learned that because of the mechanism of implant failure, the actual danger to the patient may take years to develop.

However, when a life-support system or class-III device is involved, it is of utmost importance to be able to anticipate device failure. It is therefore now generally accepted that the use of pacemakers or similar devices puts cardiologists under the obligation to maintain an up-to-date patient record and to report any adverse event.

The European and national pacemaker databases can serve as good examples of adequate co-operation between the cardiologist and the industry in terms of improving product design and developing strategies to contain patient damage. Assuming that all marketed pacemakers passed the pre-implant assessment test, large-scale structural failures of pacemaker generators and leads are not foreseen at the present time. The database, however, enables instant quick-rating, recall procedures, and risk-intensity calculations for the various strategies.

As the most significant problems with pacemakers are caused by design flaws[30], which are present in almost each product sample, a few reports and thorough failure analysis may trigger an adequate response thanks to the database, even though doctors are considered poor reporters of adverse events.[13] Sometimes, a mechanical problem can be anticipated thanks to the technical information obtained by retrieval analysis.

In the early days of implantation technology, all parties were satisfied with the rather short-term expectations on durability and effectiveness. However, due to the ageing of the population in the industrialized world, many devices will be 'outlived'. Pacemaker generators will thus have to be replaced or reloaded, and pacemaker leads might unintentionally long be exposed to the patient, sometimes for decades. Degradation of the 'plastic' coating, thrombus formation, and encapsulation may very well cause problems such as sepsis and vascular obstruction, for which heroic life-saving procedures might be needed. This shows that the very success of a device might generate life-threatening risks in the long-term.

To make the knowledge on a product's life cycle complete, implant retrieval is vital. It might confirm the preimplant expectations and validate the preimplant tests. Both for incidental and for routine implant retrieval, a consensus is required on a number of prerequisites. First of all, a research focus or problem-solving target is required. Chemical and physical analyses are extremely expensive. Therefore, before embarking on retrieval analysis, a protocol should be available on how to handle retrieved implants, describe clinical findings, make use of video or photography, and preserve and clean retrieved implants. Standards are already available, but not very well known to the clinicians. A protocol on test procedures and data interpretation should be available too. Last but not least, retrieval analysis often produces unexpected and unwelcome information, which may lead to a conflict of interest. It should be clear that the results of retrieval analysis should be shared with the retrieving doctor, and that these results should be explained to him. If necessary, the retrieving doctor may decide to obtain an expert opinion. Retrieval analysis is a matter of bioengineering, which is alien to most clinicians. Nevertheless, clinicians will have to accept that retrieval analysis, just like postmortem studies, can provide indispensable feedback for medical decision-making.

How Does the Regulatory System Work Out for the Cardiologist?

One may question whether pacemakers and cardioverter-defibrillators put special demands on the cardiac profession. The answer is yes. The use of these devices for complex cardiac disease is certainly demanding, affecting clinical decision-making where it relates to efficacy, effectiveness, and safety. Many cardiologists do not seem to be aware of the fact that high-tech hardware also requires high-tech 'software' (such as regulations, financial interest, safety trade-offs, ethics, and patient protection).[31]

Cardiologists operate in the front line of medical progress and what they are experiencing at the present time will be encountered by other specialties a few years from now. This phenomenon is not unusual and might be rather appealing. Therefore, the general conclusion is that the well-trained, well-educated, and enthusiastic cardiologist should be sufficiently equipped and organized to cope with the regulatory environment he will face.

A Faulty Pacing Component

Problems are usually all different, and problems caused by failed electromedical devices are no exception. The recent problems with the Accufix Atrial J-leads of Telectronics, Inc. were due to a fractured J-shaped retention wire. The Dutch cardiac and cardiosurgical profession received from the manufacturer relevant recall-information (dated January 23, 1995). It contained the results of ongoing studies, procedures, and also recommendations. It is noted in this document that worldwide approximately 42,421 patients carry this device, which gives a good impression of the problem's magnitude. It was also stated that 'the incidence of the fracture of these leads is significantly higher than previously reported and expected. You have not previously received this information'.

This information to doctors, with a potential impact on counselling and treating patients, was provided after close consultation of health authorities and expert panels. Based on this information, one might conclude that the manufacturer acted according to the established procedures. However, it is important that cardiologists consider the following aspects. Compared with the cardiac profession, the manufacturer has virtually a monopoly where it relates to resources, materials knowledge (via his worldwide network), comprehensive knowledge of the technical problems, and funding (put aside for imminent products liability actions). In addition, he may benefit from the generally accepted assumption that he is the best-equipped individual to carry out retrieval analysis and orchestrate risk control actions.[32]

The potential for a conflict of interest is evident and just too familiar from other cases of device failure. Not only patient welfare is important to the manufacturer, he also has to survive stiff and often killing competition[1], keep shareholders at peace, and prevent lay-offs. Because of the complex problems for the manufacturer and the patient, clarity in terms of responsibilities and visible crisis management are required. In this respect, Telectronics, Inc. did a good job so far.

For the proper use of the manufacturer information and for adequate medical care, manufacturer and patient fully rely on the response of the cardiac profession.[30] Shortcomings of the cardiologist towards the patient and manufacturer may generate liability claims in case of damage. However, it also seems justified that cardiologist and patient are financially compensated by the manufacturer when suffering damage following an unwanted and unacceptable business incident. Various case laws on failed pacemakers led to product liability of the manufacturer, but also to the obligation for cardiologists to maintain an effective patient registry, to inform and counsel the patient, and to co-operate in order to minimize the damage to the interested party, in particular the patient. In a Dutch case, the court ruled that it should be proven that the cardiologist had implanted the failed device in good faith and also on reasonable grounds.

New Technology

A problem of entirely different dimensions is caused by a very appealing and successful aspect of pacemaker technology. In two German studies, data are presented on 39 cardioverter-defibrillator implantations. These implantations were performed by using the single-incision approach or the non-thoracotomy lead system or both.[35,35] The results of these studies suggest that a life-threatening condition can be cured by implanting a small, life-sustaining device, which only requires a small surgical intervention, while the associated risk of mortality and morbidity is low (similar to the risk of pacemaker implantation). This progress, however, also has its limitations. The studied high-tech devices are extremely expensive and their clinical use is subject of reimbursement and strict indication rules.

Although long-term follow-up study results are not yet available, the medical profession can expect requests to implant these useful, patient-friendly, and low-risk devices in patients who might suffer from potentially lethal arrhythmias in case of cardiac ischaemia or heart attack or to implant them in any elderly cardiac patient. A harmless and ready-to-save-a-life device certainly appears more patient-friendly and effective than prophylactic anti-arrhythmic medication, with its limited effects and potential dangers. Apart from the problems of funding and a lacking definition of the appropriate indication to enable clinical decision-making, evidence-based medicine models still have to 'prove' which treatment is more effective. It seems safe to predict, however, that this high-tech device will become so appealing that it is already widely used when a cost-effectiveness analysis still has to be carried out.

In some countries, it is not unusual that expensive implants are leased, which can guarantee postmortem retrieval and re-use. This procedure demands a high-quality informed consent, co-operation of the relatives, and resources to reprocess the device for re-use.[36] Again, the cardiologist will play a pivotal role. He will have to cope with problems related to reimbursement, implant indication, informed consent, implant retrieval, property rights, and quality assurance of a device reprocessed for re-use.

The Biomaterials Crisis

It is most likely that during the next decade, the need for cardiovascular devices will rapidly expand. However, entrepreneurship and consumerism, which caused a booming medical-device industry in the US, also created this industry's greatest threat. Product liability is an indispensable link in the economic chain, as it hold the interests of consumers and manufacturers together in a balanced market place. Litigation actions in the USA are extremely expensive. This is due to the level of attorney's fees, punitive damages, and the necessity to claim the real material losses (due to the minimal or absent social security provisions).[21]

As most US medical device industries are only small and unable to cope with substantial liability claims, the law offers the plaintiff or patient the opportunity to also sue the supplier of the used components or raw materials. In the class-action settlement concerning the silicone breast implant, the involved suppliers of raw silicone agreed to pay billions of dollars as compensation. In the case of the failed jaw implant, the multinational DuPont de Nemours had to spend more than $10 million for legal fees, as it was sued for providing teflon. (Note that the teflon had a value of only some tens of thousands of dollars!) It seems only logic that the suppliers of the raw materials withdrew from the medical market.[37,38]

However, in the not too distant future, this development might cause a serious shortage in the supply of raw materials, thus significantly affecting the US production of medical devices. This will cause prices of medical devices to rise and, of course, an uproar in the US biomaterials industry. However, a rescue operation might be underway. A powerful Biomaterials Availability Lobby has become active, trying to preserve the current structure of the US device industry, to break-down the regulatory FDA checks, and to reduce the possibilities to correct manufacturers by means of the manufacturer's liability when delivering substandard products. The lobbyists, however, overlook one basic problem in regard to product liability: far too many of the failed devices that did not represent new technology at the time of marketing, failed due to evident flaws in design and manufacturing.

It is rather paradoxical that the FDA, a complex regulatory framework that is fully supported by the US legislation, in fact 'helped' to produce unacceptable outcomes and supervisory failures, as in the case of the Björk-Shiley convexo-concave heart valve and silicone breast implant. The FDA, as a powerful regulatory body, will be stripped of its octopus-like ambitions by the US legislature. This will leave the cardiologist with the extra obligation to carefully watch the quality of the device he may select.

Conclusion

With or without a fully present regulatory body that designs and assesses medical standards, a critical use of high-tech devices, particularly cardiac electro-medical devices, remains mandatory. This is seated in the primary duties of any cardiologist to care for the patient. After all: 'First, do no harm'.

References

1. Starr A. The thoracic-surgical industrial complex. Ann Thorac Surg 1986;42:124-133.
2. Evidence-Based Medicine Working Group. Evidence-based medicine: a new approach to teaching the practice of medicine. JAMA 1992;268:2420-5.

3. Rowdin MA. Physicians' conflict of interests. The limitations of disclosure. N Engl J Med 1989;321:1407.
4. Relman AS. Dealing with conflicts of interest. N Engl J Med 1985;313:749-51.
5. Kellie SE, Kelly JT. Medicare peer review organization preprocedure review criteria. An analysis of criteria for three procedures. JAMA 1991;265:1265-70.
6. Beauchamp TL, Childress JF. Principles of biomedical ethics. New York: Oxford University Press, 1989:342-6.
7. Gutheil TG, Bursztajn H, Brodsky A. Malpractice prevention through the sharing of uncertainty. N Engl J Med 1984;311:49-52.
8. Koornneef F, Gaalen van GL, Mol de BAJM. A risk assessment and control model for the failing Björk-Shiley convexo-concave heart valve. Int J Tech Assess Health Care (in press).
9. Lowery A, Puelo J. Good manufacturing practices. In: Gruting CW van (ed.) Medical devices. International perspectives on health and safety. Amsterdam: Elsevier, 1994:175-95.
10. Mol de BAJM, Kallewaard M, McLellan RB, Herwerden van LA, Defauw JJ, Graaf van der Y. Single-leg fractures in explanted Björk-Shiley valves. Lancet 1994;343:9-12.
11. Gerlis L. Good Clinical practice in clinical research. Lancet 1989;i:1008-9.
12. Shapiro MF, Charrow RP. The role of data audits in detecting scientific misconduct. JAMA 1989;261:2505-11.
13. Leiper JM, Lawson DH. Why do doctors not report adverse drug reactions? Neth J Med 1985;28:546-50.
14. Pollard MR. Pharmaceutical innovation in the United States. Factors affecting future performance. Int J Tech Assess Health Care 1993;9:167-73.
15. Kessler DA, Pape SM, Sundwall DN. The federal regulation of medical devices. N Engl J Med 1987;317:357-66.
16. Kessler DA. FDA's revitalization of Medical Device Review and Regulation. Biomed Instr Tech 1994:220-6.
17. Pochin EE. The acceptance of risk. Br Med Bull 1975;31:184-90.
18. Gray D, Hampton JR, Bernstein SJ, Kosecoff J, Brook RH. Audit of coronary angiography and bypass surgery. Lancet 1990;335:1317-20.
19. Brennan TA, Leape LL, Laird NM, Herbert LE, Localio AR, Lawthers AG, Newhouse JP, Weiler PC, Hiatt HH. Incidence of adverse events and negligence in hospitalized patients. Results of the Harvard Medical Practice Study I. N Engl J Med 1991;324:370-7.
20. Leape LL, Brennan TA, Laird N, Lawthers AG, Localio AR, Barnes BA, Herbert LE, Newhouse JP, Weiler PC, Hiatt HH. The nature of adverse events in hospitalized patients. Results of the Harvard Medical Practice Study II. N Engl J Med 1991;324:377-84.
21. Spencer FC. The urgent need for major reform of the professional liability system. Ann Thorac Surg 1987:44:335-7.
22. Localio AR, Lawthers AG, Brennan TA, Laird NM, Herbert LE, Peterson LM, Newhouse JP, Weiler PC, Hiatt HH. Relation between malpractice claims and adverse events due to negligence. N Engl J Med 1991;325:245-51.
23. O'Connor GT and others, on behalf of the Northern New England Cardiovascular Disease Study Group. A regional prospective study of in-hospital mortality associated with coronary artery bypass grafting. JAMA 1991;266; 803-9.
24. Williams SV, Hash DB, Goldfarb N. Differences in mortality from coronary artery bypass graft surgery at five teaching hospitals. JAMA 1991;266:810-5.
25. Hannan EL, Kilburn H, O'Donnell JF, Lukacik G, Shields EP. Adult open heart surgery in New York State. An analysis of risk factors and hospital mortality rates. JAMA 1990:264:2768-74.
26. Black N. Medical litigation and the quality of care. Lancet 1990;335:35-8.
27. Manual BM. Professional liability - A no-fault solution. N Engl J Med 1990;322:627-30.

28. Appelbaum PS, Grisso Th. Assessing patients' capacities to consent to treatment. N Engl J Med 1988;319:1635-8.
29. Freireich EJ. Should the patient know? JAMA 1979;241:928.
30. Nobel JJ. Adverse effects reporting. In: Gruting CW van (ed.), Medical devices. International perspectives on health and safety. Amsterdam: Elsevier, 1994:275-87.
31. Redelmeier DA, Tversky A. Discrepancy between medical decisions for individual patients and for groups. N Engl J Med 1990;323:1162-4.
32. Fielder JH. Getting the bad news about your artificial heart valve. Hastings Center Report 1993;23(II):22-8.
33. Sandman PM. Emerging communication responsibilities of epidemiologists. J Clin Epidemiol 1991;44(suppl.I):41S-45S.
34. Hammel D, Block M, Geiger A, Böcker D, Stadlbauer, Breithardt G, Scheld HH. Single-incision implantation of cardioverter-defibrillators using nonthoracotomy lead systems. Ann Thorac Surg 1994;58:1614-6.
35. Markewitz A, Kaulbach H, Mattke S, Dorwarth U, Weinhold Ch, Hoffman E, Steinbeck G, Reichart B. One-incision approach for insertion of implantable cardioverter-defibrillators. Ann Thorac Surg 1994;58:1609-13.
36. Kruse JM. Experiences from the re-use of implantable pulse generators. Clin Prog Electrophysiol Pacing 1985;3:61-3.
37. Hill JD. An impending crisis involving biomaterials. Ann Thorac Surg 1994;58:1571.
38. Galletti PM. Embargo on biomaterials. Science, May 20, 1994.

INDEX

A-A interval 45
AAI pacemaker 50, 60, 61
AAIR mode 51, 61
abdominal pacemaker pocket 60, 84
abnormal automaticity 170
abrupt changes in lead impedance 132
absolute refractory period 36, 133
accessory AV pathways 199, 204
ACE-inhibitor 58
active fixation 231
activity 176
advanced AV block 64
afterpotential 138
afterpotential sensing 152
age-related changes 8
air entrapment 124, 146
ambulatory ECG (Holter) monitoring 58, 59, 99, 100
aminoglycoside 88
amoxicillin 85
ampicillin 85
analysis of pacemaker malfunction 144
angina pectoris 52
anodal insulation 124
anodal pacing 170
anterior septum 6
anterograde AV conduction 202
anteroseptal accessory pathways 204
anti-theft devices 102
antiarrhythmic drug 50, 62, 176, 200, 211
antiarrhythmic drug failures 209
antibiotic prophylaxis 81, 84
antibiotic treatment 87
anticoagulant therapy 58, 60
antirheumatic drugs 60
antitachycardia devices 206
antitachycardia pacing 167
antitachycardia programs 207
arc welders 102
arm ergometry 117
aspirin 60
associated professionals 95, 115
asynchronous pacing 65, 102, 171, 206
asynchronous ventricular contraction 210
asystole 174
ATP 177
atrial anatomy 1
atrial arrhythmias 49, 73
atrial based pacing system 68
atrial-based timing systems 40
atrial chronotropic incompetence 69
atrial contraction 39, 62
atrial electrode 61, 73
atrial electrogram 76
atrial escape interval 34, 40
atrial extrasystoles 179
atrial fibrillation 52, 58, 61, 68, 78, 168, 169, 178, 179, 199, 204, 206, 207, 208, 209, 211
atrial flutter 47, 61, 75, 168, 173, 175, 178, 199
atrial inputs 4, 8
atrial lead impedance 206
atrial oversensing 145, 156
atrial pacemaker (AAI) 51, 60, 61
atrial refractory period 35, 43
atrial ring electrodes 76
atrial sensing 77, 143
atrial signals 62, 78
atrial synchronous biventricular pacing 186
atrial tachyarrhythmias 37, 45, 47
atrial undersensing 145, 157
atrial vulnerable period 45
atrioventricular node 2
atrioventricular nodal reentry tachycardia (AVNRT) 202
atrioventricular septal junction 4
atrioventricular synchrony 187
attenuation of the intracardiac electrogram 136
atypical posteroseptal accessory pathway 204
automatic mode switch 36, 52, 211
autonomic nervous system 39, 203
2:1 AV block 40
AV block 68, 199, 202, 204, 205
AV conduction 49, 51
AV conduction system 204
AV interval 51, 141

AV nodal ablation 211
AV nodal Wenckebach point 59
AV sequential pacing 47
AV synchronous pacing 62, 63
Bachmann's bundle 4
bacterial contamination 87
battery capacity 96, 97
battery depletion 95, 231
battery impedance 100
begin of life (BOL) 97
β-blocking agents 176
bicycle ergometer exercise 62, 117
bifascicular AV block 58
biopsies 208
bipolar electrogram 29
bipolar leads 231
blanking period 36, 38, 133
bradycardia-dependent QT_c prolongation 200
bundle branches 200
cancer 55, 83
capacitive effects 14
cardiac cycle 33
cardiac surgery 200
cardiomyopathy 52, 205
cardiovascular prostheses 85
cardioversion 149, 177
catheterization laboratory 83
cathether modification of the AV node 209
cathodal-myocardial interface 127
cathodal pacing 170
cause-of-death statistics 55
causes of noncapture 125
cell usage factor 119
central fibrous body 5
cephalic vein 82
cephalo sporin 82
cephazolin 86
cerebro-vascular accidents 59
chest wall stimulation 134, 138, 154, 200
children 50
chronaxy-rheobase curve 21, 108
chronic atrial fibrillation 58, 68
chronotropic incompetence 49, 59, 62
clindamycin 86
cloxacillin 84, 85
coagulase-negative staphylococci 81, 87
coagulation equipment 130
compact AV node 7
compensatory pauses 47
complete AV block 56, 58, 68, 199, 202, 204, 205, 217
component failure 124, 138
computer database 118
conductor break 146, 147, 149, 151
congenital complete AV block 217
congenital heart disease 222
congenitally corrected transposition 223
contraction synchrony 187
control of heart rate 210
coronary heart disease 200
coronary sinus 126
'corridor' operation 208, 210
corticosteroids 83, 85
cost effectiveness 69
coumarins 58, 60, 83
crest of the interventricular septum 6
cross talk 36, 138, 140, 173
culture tests 91
cytostatics 85
daily activities 50, 69, 117
data logging 100
DC countershock 127, 150, 202
DDD mode 39, 40, 206, 207, 211
DDDR 33, 61, 206, 210, 211
decubitus of the pocket 86, 87
defibrillation 149, 177
defibrillation burns 83
degaussing installations 102
detection circuitry 99
device types 229
diabetes mellitus 83, 85
diagnostic data 100
diaper rash 83
diaphragmatic stimulation 126
diastolic filling of the ventricles 64
diathermy 173
digital cardiographs 116
digital cellular telephones 102
digoxin 58
dilated cardiomyopathy 172, 187
dilating coaxial sheets 90
direct current catheter ablation 199

diuretic therapy 58
Dotter helical basket 89
double potentials 6
dual chamber pacemaker 64, 66, 138, 145
dual chamber pacing 63, 231
dual-chamber pacing with short atrioventricular delay 186
dynamic AV interval 50
dynamic AVI operation 40
dynamic AVI shortening 39
early ventricular pacing 140
echo-doppler 64, 68
echocardiography 63, 91
effective refractory period 62
efficiency constant 119
elective replacement indicator (ERI) 97, 98, 114
electrical cardioversion 65
electrocardiograph 116
electrocardiographical atrial undersensing 143
electrocautery 102, 130, 175, 178, 207
electrolyte imbalance 149, 150
electromagnetic field 130
electromagnetic interference (EMI) 100, 205
electromagnetic noise 36
electronic counter 116
electrophysiologic studies 60, 229
elgiloy 107
encainide 176
end of life indicator (EOL) 114, 207
end of service (EOS) 98
endocardial electrograms 100
endocarditis 87, 91
endogenous signals 130
energy consumption 96
energy curve 108
environmental stress cracking (ESC) 107
epicardial leads 91, 219
escape interval 129, 200
escape rhythm 200, 202
european pacemaker patient identification card 117
event marker channel 52
evoked cardiac depolarization 36
exercise 39, 62, 211
exercise test 59, 69
exit block 111, 206
exogenous signals 130
external defibrillation 124
extracardiac stimulation 107, 112
extracorporeal shock-wave lithotripsy 102
extrasystoles 40, 179
failure reporting 232
fainting spell 58
fallback 179
false inhibition 102
far-field R wave sensing 130, 156
far-field sensing 37, 75
Faraday resistance 136
fast pathway 202
field strength 19
filter 30, 99
first rib 76
flecainide 176
flucloxacillin 82, 84, 85, 86
fluid bridge 149
fluoroscopy 76
Fontan operation 224
fractional shortening 210
general pre-operative evaluation 60
health care 55
heart failure 50, 52, 60, 63, 68, 185, 209
heart valves 85
Helmholz capacitance 136
hemodynamic benefit 63, 67
hemodynamic studies 50, 52, 59, 63
hiccup 105
high lead impedance 146, 147, 149, 151, 154, 155
high output stimulation 170
His bundle 9, 52, 200
Holter monitoring 58, 59, 99, 100 (see also ambulatory ECG monitoring)
human life span 57
HV intervals 60
hyperkalemia 128
hypertrophic cardiomyopathy 52, 187
hysteresis 171
immuno-compromised patients 83
immuno-suppressive agents 85
implantable cardioverter-defibrillator 168

implantation rate 227
improper lead connection 146, 147, 149, 151
inappropriate sinus tachycardia 203
incremental atrial pacing 59
induction heaters 102
infective vegetations 91
inferior caval vein 3
infra-nodal conduction 60
inhibited pacemaker discharge 206
input amplifier 135
insulation defect 107, 125, 136, 146, 148, 149, 151, 154, 155
intercaval area 4
interface 13, 170
interference 100, 130, 173
intermediate septal accessory pathways 204
intermittent contact in conductor 154
intermittent no output 145, 147
intermittent noncapture 145, 150
internal circuit drain 119
interrogation 100
interval of follow-up 113
intraatrial conduction time 39
intracardiac electrogram 52, 133, 134, 206
intracardiac shunts 223
intracardiac tissue reaction 111
intraventricular conduction 135
intraventricular conduction tissues 8
intrinsic atrial activity 39
intrinsic negative deflection 109
irrigation of the pocket 87
ischaemic heart disease 50
J-shaped atrial lead 169
Keith 1
laboratory investigation 60
lead discontinuity 124
lead dislodgement 83, 96, 103, 126, 200
lead explantation 89, 231
lead fixation 103
lead fracture 89
lead impedance 15, 124, 146, 148, 149, 151, 154, 155, 207
lead infection 86, 89
lead insertion 231
lead position 126
lead technology 103
left bundle branches 9
left superior vena cava 222
left ventricular enddiastolic pressure 63
left ventricular diastolic function 63, 64
left ventricular systolic function 210
lesion potential 29
life expectancy 57, 67
lithium copper sulphide 113
local tissue reaction 127
local wound care 87
locking stylet 90
lone atrial fibrillation 207
long pauses 49
longevity of the pacemaker battery 25, 68, 96, 119
lower rate 34, 39, 49
lung cancer 60
magnet mode 97
magnet rate 97, 206
magnetic field 130, 173
magnetic resonance imaging 102
marker channel 138, 144, 180
maximal tracking rate 34, 43, 45
maximum sensor rate 34
maze surgery 210
mechanical AV synchrony 205, 209, 210, 211
mechanically induced arrhythmias 169
membranous septum 2
metal detectors 102
metal ion catalyzed oxidation (MIO) 107
microwave ovens 102
minimum tracking interval 34
minute ventilation 200, 206
mitral valve leaflets 6
mode switch 37, 47, 62, 75, 78, 178, 179
moderator band 11
modification of the AV node 199, 205
modified atrial-based timing systems 42
multi-polar leads 76
muscle potentials 100
muscular atrioventricular septum 6

musculus pectoralis 110
Mustard and Senning operation 223
myocardial infarction 149
myocardial perforation 126
myopotential triggering 74
myopotentials 115, 132, 173, 175
NASPE pacemaker code 35
nerve or muscle stimulators 130
neurocardiogenic syncope 233
neurological investigation 58
nodal-bundle axis 7
noise mode behaviour 133, 173, 175, 206
non-penetrating bundle 9
Ohm's law 13
open-heart surgery 208
operating room 83
organizational aspects 112
os of the coronary sinus 202
outpatients' clinic 69
oversensing 99, 123, 129, 145, 151, 153, 172
P wave detection 45, 153
P wave oversensing 131
P wave tracking 46
paced atrio-ventricular interval 34, 39
paced QRS complex 200
pacemaker bigeminy 173
pacemaker components 199
pacemaker damage 205
pacemaker dependency 113, 199, 200
pacemaker infection 81
pacemaker inhibition 132
pacemaker malfunction 144, 145, 146, 148
pacemaker mediated tachycardia 35, 36, 48, 175
pacemaker pocket 82
pacemaker programming 49, 116
pacemaker registration 227
pacemaker replacement 83
pacemaker reuse 231
pacemaker selection 55
pacemaker syndrome 77
pacing current 119
pacing failure 170, 171
pacing for dilated cardiomyopathy 187
pacing for hypertrophic cardiomyopathy 187
pacing impedance 96
pacing in children 215, 216
pacing in elderly patients 55, 56, 68
pacing modes 69, 229
pacing safety 18, 200, 239
pacing threshold 96, 207
pacing voltage on lead 119
palpitations 210
parasympathetic denervation 203
paroxysmal atrial fibrillation 61, 211
partial lead fracture 132, 136
passive fixation 231
patient's history 68
pauses 171
pectinate muscles 3
penetrating bundle 7, 9
pericardial tamponade 126
peripheral Purkinje system 11
phantom programming 102
phrenic nerve 112
platelet aggregation inhibitors 60, 83
pocket abscess 86, 87
polyurethane polymers 106
porous electrode 23
posterior septum 6
posteroseptal accessory pathway 204
postventricular atrial refractory period (PVARP) 34, 36, 48, 50, 78, 143
povidone-iodine solution 88
power plants 102
PR interval 34
preoperative evaluation 65
prevention of cross talk 158
preventive pacing 179
proarrhythmia 168
propafenone 176
prophylactic pacing 229
provocation test 115
pseudo Wenckebach behaviour 44, 45, 51
pseudofusion 110
pulse waveform analysis 107, 144
puncture of the pectoral subclavian vein 82
QT driven pacemakers 176

quality of life 59, 62, 63, 64, 199
R wave sensing 76, 152
radiation therapy 124
radiotherapy 102
rapid atrial pacing 186
rate adaptive pacing 64, 171, 200, 207, 229
rate smoothing 36, 47
recommended replacement time (RRT) 98
reed switch 138
reentrant supraventricular tachycardia 170, 199
refractory period 99, 133
relative refractory period 133
repeat pacemaker surgery 85
repolarization potentials 99
resynchronization 179
RF catheter ablation 52, 102, 124, 178, 199
RF energy 205, 207
RF energy induced AV block 200
rheobase 108
right Amplatz catheter 89
right atrial appendage 4
right atrial vestibule 3
right bundle branch 11
right ventricular outflow tract 169
rigid grasping forceps 89
risk factors for pacemaker infection 83, 85
runaway pacemaker 102, 174, 206
sedentary life 62
sensed AV interval 34, 39
sensing abnormalities 129, 172
sensing circuit 38
sensitivity threshold 99
sensor control 35
sensor implementation 69
sensors 176, 206, 207
septal AV bypasses 206
septal short atrioventricular delay pacing 186
septicemia 91
septomarginal trabeculation 9
short circuit 146, 148
sick sinus syndrome 58, 173, 218
silicone elastomer 106
single-chamber systems 145, 229
single lead DDD pacemaker 66
single lead DDDR pacemaker 67
single lead VDD pacing systems 65
sinus node 1
sinus node artery 2
sinus node dysfunction 59, 63, 68, 74
sinus node function 49, 209
sinus rhythm 41
sinus septum 3
skeletal muscle potentials 110
skin electrodes 83
skin erosion 86, 89
skin incision 82
slew rate 30, 109
slow pathway of the AVNRT circuit 202
snare catheter 89
spread of activation 2
Staphylococcus aureus 81
Stimarec Bulletin 232
stimulation threshold 108
Stokes-Adams attack 57
strength-duration curve 108
stroke 55
subclavian crush 106
sudden death 169
sunburn 83
supernormal phase 172
surgical complete AV block 217
surgical therapies for atrial fibrillation 208, 209, 210
sympathetic drive 59
syncope 58, 59
systolic heart failure 64
T wave 141
T wave oversensing 76, 130
T wave sensing 152
tachyarrhythmia detection 37
tachycardiomyopathy 209
tailored pacemaker prescription 69
Tawara 8
telemetry 69, 83, 100, 179, 206
temporary demand pacing 83, 207
temporary electrodes 81, 85
tendon of Todaro 3
terminal branches of the conduction system 11
terminal crest 2
theoretical battery capacity 119
threatening decubitus 89

threshold elevating drugs 149, 150
thromboembolic complications 210
tight clothes 83
tilt testing 233
timing intervals 33
torsades de pointes 170, 171, 200
total atrial refractory period 34, 37
total cavo-pulmonary connection 224
transcutaneous electrical nerve stimulation 102
transitional cells 7
transtelephonic monitoring 117
transthoracic defibrillation 102
treadmill 117
triangle of Koch 7
tricuspid endocarditis 91
tricuspid valve 169, 202
tricuspid valve leaflets 6
trifascicular AV block 58
triggered activity 169, 170, 171
triggered pacing mode 154
twiddlers syndrome 104
type I people 56
type II people 56
undersensing 74, 99, 124, 133, 138, 145, 154, 172
unipolar electrogram 29, 74
unipolar leads 231
unstable lead connection 154
upper rate limit 34
upper rate pacing 49, 206
upper rate timing 43
upper tracking rate 77
VA interval 34, 39, 143
vagal induced atrial arrhythmias 49
valve prosthesis 60
VDD pacing 73
VDDR pacing 211
ventricular atrial interval 34
ventricular-based timing systems 39
ventricular blanking period 138, 141
ventricular escape interval 34
ventricular fibrillation 206
ventricular myocardium 200
ventricular oversensing 143, 145, 158
ventricular oversensing during AV interval 145, 159
ventricular oversensing during VA interval 145, 159
ventricular refractory period 38
ventricular safety pacing 38, 139, 140, 141, 145, 158
ventricular systolic function 210
ventricular tachycardia 199, 200
ventricular undersensing during AV interval 145, 160, 161
ventricular undersensing during VA interval 145, 162, 163
vulnerable period 171
VVI pacing 206, 207
VVIR pacing 61, 73, 210, 211
Wenckebach pattern 44
working myocardial cells 7

Developments in Cardiovascular Medicine

1. Ch.T. Lancée (ed.): *Echocardiology*. 1979 ISBN 90-247-2209-8
2. J. Baan, A.C. Arntzenius and E.L. Yellin (eds.): *Cardiac Dynamics*. 1980 ISBN 90-247-2212-8
3. H.J.Th. Thalen and C.C. Meere (eds.): *Fundamentals of Cardiac Pacing*. 1979 ISBN 90-247-2245-4
4. H.E. Kulbertus and H.J.J. Wellens (eds.): *Sudden Death*. 1980 ISBN 90-247-2290-X
5. L.S. Dreifus and A.N. Brest (eds.): *Clinical Applications of Cardiovascular Drugs*. 1980 ISBN 90-247-2295-0
6. M.P. Spencer and J.M. Reid: *Cerebrovascular Evaluation with Doppler Ultrasound*. With contributions by E.C. Brockenbrough, R.S. Reneman, G.I. Thomas and D.L. Davis. 1981 ISBN 90-247-2384-1
7. D.P. Zipes, J.C. Bailey and V. Elharrar (eds.): *The Slow Inward Current and Cardiac Arrhythmias*. 1980 ISBN 90-247-2380-9
8. H. Kesteloot and J.V. Joossens (eds.): *Epidemiology of Arterial Blood Pressure*. 1980 ISBN 90-247-2386-8
9. F.J.Th. Wackers (ed.): *Thallium-201 and Technetium-99m-Pyrophosphate. Myocardial Imaging in the Coronary Care Unit*. 1980 ISBN 90-247-2396-5
10. A. Maseri, C. Marchesi, S. Chierchia and M.G. Trivella (eds.): *Coronary Care Units*. Proceedings of a European Seminar (1978). 1981 ISBN 90-247-2456-2
11. J. Morganroth, E.N. Moore, L.S. Dreifus and E.L. Michelson (eds.): *The Evaluation of New Antiarrhythmic Drugs*. Proceedings of the First Symposium on New Drugs and Devices, held in Philadelphia, Pa., U.S.A. (1980). 1981 ISBN 90-247-2474-0
12. P. Alboni: *Intraventricular Conduction Disturbances*. 1981 ISBN 90-247-2483-X
13. H. Rijsterborgh (ed.): *Echocardiology*. 1981 ISBN 90-247-2491-0
14. G.S. Wagner (ed.): *Myocardial Infarction*. Measurement and Intervention. 1982 ISBN 90-247-2513-5
15. R.S. Meltzer and J. Roelandt (eds.): *Contrast Echocardiography*. 1982 ISBN 90-247-2531-3
16. A. Amery, R. Fagard, P. Lijnen and J. Staessen (eds.): *Hypertensive Cardiovascular Disease*. Pathophysiology and Treatment. 1982 IBSN 90-247-2534-8
17. L.N. Bouman and H.J. Jongsma (eds.): *Cardiac Rate and Rhythm*. Physiological, Morphological and Developmental Aspects. 1982 ISBN 90-247-2626-3
18. J. Morganroth and E.N. Moore (eds.): *The Evaluation of Beta Blocker and Calcium Antagonist Drugs*. Proceedings of the 2nd Symposium on New Drugs and Devices, held in Philadelphia, Pa., U.S.A. (1981). 1982 ISBN 90-247-2642-5
19. M.B. Rosenbaum and M.V. Elizari (eds.): *Frontiers of Cardiac Electrophysiology*. 1983 ISBN 90-247-2663-8
20. J. Roelandt and P.G. Hugenholtz (eds.): *Long-term Ambulatory Electrocardiography*. 1982 ISBN 90-247-2664-6
21. A.A.J. Adgey (ed.): *Acute Phase of Ischemic Heart Disease and Myocardial Infarction*. 1982 ISBN 90-247-2675-1
22. P. Hanrath, W. Bleifeld and J. Souquet (eds.): *Cardiovascular Diagnosis by Ultrasound*. Transesophageal, Computerized, Contrast, Doppler Echocardiography. 1982 ISBN 90-247-2692-1
23. J. Roelandt (ed.): *The Practice of M-Mode and Two-dimensional Echocardiography*. 1983 ISBN 90-247-2745-6
24. J. Meyer, P. Schweizer and R. Erbel (eds.): *Advances in Noninvasive Cardiology*. Ultrasound, Computed Tomography, Radioisotopes, Digital Angiography. 1983 ISBN 0-89838-576-8
25. J. Morganroth and E.N. Moore (eds.): *Sudden Cardiac Death and Congestive Heart Failure*. Diagnosis and Treatment. Proceedings of the 3rd Symposium on New Drugs and Devices, held in Philadelphia, Pa., U.S.A. (1982). 1983 ISBN 0-89838-580-6
26. H.M. Perry Jr. (ed.): *Lifelong Management of Hypertension*. 1983 ISBN 0-89838-582-2
27. E.A. Jaffe (ed.): *Biology of Endothelial Cells*. 1984 ISBN 0-89838-587-3

Developments in Cardiovascular Medicine

28. B. Surawicz, C.P. Reddy and E.N. Prystowsky (eds.): *Tachycardias*. 1984 ISBN 0-89838-588-1
29. M.P. Spencer (ed.): *Cardiac Doppler Diagnosis*. Proceedings of a Symposium, held in Clearwater, Fla., U.S.A. (1983). 1983 ISBN 0-89838-591-1
30. H. Villarreal and M.P. Sambhi (eds.): *Topics in Pathophysiology of Hypertension*. 1984 ISBN 0-89838-595-4
31. F.H. Messerli (ed.): *Cardiovascular Disease in the Elderly*. 1984 Revised edition, 1988: see below under Volume 76
32. M.L. Simoons and J.H.C. Reiber (eds.): *Nuclear Imaging in Clinical Cardiology*. 1984 ISBN 0-89838-599-7
33. H.E.D.J. ter Keurs and J.J. Schipperheyn (eds.): *Cardiac Left Ventricular Hypertrophy*. 1983 ISBN 0-89838-612-8
34. N. Sperelakis (ed.): *Physiology and Pathology of the Heart*. 1984 Revised edition, 1988: see below under Volume 90
35. F.H. Messerli (ed.): *Kidney in Essential Hypertension*. Proceedings of a Course, held in New Orleans, La., U.S.A. (1983). 1984 ISBN 0-89838-616-0
36. M.P. Sambhi (ed.): *Fundamental Fault in Hypertension*. 1984 ISBN 0-89838-638-1
37. C. Marchesi (ed.): *Ambulatory Monitoring*. Cardiovascular System and Allied Applications. Proceedings of a Workshop, held in Pisa, Italy (1983). 1984 ISBN 0-89838-642-X
38. W. Kupper, R.N. MacAlpin and W. Bleifeld (eds.): *Coronary Tone in Ischemic Heart Disease*. 1984 ISBN 0-89838-646-2
39. N. Sperelakis and J.B. Caulfield (eds.): *Calcium Antagonists*. Mechanism of Action on Cardiac Muscle and Vascular Smooth Muscle. Proceedings of the 5th Annual Meeting of the American Section of the I.S.H.R., held in Hilton Head, S.C., U.S.A. (1983). 1984 ISBN 0-89838-655-1
40. Th. Godfraind, A.G. Herman and D. Wellens (eds.): *Calcium Entry Blockers in Cardiovascular and Cerebral Dysfunctions*. 1984 ISBN 0-89838-658-6
41. J. Morganroth and E.N. Moore (eds.): *Interventions in the Acute Phase of Myocardial Infarction*. Proceedings of the 4th Symposium on New Drugs and Devices, held in Philadelphia, Pa., U.S.A. (1983). 1984 ISBN 0-89838-659-4
42. F.L. Abel and W.H. Newman (eds.): *Functional Aspects of the Normal, Hypertrophied and Failing Heart*. Proceedings of the 5th Annual Meeting of the American Section of the I.S.H.R., held in Hilton Head, S.C., U.S.A. (1983). 1984 ISBN 0-89838-665-9
43. S. Sideman and R. Beyar (eds.): [3-D] *Simulation and Imaging of the Cardiac System*. State of the Heart. Proceedings of the International Henry Goldberg Workshop, held in Haifa, Israel (1984). 1985 ISBN 0-89838-687-X
44. E. van der Wall and K.I. Lie (eds.): *Recent Views on Hypertrophic Cardiomyopathy*. Proceedings of a Symposium, held in Groningen, The Netherlands (1984). 1985 ISBN 0-89838-694-2
45. R.E. Beamish, P.K. Singal and N.S. Dhalla (eds.), *Stress and Heart Disease*. Proceedings of a International Symposium, held in Winnipeg, Canada, 1984 (Vol. 1). 1985 ISBN 0-89838-709-4
46. R.E. Beamish, V. Panagia and N.S. Dhalla (eds.): *Pathogenesis of Stress-induced Heart Disease*. Proceedings of a International Symposium, held in Winnipeg, Canada, 1984 (Vol. 2). 1985 ISBN 0-89838-710-8
47. J. Morganroth and E.N. Moore (eds.): *Cardiac Arrhythmias*. New Therapeutic Drugs and Devices. Proceedings of the 5th Symposium on New Drugs and Devices, held in Philadelphia, Pa., U.S.A. (1984). 1985 ISBN 0-89838-716-7
48. P. Mathes (ed.): *Secondary Prevention in Coronary Artery Disease and Myocardial Infarction*. 1985 ISBN 0-89838-736-1
49. H.L. Stone and W.B. Weglicki (eds.): *Pathobiology of Cardiovascular Injury*. Proceedings of the 6th Annual Meeting of the American Section of the I.S.H.R., held in Oklahoma City, Okla., U.S.A. (1984). 1985 ISBN 0-89838-743-4

Developments in Cardiovascular Medicine

50. J. Meyer, R. Erbel and H.J. Rupprecht (eds.): *Improvement of Myocardial Perfusion.* Thrombolysis, Angioplasty, Bypass Surgery. Proceedings of a Symposium, held in Mainz, F.R.G. (1984). 1985 ISBN 0-89838-748-5
51. J.H.C. Reiber, P.W. Serruys and C.J. Slager (eds.): *Quantitative Coronary and Left Ventricular Cineangiography.* Methodology and Clinical Applications. 1986 ISBN 0-89838-760-4
52. R.H. Fagard and I.E. Bekaert (eds.): *Sports Cardiology.* Exercise in Health and Cardiovascular Disease. Proceedings from an International Conference, held in Knokke, Belgium (1985). 1986 ISBN 0-89838-782-5
53. J.H.C. Reiber and P.W. Serruys (eds.): *State of the Art in Quantitative Cornary Arteriography.* 1986 ISBN 0-89838-804-X
54. J. Roelandt (ed.): *Color Doppler Flow Imaging and Other Advances in Doppler Echocardiography.* 1986 ISBN 0-89838-806-6
55. E.E. van der Wall (ed.): *Noninvasive Imaging of Cardiac Metabolism.* Single Photon Scintigraphy, Positron Emission Tomography and Nuclear Magnetic Resonance. 1987 ISBN 0-89838-812-0
56. J. Liebman, R. Plonsey and Y. Rudy (eds.): *Pediatric and Fundamental Electrocardiography.* 1987 ISBN 0-89838-815-5
57. H.H. Hilger, V. Hombach and W.J. Rashkind (eds.), *Invasive Cardiovascular Therapy.* Proceedings of an International Symposium, held in Cologne, F.R.G. (1985). 1987 ISBN 0-89838-818-X
58. P.W. Serruys and G.T. Meester (eds.): *Coronary Angioplasty.* A Controlled Model for Ischemia. 1986 ISBN 0-89838-819-8
59. J.E. Tooke and L.H. Smaje (eds.): *Clinical Investigation of the Microcirculation.* Proceedings of an International Meeting, held in London, U.K. (1985). 1987 ISBN 0-89838-833-3
60. R.Th. van Dam and A. van Oosterom (eds.): *Electrocardiographic Body Surface Mapping.* Proceedings of the 3rd International Symposium on B.S.M., held in Nijmegen, The Netherlands (1985). 1986 ISBN 0-89838-834-1
61. M.P. Spencer (ed.): *Ultrasonic Diagnosis of Cerebrovascular Disease.* Doppler Techniques and Pulse Echo Imaging. 1987 ISBN 0-89838-836-8
62. M.J. Legato (ed.): *The Stressed Heart.* 1987 ISBN 0-89838-849-X
63. M.E. Safar (ed.): *Arterial and Venous Systems in Essential Hypertension.* With Assistance of G.M. London, A.Ch. Simon and Y.A. Weiss. 1987 ISBN 0-89838-857-0
64. J. Roelandt (ed.): *Digital Techniques in Echocardiography.* 1987 ISBN 0-89838-861-9
65. N.S. Dhalla, P.K. Singal and R.E. Beamish (eds.): *Pathology of Heart Disease.* Proceedings of the 8th Annual Meeting of the American Section of the I.S.H.R., held in Winnipeg, Canada, 1986 (Vol. 1). 1987 ISBN 0-89838-864-3
66. N.S. Dhalla, G.N. Pierce and R.E. Beamish (eds.): *Heart Function and Metabolism.* Proceedings of the 8th Annual Meeting of the American Section of the I.S.H.R., held in Winnipeg, Canada, 1986 (Vol. 2). 1987 ISBN 0-89838-865-1
67. N.S. Dhalla, I.R. Innes and R.E. Beamish (eds.): *Myocardial Ischemia.* Proceedings of a Satellite Symposium of the 30th International Physiological Congress, held in Winnipeg, Canada (1986). 1987 ISBN 0-89838-866-X
68. R.E. Beamish, V. Panagia and N.S. Dhalla (eds.): *Pharmacological Aspects of Heart Disease.* Proceedings of an International Symposium, held in Winnipeg, Canada (1986). 1987 ISBN 0-89838-867-8
69. H.E.D.J. ter Keurs and J.V. Tyberg (eds.): *Mechanics of the Circulation.* Proceedings of a Satellite Symposium of the 30th International Physiological Congress, held in Banff, Alberta, Canada (1986). 1987 ISBN 0-89838-870-8
70. S. Sideman and R. Beyar (eds.): *Activation, Metabolism and Perfusion of the Heart.* Simulation and Experimental Models. Proceedings of the 3rd Henry Goldberg Workshop, held in Piscataway, N.J., U.S.A. (1986). 1987 ISBN 0-89838-871-6

Developments in Cardiovascular Medicine

71. E. Aliot and R. Lazzara (eds.): *Ventricular Tachycardias*. From Mechanism to Therapy. 1987 ISBN 0-89838-881-3
72. A. Schneeweiss and G. Schettler: *Cardiovascular Drug Therapoy in the Elderly*. 1988 ISBN 0-89838-883-X
73. J.V. Chapman and A. Sgalambro (eds.): *Basic Concepts in Doppler Echocardiography*. Methods of Clinical Applications based on a Multi-modality Doppler Approach. 1987 ISBN 0-89838-888-0
74. S. Chien, J. Dormandy, E. Ernst and A. Matrai (eds.): *Clinical Hemorheology*. Applications in Cardiovascular and Hematological Disease, Diabetes, Surgery and Gynecology. 1987 ISBN 0-89838-807-4
75. J. Morganroth and E.N. Moore (eds.): *Congestive Heart Failure*. Proceedings of the 7th Annual Symposium on New Drugs and Devices, held in Philadelphia, Pa., U.S.A. (1986). 1987 ISBN 0-89838-955-0
76. F.H. Messerli (ed.): *Cardiovascular Disease in the Elderly*. 2nd ed. 1988 ISBN 0-89838-962-3
77. P.H. Heintzen and J.H. Bürsch (eds.): *Progress in Digital Angiocardiography*. 1988 ISBN 0-89838-965-8
78. M.M. Scheinman (ed.): *Catheter Ablation of Cardiac Arrhythmias*. Basic Bioelectrical Effects and Clinical Indications. 1988 ISBN 0-89838-967-4
79. J.A.E. Spaan, A.V.G. Bruschke and A.C. Gittenberger-De Groot (eds.): *Coronary Circulation*. From Basic Mechanisms to Clinical Implications. 1987 ISBN 0-89838-978-X
80. C. Visser, G. Kan and R.S. Meltzer (eds.): *Echocardiography in Coronary Artery Disease*. 1988 ISBN 0-89838-979-8
81. A. Bayés de Luna, A. Betriu and G. Permanyer (eds.): *Therapeutics in Cardiology*. 1988 ISBN 0-89838-981-X
82. D.M. Mirvis (ed.): *Body Surface Electrocardiographic Mapping*. 1988 ISBN 0-89838-983-6
83. M.A. Konstam and J.M. Isner (eds.): *The Right Ventricle*. 1988 ISBN 0-89838-987-9
84. C.T. Kappagoda and P.V. Greenwood (eds.): *Long-term Management of Patients after Myocardial Infarction*. 1988 ISBN 0-89838-352-8
85. W.H. Gaasch and H.J. Levine (eds.): *Chronic Aortic Regurgitation*. 1988 ISBN 0-89838-364-1
86. P.K. Singal (ed.): *Oxygen Radicals in the Pathophysiology of Heart Disease*. 1988 ISBN 0-89838-375-7
87. J.H.C. Reiber and P.W. Serruys (eds.): *New Developments in Quantitative Coronary Arteriography*. 1988 ISBN 0-89838-377-3
88. J. Morganroth and E.N. Moore (eds.): *Silent Myocardial Ischemia*. Proceedings of the 8th Annual Symposium on New Drugs and Devices (1987). 1988 ISBN 0-89838-380-3
89. H.E.D.J. ter Keurs and M.I.M. Noble (eds.): *Starling's Law of the Heart Revisted*. 1988 ISBN 0-89838-382-X
90. N. Sperelakis (ed.): *Physiology and Pathophysiology of the Heart*. Rev. ed. 1988 3rd, revised edition, 1994: see below under Volume 151
91. J.W. de Jong (ed.): *Myocardial Energy Metabolism*. 1988 ISBN 0-89838-394-3
92. V. Hombach, H.H. Hilger and H.L. Kennedy (eds.): *Electrocardiography and Cardiac Drug Therapy*. Proceedings of an International Symposium, held in Cologne, F.R.G. (1987). 1988 ISBN 0-89838-395-1
93. H. Iwata, J.B. Lombardini and T. Segawa (eds.): *Taurine and the Heart*. 1988 ISBN 0-89838-396-X
94. M.R. Rosen and Y. Palti (eds.): *Lethal Arrhythmias Resulting from Myocardial Ischemia and Infarction*. Proceedings of the 2nd Rappaport Symposium, held in Haifa, Israel (1988). 1988 ISBN 0-89838-401-X
95. M. Iwase and I. Sotobata: *Clinical Echocardiography*. With a Foreword by M.P. Spencer. 1989 ISBN 0-7923-0004-1

Developments in Cardiovascular Medicine

96. I. Cikes (ed.): *Echocardiography in Cardiac Interventions.* 1989 ISBN 0-7923-0088-2
97. E. Rapaport (ed.): *Early Interventions in Acute Myocardial Infarction.* 1989 ISBN 0-7923-0175-7
98. M.E. Safar and F. Fouad-Tarazi (eds.): *The Heart in Hypertension.* A Tribute to Robert C. Tarazi (1925-1986). 1989 ISBN 0-7923-0197-8
99. S. Meerbaum and R. Meltzer (eds.): *Myocardial Contrast Two-dimensional Echocardiography.* 1989 ISBN 0-7923-0205-2
100. J. Morganroth and E.N. Moore (eds.): *Risk/Benefit Analysis for the Use and Approval of Thrombolytic, Antiarrhythmic, and Hypolipidemic Agents.* Proceedings of the 9th Annual Symposium on New Drugs and Devices (1988). 1989 ISBN 0-7923-0294-X
101. P.W. Serruys, R. Simon and K.J. Beatt (eds.): *PTCA - An Investigational Tool and a Non-operative Treatment of Acute Ischemia.* 1990 ISBN 0-7923-0346-6
102. I.S. Anand, P.I. Wahi and N.S. Dhalla (eds.): *Pathophysiology and Pharmacology of Heart Disease.* 1989 ISBN 0-7923-0367-9
103. G.S. Abela (ed.): *Lasers in Cardiovascular Medicine and Surgery.* Fundamentals and Technique. 1990 ISBN 0-7923-0440-3
104. H.M. Piper (ed.): *Pathophysiology of Severe Ischemic Myocardial Injury.* 1990 ISBN 0-7923-0459-4
105. S.M. Teague (ed.): *Stress Doppler Echocardiography.* 1990 ISBN 0-7923-0499-3
106. P.R. Saxena, D.I. Wallis, W. Wouters and P. Bevan (eds.): *Cardiovascular Pharmacology of 5-Hydroxytryptamine.* Prospective Therapeutic Applications. 1990 ISBN 0-7923-0502-7
107. A.P. Shepherd and P.A. Öberg (eds.): *Laser-Doppler Blood Flowmetry.* 1990 ISBN 0-7923-0508-6
108. J. Soler-Soler, G. Permanyer-Miralda and J. Sagristà-Sauleda (eds.): *Pericardial Disease.* New Insights and Old Dilemmas. 1990 ISBN 0-7923-0510-8
109. J.P.M. Hamer: *Practical Echocardiography in the Adult.* With Doppler and Color-Doppler Flow Imaging. 1990 ISBN 0-7923-0670-8
110. A. Bayés de Luna, P. Brugada, J. Cosin Aguilar and F. Navarro Lopez (eds.): *Sudden Cardiac Death.* 1991 ISBN 0-7923-0716-X
111. E. Andries and R. Stroobandt (eds.): *Hemodynamics in Daily Practice.* 1991 ISBN 0-7923-0725-9
112. J. Morganroth and E.N. Moore (eds.): *Use and Approval of Antihypertensive Agents and Surrogate Endpoints for the Approval of Drugs affecting Antiarrhythmic Heart Failure and Hypolipidemia.* Proceedings of the 10th Annual Symposium on New Drugs and Devices (1989). 1990 ISBN 0-7923-0756-9
113. S. Iliceto, P. Rizzon and J.R.T.C. Roelandt (eds.): *Ultrasound in Coronary Artery Disease.* Present Role and Future Perspectives. 1990 ISBN 0-7923-0784-4
114. J.V. Chapman and G.R. Sutherland (eds.): *The Noninvasive Evaluation of Hemodynamics in Congenital Heart Disease.* Doppler Ultrasound Applications in the Adult and Pediatric Patient with Congenital Heart Disease. 1990 ISBN 0-7923-0836-0
115. G.T. Meester and F. Pinciroli (eds.): *Databases for Cardiology.* 1991 ISBN 0-7923-0886-7
116. B. Korecky and N.S. Dhalla (eds.): *Subcellular Basis of Contractile Failure.* 1990 ISBN 0-7923-0890-5
117. J.H.C. Reiber and P.W. Serruys (eds.): *Quantitative Coronary Arteriography.* 1991 ISBN 0-7923-0913-8
118. E. van der Wall and A. de Roos (eds.): *Magnetic Resonance Imaging in Coronary Artery Disease.* 1991 ISBN 0-7923-0940-5
119. V. Hombach, M. Kochs and A.J. Camm (eds.): *Interventional Techniques in Cardiovascular Medicine.* 1991 ISBN 0-7923-0956-1
120. R. Vos: *Drugs Looking for Diseases.* Innovative Drug Research and the Development of the Beta Blockers and the Calcium Antagonists. 1991 ISBN 0-7923-0968-5

Developments in Cardiovascular Medicine

121. S. Sideman, R. Beyar and A.G. Kleber (eds.): *Cardiac Electrophysiology, Circulation, and Transport.* Proceedings of the 7th Henry Goldberg Workshop (Berne, Switzerland, 1990). 1991 ISBN 0-7923-1145-0
122. D.M. Bers: *Excitation-Contraction Coupling and Cardiac Contractile Force.* 1991 ISBN 0-7923-1186-8
123. A.-M. Salmasi and A.N. Nicolaides (eds.): *Occult Atherosclerotic Disease.* Diagnosis, Assessment and Management. 1991 ISBN 0-7923-1188-4
124. J.A.E. Spaan: *Coronary Blood Flow.* Mechanics, Distribution, and Control. 1991 ISBN 0-7923-1210-4
125. R.W. Stout (ed.): *Diabetes and Atherosclerosis.* 1991 ISBN 0-7923-1310-0
126. A.G. Herman (ed.): *Antithrombotics.* Pathophysiological Rationale for Pharmacological Interventions. 1991 ISBN 0-7923-1413-1
127. N.H.J. Pijls: *Maximal Myocardial Perfusion as a Measure of the Functional Significance of Coronary Arteriogram.* From a Pathoanatomic to a Pathophysiologic Interpretation of the Coronary Arteriogram. 1991 ISBN 0-7923-1430-1
128. J.H.C. Reiber and E.E. v.d. Wall (eds.): *Cardiovascular Nuclear Medicine and MRI.* Quantitation and Clinical Applications. 1992 ISBN 0-7923-1467-0
129. E. Andries, P. Brugada and R. Stroobrandt (eds.): *How to Face 'the Faces' of Cardiac Pacing.* 1992 ISBN 0-7923-1528-6
130. M. Nagano, S. Mochizuki and N.S. Dhalla (eds.): *Cardiovascular Disease in Diabetes.* 1992 ISBN 0-7923-1554-5
131. P.W. Serruys, B.H. Strauss and S.B. King III (eds.): *Restenosis after Intervention with New Mechanical Devices.* 1992 ISBN 0-7923-1555-3
132. P.J. Walter (ed.): *Quality of Life after Open Heart Surgery.* 1992 ISBN 0-7923-1580-4
133. E.E. van der Wall, H. Sochor, A. Righetti and M.G. Niemeyer (eds.): *What's new in Cardiac Imaging*? SPECT, PET and MRI. 1992 ISBN 0-7923-1615-0
134. P. Hanrath, R. Uebis and W. Krebs (eds.): *Cardiovascular Imaging by Ultrasound.* 1992 ISBN 0-7923-1755-6
135. F.H. Messerli (ed.): *Cardiovascular Disease in the Elderly.* 3rd ed. 1992 ISBN 0-7923-1859-5
136. J. Hess and G.R. Sutherland (eds.): *Congenital Heart Disease in Adolescents and Adults.* 1992 ISBN 0-7923-1862-5
137. J.H.C. Reiber and P.W. Serruys (eds.): *Advances in Quantitative Coronary Arteriography.* 1993 ISBN 0-7923-1863-3
138. A.-M. Salmasi and A.S. Iskandrian (eds.): *Cardiac Output and Regional Flow in Health and Disease.* 1993 ISBN 0-7923-1911-7
139. J.H. Kingma, N.M. van Hemel and K.I. Lie (eds.): *Atrial Fibrillation, a Treatable Disease?* 1992 ISBN 0-7923-2008-5
140. B. Ostadel and N.S. Dhalla (eds.): *Heart Function in Health and Disease.* Proceedings of the Cardiovascular Program (Prague, Czechoslovakia, 1991). 1992 ISBN 0-7923-2052-2
141. D. Noble and Y.E. Earm (eds.): *Ionic Channels and Effect of Taurine on the Heart.* Proceedings of an International Symposium (Seoul, Korea , 1992). 1993 ISBN 0-7923-2199-5
142. H.M. Piper and C.J. Preusse (eds.): *Ischemia-reperfusion in Cardiac Surgery.* 1993 ISBN 0-7923-2241-X
143. J. Roelandt, E.J. Gussenhoven and N. Bom (eds.): *Intravascular Ultrasound.* 1993 ISBN 0-7923-2301-7
144. M.E. Safar and M.F. O'Rourke (eds.): *The Arterial System in Hypertension.* 1993 ISBN 0-7923-2343-2
145. P.W. Serruys, D.P. Foley and P.J. de Feyter (eds.): *Quantitative Coronary Angiography in Clinical Practice.* With a Foreword by Spencer B. King III. 1994 ISBN 0-7923-2368-8

Developments in Cardiovascular Medicine

146. J. Candell-Riera and D. Ortega-Alcalde (eds.): *Nuclear Cardiology in Everyday Practice.* 1994 (in prep.) ISBN 0-7923-2374-2
147. P. Cummins (ed.): *Growth Factors and the Cardiovascular System.* 1993 ISBN 0-7923-2401-3
148. K. Przyklenk, R.A. Kloner and D.M. Yellon (eds.): *Ischemic Preconditioning: The Concept of Endogenous Cardioprotection.* 1993 ISBN 0-7923-2410-2
149. T.H. Marwick: *Stress Echocardiography.* Its Role in the Diagnosis and Evaluation of Coronary Artery Disease. 1994 ISBN 0-7923-2579-6
150. W.H. van Gilst and K.I. Lie (eds.): *Neurohumoral Regulation of Coronary Flow.* Role of the Endothelium. 1993 ISBN 0-7923-2588-5
151. N. Sperelakis (ed.): *Physiology and Pathophysiology of the Heart.* 3rd rev. ed. 1994 ISBN 0-7923-2612-1
152. J.C. Kaski (ed.): *Angina Pectoris with Normal Coronary Arteries: Syndrome X.* 1994 ISBN 0-7923-2651-2
153. D.R. Gross: *Animal Models in Cardiovascular Research.* 2nd rev. ed. 1994 ISBN 0-7923-2712-8
154. A.S. Iskandrian and E.E. van der Wall (eds.): *Myocardial Viability.* Detection and Clinical Relevance. 1994 ISBN 0-7923-2813-2
155. J.H.C. Reiber and P.W. Serruys (eds.): *Progress in Quantitative Coronary Arteriography.* 1994 ISBN 0-7923-2814-0
156. U. Goldbourt, U. de Faire and K. Berg (eds.): *Genetic Factors in Coronary Heart Disease.* 1994 ISBN 0-7923-2752-7
157. G. Leonetti and C. Cuspidi (eds.): *Hypertension in the Elderly.* 1994 ISBN 0-7923-2852-3
158. D. Ardissino, S. Savonitto and L.H. Opie (eds.): *Drug Evaluation in Angina Pectoris.* 1994 ISBN 0-7923-2897-3
159. G. Bkaily (ed.): *Membrane Physiopathology.* 1994 ISBN 0-7923-3062-5
160. R.C. Becker (ed.): *The Modern Era of Coronary Thrombolysis.* 1994 ISBN 0-7923-3063-3
161. P.J. Walter (ed.): *Coronary Bypass Surgery in the Elderly.* Ethical, Economical and Quality of Life Aspects. With a foreword by N.K. Werger. 1995 ISBN 0-7923-3188-5
162. J.W. de Jong and R. Ferrari (eds.), *The Carnitine System.* A New Therapeutical Approach to Cardiovascular Diseases. 1995 ISBN 0-7923-3318-7
163. C.A. Neill and E.B. Clark: *The Developing Heart: A 'History' of Pediatric Cardiology.* 1995 ISBN 0-7923-3375-6
164. N. Sperelakis: *Electrogenesis of Biopotentials in the Cardiovascular System.* 1995 ISBN 0-7923-3398-5
165. M. Schwaiger (ed.): *Cardiac Positron Emission Tomography.* 1995 ISBN 0-7923-3417-5
166. E.E. van der Wall, P.K. Blanksma, M.G. Niemeyer and A.M.J. Paans (eds.): *Cardiac Positron Emission Tomography.* Viability, Perfusion, Receptors and Cardiomyopathy. 1995 ISBN 0-7923-3472-8
167. P.K. Singal, I.M.C. Dixon, R.E. Beamish and N.S. Dhalla (eds.): *Mechanism of Heart Failure.* 1995 ISBN 0-7923-3490-6
168. N.S. Dhalla, P.K. Singal, N. Takeda and R.E. Beamish (eds.): *Pathophysiology of Heart Failure.* 1995 ISBN 0-7923-3571-6
169. N.S. Dhalla, G.N. Pierce, V. Panagia and R.E. Beamish (eds.): *Heart Hypertrophy and Failure.* 1995 ISBN 0-7923-3572-4
170. S.N. Willich and J.E. Muller (eds.): *Triggering of Acute Coronary Syndromes:* Implications for Prevention. 1995 ISBN 0-7923-3605-4
171. E.E. van der Wall, T.H. Marwick and J.H.C. Reiber (eds.): *Advances in Imaging Techniques in Ischemic Heart Disease.* 1995 ISBN 0-7923-3620-8
172. B. Swynghedauw: *Molecular Cardiology for the Cardiologist.* ISBN 0-7923-3622-4
173. C.A. Niember and U. Sechtem (eds.): *Imaging and Intervention in Cardiology.* ISBN 0-7923-3649-6

Developments in Cardiovascular Medicine

174. Not yet published.
175. N.M. van Hemel, F.H.M. Wittkampf and H. Ector (eds.): *The Pacemaker Clinic of the 90's*. Essentials in Brady-Pacing. 1995 ISBN 0-7923-3688-7

Previous volumes are still available

KLUWER ACADEMIC PUBLISHERS – DORDRECHT / BOSTON / LONDON